Applications of Three-dimensional Imaging for Craniofacial Region

Shailendra Singh Rana
Prabhat Kumar Chaudhari
Abhishek Gupta
Editors

Applications of Three-dimensional Imaging for Craniofacial Region

Springer

Editors
Shailendra Singh Rana
Department of Dentistry
All India Institute of Medical Sciences
Bathinda, Punjab, India

Abhishek Gupta
Biomedical Applications Division
CSIR-Central Scientific Instruments
Organisation
Chandigarh, India

Prabhat Kumar Chaudhari
Division of Orthodontics and
Dentofacial Deformities, Centre for
Dental Education and Research (CDER)
All India Institute of Medical Sciences
New Delhi, Delhi, India

ISBN 978-981-97-4610-1 ISBN 978-981-97-4608-8 (eBook)
https://doi.org/10.1007/978-981-97-4608-8

This Springer imprint is published by the registered company Springer Nature Singapore Pte Ltd.
The registered company address is: 152 Beach Road, #21-01/04 Gateway East, Singapore 189721, Singapore

Contents

About the Editors

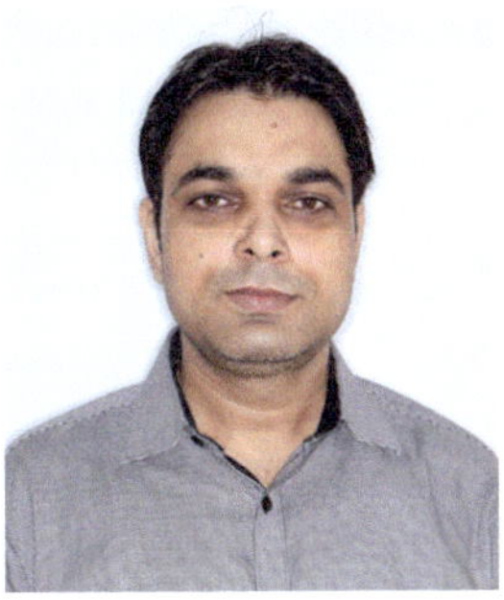

Shailendra Singh Rana, MDS, MAMS, MFDS RCPS (Glasg) completed his postgraduation in Orthodontics in 2014 from the prestigious All India Institute of Medical Sciences, New Delhi. He continued working as a Senior Resident for 3 years and as a cleft fellow at AIIMS, New Delhi till 2019. Currently, he is working as Associate Professor at AIIMS, Bathinda, Punjab. He is also a life member of various societies like the National Academy of Medical Sciences (India), the Indian Orthodontic Society, the Indian Society for Dental Research, the International Association of Dental Research, the Indian Society of Cleft Lip, Palate and Craniofacial Anomalies, fellow-Member of the World Federation of Orthodontists and the Indian Dental Association. He has presented various papers at national and international conferences and symposiums. He has over 20 publications in national and international journals and 8 book chapters to his name. He has filed four patents in India. He was awarded the *prestigious S. S. Sidhu Award in 2023 by the National Academy of Medical Sciences.* He is actively involved in teaching and training in Master of Dental Surgery (MDS) program. His current interest areas are orthodontic treatment in cleft lip and palate patients, Artificial Intelligence, miniscrew implants for orthodontic anchorage, 3D printing, and procedures that shorten orthodontic treatment duration. Lastly, he is also the Principal Investigator of several research projects funded by national agencies such as ICMR and SERB. Through his clinical and research work he aims to simplify orthodontic treatment as per the needs of our country.

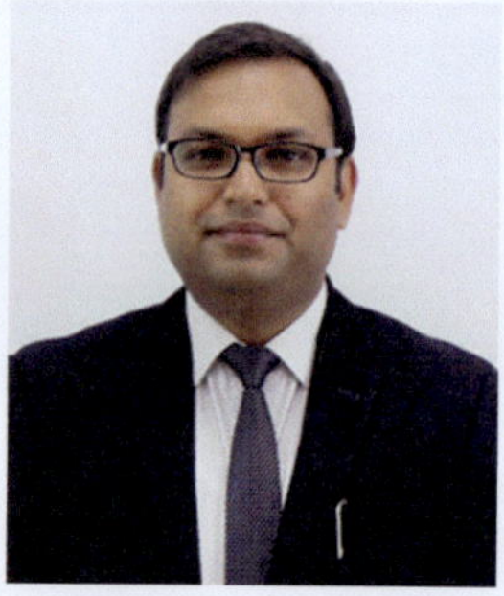

Prabhat Kumar Chaudhari, MDS, FAMS, FDS RCPS (Glasg) completed his degree in dental surgery in 2008, with specific training in orthodontics and dentofacial orthopedics in 2011 from Aligarh Muslim University, Aligarh, India. Currently, he is an additional professor at the Division of Orthodontics and Dentofacial Deformities at the Centre for Dental Education and Research, All India Institute of Medical Sciences (AIIMS), New Delhi, India. Dr Chaudhari's research interests include orthodontic care of children with and without cleft lip and palate, the application of 3D printing and non-ionizing surface imaging in oral health science in general and in orthodontics in particular along with the application of artificial intelligence-based deep neural networks for dental application. He has published several papers in peer-reviewed journals and some book chapters. Dr Chaudhari is involved in teaching and training in cleft and craniofacial orthodontic fellowship program, Master of Dental Surgery (MDS) program, and bachelor of science in Dental Operating Room Assistant (BSc DORA) program. He is a fellow of the National Academy of Medical Sciences (India), a member of the National Academy of Sciences, India (NASI), and a member of the topic group "Dental Diagnostics and Digital Dentistry" (TG-Dental) as part of the International Telecommunication Union and the World Health Organization (ITU/WHO) Focus Group on Artificial Intelligence for Health (FG-AI4H). Dr Chaudhari is an associate editor of BMC Oral Health (digital dentistry section) and section editor for the *Journal of Oral Biology and Craniofacial Research*.

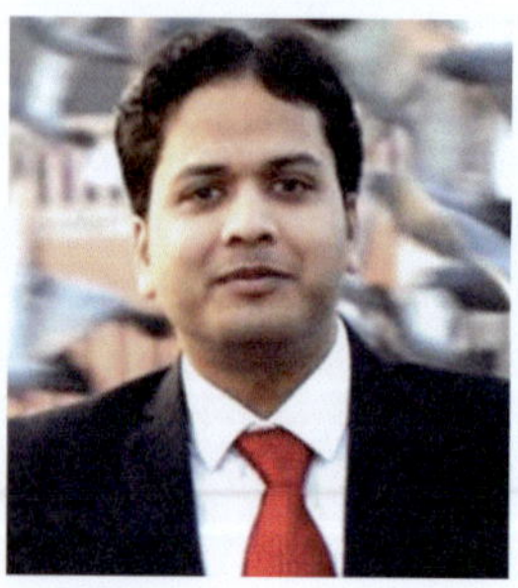

Abhishek Gupta, PhD, M.E., B.E. is currently working as Senior Scientist at CSIR-Central Scientific Instruments Organisation, Chandigarh, India. He has completed BE (CSE), ME (CSE), and PhD (Engineering) in computer science and engineering. He is working in the field of computational dentistry and medical image processing. His research areas are medical/dental imaging, computer vision, and artificial intelligence. He has worked widely in the area of computational dentistry. He has filed eight patents in India and in the USA. Out of them two US patents and two Indian patents have been granted in his credit. He has authored around 30 articles in SCI journals and authored several other articles in conferences and other journals with reputed indexing. He has guided three PhD theses, seven MTech dissertations, and several BTech projects. He has served as a lead guest editor of many reputed SCI journals published by Springer and Wiley. Currently, he is serving as associate editor for the *Journal of Multimedia Tools and Applications* in medical imaging theme. Recently, in 2024, he has been recognized under the "WORLD RANKING OF TOP 2% SCIENTISTS" as per the report published by Stanford University, USA.

An Overview of 3D Craniofacial Imaging

1

Abirami Rajasekaran, Shalini Gupta,
Ahmad Al-Hassiny, Shailendra Singh Rana,
and Prabhat Kumar Chaudhari

1.1 Introduction

The evolution of craniofacial assessment methods from craniometry, anthropometry, and two-dimensional (2D) imaging to three-dimensional (3D) imaging has significantly enhanced our potential in interpreting complex anatomy. Contemporary 3D imaging techniques are advanced aids to facilitate the comprehensive evaluation of craniofacial components and its interrelationships for diagnosis, treatment planning, virtual simulation, and fabrication of customized medical devices/prostheses [1]. It enables the integration of state-of-the-art computational methods like artificial intelligence, finite element analysis, bioinformatics, and radiomics, also improving patient education and motivation.

A. Rajasekaran · P. K. Chaudhari
Division of Orthodontics and Dentofacial Deformities, Centre for Dental Education and Research (CDER), All India Institute of Medical Sciences (AIIMS), New Delhi, India

S. Gupta (✉)
Division of Orthodontics and Dentofacial Deformities, Centre for Dental Education and Research (CDER), All India Institute of Medical Sciences, New Delhi, Delhi, India

A. Al-Hassiny
Institute of Digital Dentistry, Wellington, New Zealand

S. S. Rana
Department of Dentistry, All India Institute of Medical Sciences, Bathinda, Punjab, India

1.2 What Is 3D Imaging?

The National Library of Medicine's MeSH (Medical Subject Headings; MeSH Unique ID: D003952) defines medical imaging (*or diagnostic imaging*) as 'any visual display of structural or functional patterns of organs or tissues (*for diagnostic evaluation*)' [2]. It defines three-dimensional imaging (MeSH Unique ID: D021621) as 'the process of generating three-dimensional images by electronic, photographic, or other methods. For example, 3D images can be generated by assembling multiple tomographic images with the aid of a computer, while photographic 3D images (holography) can be made by exposing the film to the interference pattern created when two laser light sources shine on an object' [3].

The 'reconstruction algorithm' to merge the multiple 2D slices/images constitutes the basis of all ionizing and non-ionizing 3D imaging techniques. Pertaining to geometry, conventional 2D imaging is based on two spatial coordinates, i.e. along *x*- and *y*-axes. While in 3D imaging, the addition of the third axis (z-axis) representing the depth of the intended field of view contributes to the 3D representation of that object/subject [4].

S. S. Rana et al. (eds.), *Applications of Three-dimensional Imaging for Craniofacial Region*,
https://doi.org/10.1007/978-981-97-4608-8_1

Their corresponding perpendicular surfaces define the object in all three planes of space, i.e. sagittal, coronal, and axial.

1.3 A Brief History of the Development of 3D Craniofacial Imaging

The end of the nineteenth century marks an eminent discovery in medical radio diagnostics with the presentation of a new kind of ray by Wilhelm Conrad Roentgen, a German experimental physicist (1895). For the sake of brevity, the discoverer called it an 'X-ray,' which had the property to penetrate black cardboard, and even a 15 mm thick aluminium sheet [5]. It is electromagnetic radiation that works by the principle of 'attenuation,' i.e. reduction of beam intensity as it traverses through the matter by deflection or absorption.

The potentiality of X-rays has been utilized in the field of dentistry thereafter. In the earlier days, Dr. Edmund Kells referred to dental radiographs as 'skiagraphs' (i.e. shadow pictures) [6]. The possibility to capture the maxillary and mandibular dentition in a single film has been attempted with the great minds of H. Numata and Y.V. Paatero [7, 8]. This led to the technique called 'parablography,' which was later refined to 'orthoradial pantomography' shortly called 'orthopantomography' [9].

Intending to evaluate the effects of orthodontic treatment, Broadbent and Todd superimposed serial skull radiographs and realized the lack of standardization. This eventually led to the development of the 'Broadbent-Bolton cephalometer.' It had 2 X-ray sources to take a pair of 2D images from posteroanterior and lateral perspectives followed by the mathematical method of deriving 3D measurements. However, the conditions were not suited for routine usage in clinical settings [10].

The collaborative efforts in science and technology to promote the integration of radiographic imaging with personal computing set the pace in history with the following developments.

1.3.1 Computed Tomography (CT)

The mathematical fundamentals laid down by John Radon [11] and the prototype model by William H. Oldendorf [12] constitute the preliminary efforts to establish computed tomographic scanning. From a physics background, Allan M. Cormack of Tufts University, Massachusetts, successfully formulated desktop calculations and subsequently published his initial work in 1963 [13]. However, there was a lack of radiographic equipment to test his equations [14].

With the integrative financial support extended by Electric and Musical Industries (EMI) and the British Department of Health and Social Security (DHSS), an electronics engineer employed in research at EMI named 'Godfrey N. Hounsfield' was credited for developing the 'EMI scanner.' The first scientific work from Central Research Laboratories (CRL) of EMI Ltd., titled 'Computerized transverse axial scanning (tomography)' was presented in 1972 and published in the year 1973 [15]. The independent efforts of Hounsfield and Cormack for the revolutionary invention of CT were honoured with the prestigious Nobel prize in 1979.

1.3.2 Magnetic Resonance Imaging (MRI)

The discovery of magnetic field by Nikolas Tesla, 'the spin theory' by Rabi et al. [16], and its demonstration in solids-liquids by Bloch et al. [17, 18], as well as Purcell et al. [19], were recognized as the basis of nuclear magnetic resonance (NMR) imaging. It was considered a spectroscopic technique to study molecular characteristics at the atomic level. The extension of NMR for medical diagnostic application was pioneered by Dr. Damadian's observation that the relaxation time of malignant tissue was different as compared to the normal tissue in rats [20]. This eventually led to the 'magnetic resonance imaging' (MRI) in medical diagnostics.

Though NMR and MRI are similar regarding their basic physical phenomenon being 'magnetic resonance,' they differ based on the sample type and magnetic field strength. The Nobel laureates—Paul Lauterbur and Peter Mansfield—were known for the first acknowledged imaging [21] and 'echo planar imaging' in functional neuroimaging [22, 23], respectively. The acquisition of the first 3D-MRI was reported by Kramer in 1981 [24].

1.3.3 Ultrasonography (USG)

The contextual ideology from the experiments on bat navigation by Spallanzani [25], submarine, spotting the iceberg aftermath of the Titanic sink, and the development of piezoelectric crystals formed the nidus for practical applications of ultrasonography [26]. The landmark paper that drew the attention of medical diagnostics was by Dr. Ivan Donald [27]. The authors had reported the evaluation of an abdominal mass using A-scan with the shift of provisional diagnosis from ascites to ovarian cyst [28]. Thus, an imaging modality using sound waves which is non-ionizing was greatly appreciated.

The Doppler effect, the transmission of sound through water, a transducer made up of an array of piezoelectric crystals and echoes, constitute its principal background. The first 3D reconstruction was reported by a Japanese team led by Dr. Kazunori Baba in 1989 [29].

1.3.4 Cone Beam Computed Tomography (CBCT)

The rational algorithm formulation for a cone-beam geometry of irradiation by Feldkemp et al. in 1984 was a practical way of reconstruction besides the pre-existing fan-beam geometry of CT [30]. The Italian team led by Mozzo presented their new cone-beam CT (CBCT) for dentomaxillofacial imaging in the year 1998. The authors claimed the radiation dose to be one-sixth of the conventional CT unit [31].

1.3.5 Digital Dental Scanning

The prospect of scanning the dental arch emerged as a surplus outcome from the development of automated dental prosthesis by 'CAD/CAM,' i.e. computer-aided designing and manufacturing [32]. The research output of the thesis 'The Optical Impression' by Dr. Duret (1970–1973) yielded a French system having a handheld optical probe with a laser source for dental scanning [33, 34]. The availability of its prototype in 1983 and the public presentation in 1985 were considered to be noteworthy landmarks [35]. Parallelly, Dr. Werner Mörmann, and Marco Brandestini developed the Swiss system marketed as CEREC (Chairside Economical Restoration of Esthetic Ceramic) which utilized a three-dimensional camera for optical tomographic scanning [32, 36]. From there on, various dental scanners were launched based on optical principles like parallel confocal microscopy, accordion fringe interferometry, 3D in-motion video, and structured light technique with active triangulation [37].

1.3.6 Facial Scanning

The thesis work submitted by Thalmann-Degan in 1944 at the University of Zurich titled 'Die Stereophotogrammetrie, ein diagnostisches Hilfsmittel in der Kieferorthopädie' (Translation: Stereophotogrammetry, a diagnostic tool in orthodontics) is a special mention in the historical timeline of facial scanning [38]. However, Moss et al. have been entailed as the first to employ 3D laser scanning for monitoring growth at the Department of Orthodontics at University

College in London [39]. It has been reported that Cacou in 1995 integrated laser scanners with electromyography for evaluation of facial muscle function [38]. Contemporarily, higher-end mobile phones and tablets with depth sensors form the affordable solutions to accomplish facial scanning.

1.4 Various 3D Imaging Modalities for Craniofacial Applications

The term 'tomography' derived its origin from the Greek words *tomos* (slice, section) and *graphia* (writing, describing). Computed tomography (CT) is a non-destructive tomographic scan using X-ray transmission and a computer algorithm to reconstruct the image [40]. Based on the source-detector movement, number of detectors, and X-ray beam geometry, the different generations came into existence. The first to the fourth generation of CT scanners are employed in craniofacial 3D imaging modality; the modern systems offer mechanical simplicity and speed of acquisition.

Translation of radiation beam geometry from parallel/fan shape to cone shape has yielded 'CBCT.' To fulfil the need for greater resolution, the improvements brought about 'micro-CT' [41], 'nano-CT' [42], and 'X-ray microscopy' [43]. The variation in the path of the beam from the earlier stepwise (stop and shoot) method to the helical pattern has formed the basis for 'helical/spiral CT.' The use of a laser beam followed by fringe detection resulted in 'optical coherence tomography' (OCT) [44].

Nuclear imaging techniques like 'positron emission tomography' (PET) and 'single photon emission tomography' (SPECT) enable in vivo quantification of radioactivity and provide metabolic and functional information. The integration of CT along with these systems imparts greater resolution for detailed anatomy.

Magnetic resonance imaging (MRI) utilizes the resonance signal of hydrogen atoms from tissues inherent to the human body to be detected by the scanner. It provides excellent soft tissue contrast, and its most common sequences are T1- and T2-weighted images. A specialized form of MRI termed functional MRI (fMRI) can record brain activity during critical functions. An ultrafast technique by turbo fast low-angle shot (FLASH) has a scanning time of about 1 s [45].

Ultrasonography makes use of high-frequency sound waves to produce dynamic images (sonograms) of the internal organs, tissues, or blood flow. The different densities of the tissues—anechoic, hypoechoic, isoechoic, and hyperechoic—result in sonograms. Colour Doppler enables the evaluation of vascularity by illustrating the direction and velocity of flow within a user-defined field of view.

Facial scanners employ different scanning methods like stereophotogrammetry, structured light scanning, and laser scanning. The cameras from different viewpoints capture the subject followed by computer processing for stereophotogrammetry. A pattern of light projected over the subject is captured by the camera followed by computer processing for structured light scanning technique, while the laser beam is projected instead of structured light and captured by camera/sensor followed by computer processing in laser scanning technique [38].

Acquiring data from the dental arch and associated structures has been made possible via indirect and direct techniques. The indirect technique involves the use of desktop scanners for the digitization of the plaster model obtained from traditional alginate/elastomeric impressions. However, the direct technique involves the use of intraoral scanners for obtaining data from the patients without the need for laboratory procedures.

1.5 Contemporary Applications of 3D Craniofacial Imaging

3D craniofacial imaging techniques allow qualitative (i.e. visual) as well as quantitative inspection and evaluation of internal and external anatomy. It bestows a multitude of purposes encompassing screening, diagnostics, treatment planning, interventional, and progress follow-up.

Tomographic imaging techniques like spiral CT and CBCT have been employed in the craniofacial region for hard tissue imaging. CBCT can collimate the X-ray beam to the limited region of interest by opting for a different field of view (FOV). It helps to locate and determine the extent of pathological lesions, fractures, impacted teeth, bone grafting sites, airway, temporomandibular joint, and paranasal air sinuses three-dimensionally. It has been used to assess implant placement sites in terms of bone density, height, depth, and width and to identify the contiguous vital structures by nerve mapping ensuring safer insertion. Thus, it facilitates clinical procedures directly by DNGS (Dynamic Navigation-Guided Surgeries) or indirectly by fabricating implant placement guides [46]. Image-guided radiotherapy is also considered an advanced application in terms of intervention.

From the 3D imaging datasets, virtual planning of orthognathic surgery, orthomorphic surgery, tumour resection, joint reconstruction, and distraction osteogenesis are also undertaken. With additive manufacturing technology, patient-specific implants, surgical guides, and prostheses have been customized contemporarily.

Advanced high-resolution modalities like micro-CT and nano-CT have greater potential in research by imparting greater accuracy. Current applications include the evaluation of root canal morphology, enamel thickness, and bone remodeling (especially mandibular condyle and alveolar bone healing following periodontal/endodontic therapy). It forms a vital source for generating complex models based on a patient's geometry for finite element analysis. Stress associated with cavity preparation, nickel-titanium rotary file deformation, resistance limits of the mandibular condyle, and the relation between third molar to angle fracture has been studied intricately [47].

Optical coherence tomography (OCT) has been employed in the diagnosis of oral cancer, the fit of a restoration or prosthesis, the detection of enamel defects/cracks/caries, and periodontal tissue evaluation [48].

3D cephalometrics overcome the bilateral overlapping of anatomical structures and nonlinear magnification associated with 2D cephalograms. It benefits in landmark plotting verified on all three dimensions (multi-planar reconstruction, and volume-based verification), detailed evaluation of facial asymmetry, and 3D virtual orthognathic planning. Moreover, 2D cephalograms can be derived with varied principles (ray sum, maximum intensity projection, hemifacial projection), if deemed necessary.

The excellent soft-tissue contrast of MRI gains its application in the evaluation of internal anatomy in temporomandibular joint disorders (TMD), glenoid fossa-articular disc-condyle complex relationship following orthopaedic/functional appliance treatment in dentofacial orthopaedics, airway morphology, masticatory/facial muscle pathology, and diagnosis of salivary gland tumours. Functional MRI (fMRI) has been acquired to quantify brain activity changes with occlusal interference [49], dental pain [50], and removable functional appliances [51]. Dynamic MRI has been employed in the investigation of airway characteristics (i.e. site of obstruction) in obstructive sleep apnoea [52].

USG merits in the evaluation of pathologies related to major salivary glands, articular disc displacement, peri-implant tissue, periapical lesion detection, thickness changes of oral mucosa with periodontal surgery, cervical lymph nodes, early caries detection (with high frequency-ultra sound), follow-up of root end surgery especially anterior part of both the jaws and masticatory muscle health with orthodontic, orthognathic treatment, and prosthetic rehabilitation [53].

Though USG has been the standard line of investigation in foetal screening for orofacial malformations, a recent systematic review has comprehended that foetal MRI could be a valuable second line of investigation [54]. The reason is that the amniotic fluid volume, foetal position, or maternal obesity will not influence imaging quality with MRI.

The desktop and intraoral scanners create digital dental models that allow easier recording, transfer, storage, evaluation, and treatment planning. It facilitates the computer-aided designing and manufacturing of appliances, indirect restoration, and prostheses. Software modules for virtual face bow transfer and virtual articulations allow the clinician to evaluate the occlusion and motion path of the mandible three-dimensionally, thereby having potential application in full-mouth rehabilitation as well as TMDs. On an advance note, intraoral scanners with near-infrared transillumination (NIRI) technology allow the detection of caries by characterizing the internal anatomy of the tooth [55].

By combining the digital imaging and communications in medicine (DICOM) dataset of CT/CBCT/MRI, the object (OBJ) file of the facial scanner, and the standard tessellation language (STL) dataset of the intraoral/desktop scanner, the creation of a virtual patient is a current reality.

Facial scanning further forms the datasets for machine learning to screen obstructive sleep apnoea patients in external settings, for smile designing, for customization of extraoral appliances like continuous positive airway and pressure (CPAP), and aesthetic evaluation with treatment [38].

References

1. Vandenberghe B. The digital patient–imaging science in dentistry. J Dent. 2018;1(74):S21–6.
2. https://www.ncbi.nlm.nih.gov/mesh/68003952. Accessed 11 May 2023.
3. https://www.ncbi.nlm.nih.gov/mesh/68021621. Accessed 11 May 2023.
4. Hajeer MY, Millett DT, Ayoub AF, Siebert JP. Current products and practices: applications of 3D imaging in orthodontics: part I. J Orthod. 2004;31(1):62–70.
5. Röntgen WC. On a new kind of rays. Science. 1896;3(59):227–31.
6. Kells CE. The X-ray in dental practice. J Natl Dent Assoc. 1920;7(3):241–72.
7. Hallikainen D. History of panoramic radiography. Acta Radiol. 1996;37(3):441–5.
8. Paatero YV. A new tomographical method for radiographing curved outer surfaces. Acta Radiol. 1949;32(2–3):177–84.
9. Tammisalo EH. Professor Yrjö V. Paatero—The pioneer of panoramic oral tomography. Dentomaxillofac Radiol. 1975;4(1):53–6.
10. Hans MG, Palomo JM, Valiathan M. History of imaging in orthodontics from Broadbent to cone-beam computed tomography. Am J Orthod Dentofacial Orthop. 2015;148(6):914–21.
11. Radon J. On the determination of functions from their integral values along certain manifolds. IEEE Trans Med Imaging. 1986;5(4):170–6.
12. Oldendorf WH. Isolated flying spot detection of radiodensity dis-continuities-displaying the internal structural pattern of a complex object. IRE Trans Biomed Electron. 1961;8(1):68–72.
13. Cormack AM. Representation of a function by its line integrals, with some radiological applications. J Appl Phys. 1963;34(9):2722–7.
14. Raju TN. The nobel chronicles. Lancet. 1999;354(9175):347.
15. Hounsfield GN. Computerized transverse axial scanning (tomography): part 1. Description of system. Br J Radiol. 1973;46(552):1016–22.
16. Rabi II, Zacharias JR, Millman S, Kusch P. A new method of measuring nuclear magnetic moment. Phys Rev. 1938;53(4):318.
17. Bloch F. Nuclear induction. Phys Rev. 1946;70(7–8):460–74.
18. Bloch F, Hansen WW, Packard M. The nuclear induction experiment. Phys Rev. 1946;70(7–8):474–85.
19. Purcell EM, Torrey HC, Pound RV. Resonance absorption by nuclear magnetic moments in a solid. Phys Rev. 1946;69(1–2):37–8.
20. Damadian R. Tumor detection by nuclear magnetic resonance. Science. 1971;171(3976):1151–3.
21. Lauterbur PC. Magnetic resonance zeugmatography. Pure Appl Chem. 1974;40(1–2):149–57.
22. Mansfield P. Multi-planar image formation using NMR spin echoes. J Phys C Solid State Phys. 1977;10(3):L55–8.
23. Mansfield P, Pykett IL. Biological and medical imaging by NMR. J Magn Reson. 2011;213(2):513–31.
24. Kramer DM, Schneider JS, Rudin AM, Lauterbur PC. True three-dimensional nuclear magnetic resonance zeugmatographic images of a human brain. Neuroradiology. 1981;21(5):239–44.
25. Dijkgraaf S. Spallanzani's unpublished experiments on the sensory basis of object perception in bats. Isis. 1960;51(1):9–20.
26. Newman PG, Rozycki GS. The history of ultrasound. Surg Clin N Am. 1998;78(2):179–95.
27. Donald I, Macvicar J, Brown TG. Investigation of abdominal masses by pulsed ultrasound. Lancet. 1958;271(7032):1188–95.
28. Donald I. Sonar—the story of an experiment. Ultrasound Med Biol. 1974;1(2):109–17.
29. Baba K, Satoh K, Sakamoto S, Okai T, Ishii S. Development of an ultrasonic system for three-dimensional reconstruction of the fetus. J Perinat Med. 1989;17(1):19–24.
30. Feldkamp LA, Davis LC, Kress JW. Practical cone-beam algorithm. J Opt Soc Am A. 1984;1(6):612.

31. Mozzo P, Procacci C, Tacconi A, Tinazzi Martini P, Bergamo Andreis IA. A new volumetric CT machine for dental imaging based on the cone-beam technique: preliminary results. Eur Radiol. 1998;8(9):1558–64.
32. Rekow D. Computer-aided design and manufacturing in dentistry: a review of the state of the art. J Prosthet Dent. 1987;58(4):512–6.
33. Duret F. Optical impression: thesis. University Claude-Bernard—Lyon. 1973. https://www.francois-duret.com/thesis-ref-doc/. Accessed 11 May 2023.
34. Martin CB, Chalmers EV, McIntyre GT, Cochrane H, Mossey PA. Orthodontic scanners: what's available? J Orthod. 2015;42(2):136–43.
35. Duret F, Blouin J-L, Duret B. CAD-CAM in dentistry. J Am Dent Assoc. 1988;117(6):715–20.
36. Mörmann WH. The evolution of the CEREC system. J Am Dent Assoc. 2006;1(137):7S–13S.
37. Chaudhari PK, Bhatia D, Sharan J, editors. 3D printing in oral health science: applications and future directions. Cham: Springer International Publishing; 2022. https://link.springer.com/10.1007/978-3-031-07369-4. Accessed 6 March 2023
38. Lee JD, Nguyen O, Lin Y-C, et al. Facial scanners in dentistry: an overview. PRO. 2022;4(4):664–78.
39. Jacobson A. Methods of three dimensional analysis of patients with asymmetry of the face. Am J Orthod Dentofac Orthop. 1992;102(3):289.
40. https://www.ncbi.nlm.nih.gov/mesh/68014057. Accessed 11 May 2023.
41. Elliott JC, Dover SD. X-ray microtomography. J Microsc. 1982;126(2):211–3.
42. Sasov A. X-ray nanotomography. In Developments in X-ray Tomography IV, vol. 5535; 2004. p. 201–11.
43. Niemann B, Rudolph D, Schmahl G. X-ray microscopy with synchrotron radiation. Appl Opt. 1976;15(8):1883–4.
44. Huang D, Swanson EA, Lin CP, Schuman JS, Stinson WG, Chang W, et al. Optical coherence tomography. Science. 1991;254(5035):1178–81.
45. Suto Y, Matsuo T, Kato T, et al. Evaluation of the pharyngeal airway in patients with sleep apnea: value of ultrafast MR imaging. Am J Roentgenol. 1993;160(2):311–4.
46. Venkatesh E, Elluru SV. Cone beam computed tomography: basics and applications in dentistry. J Istanb Univ Fac Dent. 2017;51(3 Suppl 1):S102.
47. Swain MV, Xue J. State of the art of micro-CT applications in dental research. Int J Oral Sci. 2009;1(4):177–88.
48. Machoy M, Seeliger J, Szyszka-Sommerfeld L, Koprowski R, Gedrange T, Woźniak K. The use of optical coherence tomography in dental diagnostics: a state-of-the-art review. J Healthc Eng. 2017;2017:1–31.
49. Niraj LK, Patthi B, Singla A, Gupta R, Ali I, Dhama K, Kumar JK, Prasad M. MRI in dentistry-A future towards radiation free imaging–systematic review. J Clin Diagn Res. 2016;10(10):ZE14.
50. Lin CS, Niddam DM, Hsu ML. Meta-analysis on brain representation of experimental dental pain. J Dent Res. 2014;93(2):126–33.
51. Ozdiler O, Orhan K, Cesur E, Köklü A, Algın O. Evaluation of temporomandibular joint, masticatory muscle, and brain cortex activity in patients treated by removable functional appliances: a prospective fMRI study. Dentomaxillofac Radiol. 2019;48(7):20190216.
52. Volner K, Chao S, Camacho M. Dynamic sleep MRI in obstructive sleep apnea: a systematic review and meta-analysis. Eur Arch Otorrinolaringol. 2022;279(2):595–607.
53. Reda R, Zanza A, Cicconetti A, et al. Ultrasound imaging in dentistry: a literature overview. J Imaging. 2021;7(11):238.
54. Tonni G, Peixoto AB, Werner H, et al. Ultrasound and fetal magnetic resonance imaging: clinical performance in the prenatal diagnosis of orofacial clefts and mandibular abnormalities. J Clin Ultrasound. 2023;51(2):346–61.
55. Sebastian N, Singh A, Gehlot PM, Mariswamy AB. Role of intraoral scanners in the detection of dental caries: a review. J Clin Diagn Res. 2022;16(10):ZE07–10.

Computed Tomography Imaging for Craniofacial and Dental Applications

2

Sameer Peer, Paramdeep Singh, Shailendra Singh Rana, and Tarun Kumar Singh

2.1 Introduction

Cone-beam computed tomography (CBCT) is a current technological advancement in the ever-evolving field of computed tomography (CT). CBCT allows high-resolution imaging of the craniofacial region with reduced radiation dose in comparison to conventional CT. The adoption of CBCT in clinical practice has taken a few decades since its first described use in angiography in the year 1982 [1]. With the advancement in flat panel detector technology, computing efficiency of the latest computer systems, and X-ray tube technology, it has been possible to incorporate compact CBCT systems into clinical use in outpatient departments and dental clinics [2]. Although both CBCT and conventional CT have similar fundamental principles, they differ in terms of the geometry of the X-ray beam, radiation dose delivered, and image reconstruction algorithms [3].

Micro-CT is a non-destructive technique to examine the internal structure of materials which may be utilized for imaging in vivo and ex vivo. The first micro-CT system was developed by Feldkamp in the early 1980s to study the internal structure of ceramics. In medicine, micro-CT has found applications in dental and maxillofacial research. Although micro-CT has a higher spatial resolution than CT and CBCT, its widespread use is restricted by its relatively greater radiation dose and the large volume of data generated, which puts constrain on computational systems and storage systems [4].

In this chapter, the physical concepts behind CT, CBCT, and micro-CT are briefly described, followed by a review of the clinical uses of CBCT and micro-CT in craniofacial and dental imaging.

2.2 Basic Physics of CT

CT has been considered one of the landmark inventions in the field of medicine. In 1967, Alan Cormack and Sir Godfrey Hounsfield developed the very first CT scanner [5]. The first generation of CT scanners was based on the pencil-beam geometry of X-rays, where the X-rays were directed from the source to detectors placed diametrically opposite to the source. The intensity of X-rays that were transmitted was measured by the detectors. This was followed by rotation and translation of the X-ray source and detectors to obtain images for a different projection. This procedure was repeated many times to acquire multiple projections of X-ray, which would then be used to create an axial image of the object scanned using a reconstruction algorithm [6].

S. Peer · P. Singh
Department of Radiology, All India Institute of Medical Sciences, Bathinda, Punjab, India

S. S. Rana · T. K. Singh (✉)
Department of Dentistry, All India Institute of Medical Sciences, Bathinda, Punjab, India

S. S. Rana et al. (eds.), *Applications of Three-dimensional Imaging for Craniofacial Region*, https://doi.org/10.1007/978-981-97-4608-8_2

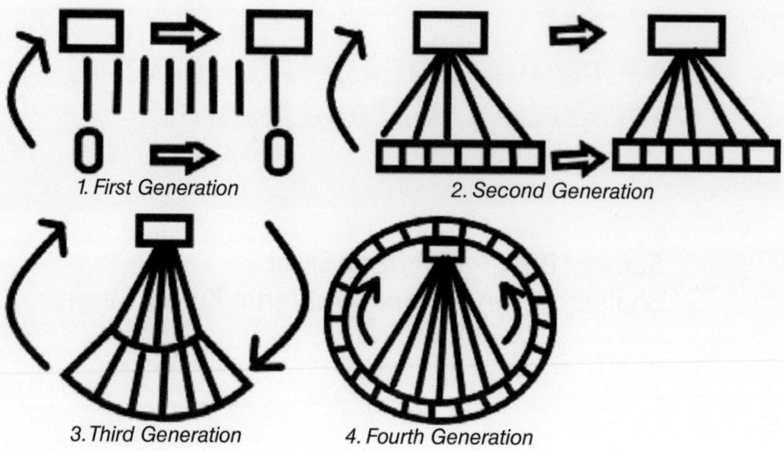

Fig. 2.1 Schematic representation of the geometry of X-ray beam and detectors in various generations of CT scanners. (1) In first-generation CT scanners, a pencil-thin beam falls on the detector, followed by a translation of the whole detector-tube assembly and small incremental rotation. (2) Second-generation CT scanner had a fan beam geometry with rotation of the detector-tube assembly and then small incremental angular rotation. (3) Third-generation CT scanners had a rotate-rotate detector-tube configuration with multiple arrays of detectors. (4) Fourth-generation CT scanners had a complete ring of detectors that remained static followed by complete rotation of the detector

X-rays undergo attenuation once they pass through an object. For a mono-energetic X-ray beam passing through a homogenous object, the expression of transmitted X-ray intensity obeys 'the Lambert-beer law', which is given by the expression:

$$I = I_0 e^{-\mu x}$$

Here, I indicates the intensity of the transmitted X-Ray, μ indicates the linear attenuation coefficient, x indicates the path length of the X-Ray and I_0 indicates the intensity of the incident X-Ray.

For inhomogeneous objects, such as human tissues, the expression is modified as:

$$I = I_0 e^{-\int \mu x dX}$$

The negative logarithm of this expression provides us with line integrals of 'linear attenuation coefficients' (μ). The ray sum is a line integral of μ at any angle θ, and a set of ray sums at angle θ is a projection [7]. The computation of μ follows Radon's theory, which essentially deals with the calculation of μ at a given point from many projections, which are obtained by varying the angle θ at that point [8].

Over the years, CT scanners have undergone various technical modifications which are described in terms of generations. As mentioned previously, the first-generation CT scanners use a pencil beam geometry of X-Ray with the translate-rotate configuration of source and detector. The second generation utilized a fan beam geometry and a single array of detectors with rotate-rotate configuration. The third generation utilized a fan beam geometry and an arc of detectors. The fourth generation utilized fan beam geometry with a complete ring of detectors. Currently, multi-detector row CT (MDCT) is in vogue which utilizes a fan beam geometry and an arch of multiple rows of detectors, a concept based on third-generation CT scanners [9]. Salient features of various generations of CT are shown as line diagrams Fig. 2.1.

2.3 CBCT Data Acquisition

Cone-beam CT, as the name suggests, utilizes the 'cone-beam' geometry of X-rays as opposed to fan beam geometry used in conventional MDCT. Collimation of X-ray beam in MDCT limits z-axis coverage of detectors by the X-ray beam. Thus, the object to be scanned needs to be moved along the z-axis to obtain multiple slices of data which are then reconstructed into a volumetric dataset. In contrast, the conical geometry of the X-ray beam ensures complete volumetric acquisition of data in a single rotation, without the need for translation along the z-axis. In modern CT scanners with multiple rows and multiple detectors, the acquisition geometry closely approximates a cone-beam geometry [10]. Figure 2.2 demonstrates a "schematic representation of image acquisition" using CBCT and how it differs from MDCT. CBCT system (NewTom GiANO HR) is shown in Fig. 2.3.

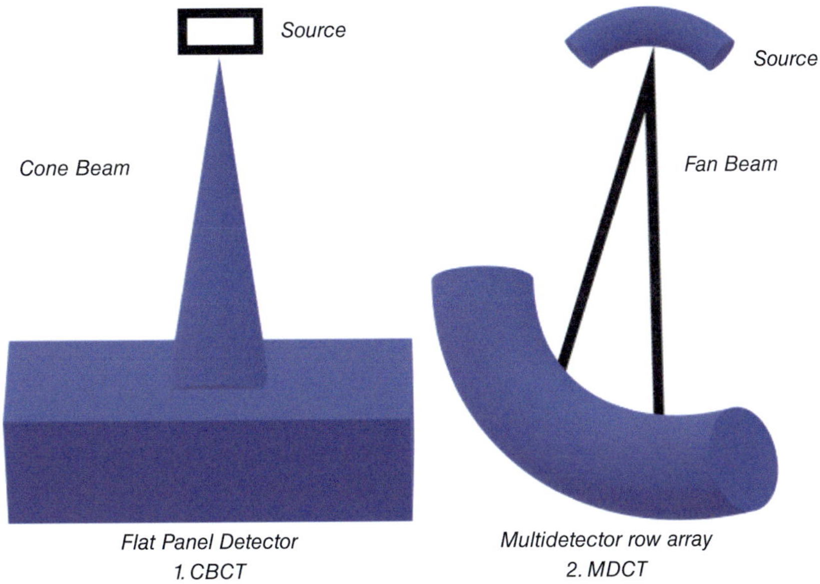

Fig. 2.2 Schematic representation of image acquisition in CBCT and MDCT

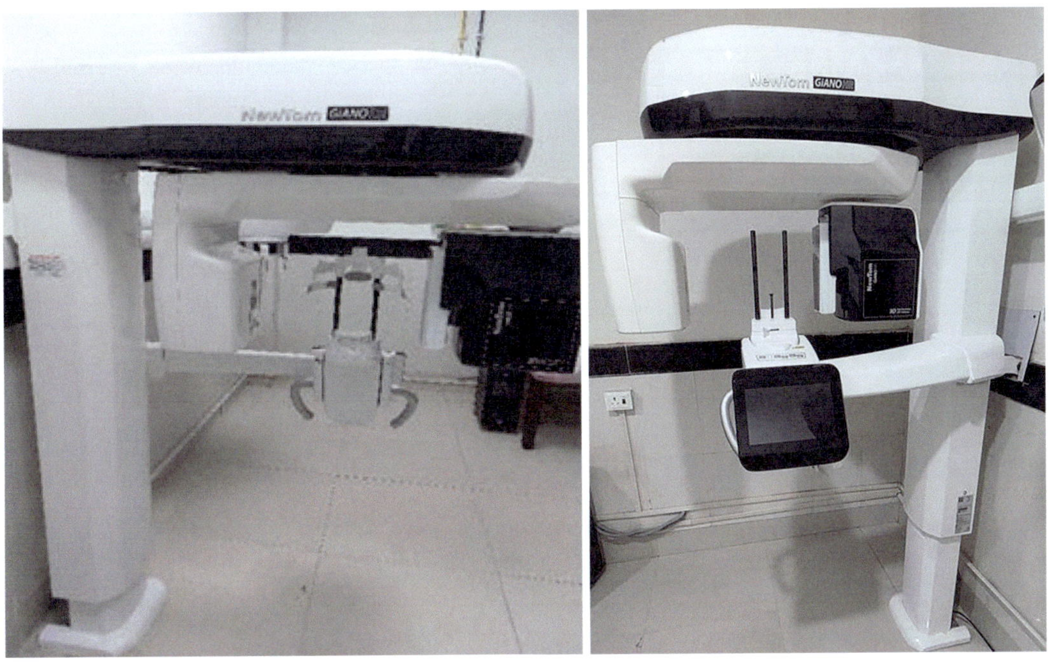

Fig. 2.3 (NewTomGiANO HR system)

2.4 Flat Panel Detectors (FPD)

FPDs convert the energy of incident X-ray photons to digital signals. FPDs consist of an array of scintillating crystals developed over a matrix of photodiodes which are inserted within a solid-state amorphous selenium or silicon layer [11]. Once the X-ray photons strike the scintillator crystals, the energy of the incident X-ray photon is converted into light, which is directed to a photo-diode array where the energy is stored as an electric charge. Then the transistors embedded within the amorphous silicon/selenium layer relay a signal intensity, which is associated with the charge stored within the photodiode and is proportional to the energy of incident X-ray photons. CsI (cesium iodide) scintillator crystals enable high spatial resolution imaging due to their linear fibre-optic cable-like structure, which reduces lateral transmission and dissipation of light [12]. In comparison with X-ray intensifying screens and charge-coupled devices (CCD), the FPDs allow for much higher spatial resolution of images [13]. Figure 2.4 depicts the schematic representation of Si: H-based FPD.

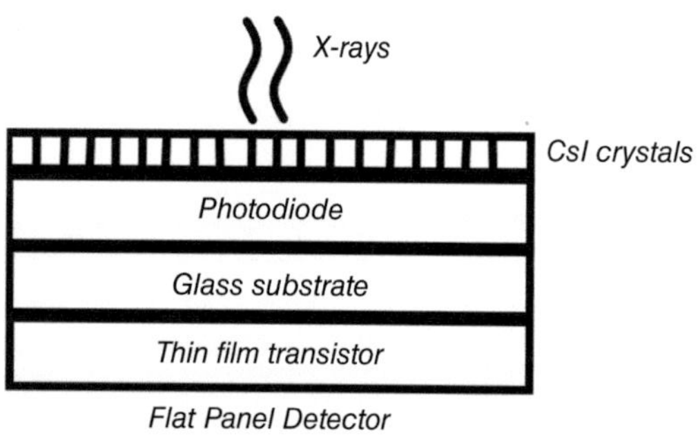

Fig. 2.4 Schematic representation of the construction of a flat panel detector (FPD)

2.5 Image Reconstruction Algorithms in CBCT

In tomography, the raw data is in the form of multiple one-dimensional projections, which need to be reconstructed into a 2D or 3D image. This process involves solving an inversion problem. CBCT utilizes the Feldkamp algorithm for the reconstruction of projection data [10, 14]. This includes the use of a kernel or a mathematical filter to the raw data before it is being projected and, thus, creating high-resolution 3D images. The process of filtering or application of kernel reduces the blur, which otherwise is an integral part of back projection [15]. In essence, the 'Feldkamp algorithm is an adaption of 3D filtered back projection' method found in MDCT reconstruction algorithms. While early CBCT systems utilized the Feldkamp algorithm for the complete circumference of the cone beam at the vertex, recent technologies use what is known as the modified Feldkamp algorithm which utilizes small arcs of the circumference for reconstruction [10].

Using a CBCT system with a modified Feldkamp reconstruction algorithm, an isotropic voxel of size $150 \times 150 \times 150\ \mu m^3$ can be obtained which improves the quality of reconstruction in any plane with a reduction of partial volume artifacts. In contrast, MDCT can achieve an in-plane resolution of $500 \times 500\ \mu m^2$ and a resolution of 500–1000 μm along the z-axis [13].

2.6 Image Quality in CBCT

Many physical parameters determine the image quality obtained in CBCT. Among these, contrast and spatial resolution, quantum noise, and DQE

('Detector quantum efficiency') are of specific importance in CBCT [16]. In CBCT, spatial resolution is excellent on account of the construction of the FPDs, in particular the tunnel-like transmission of photons within the scintillating crystals. In contrast, the contrast resolution of FPDs is hampered by increased scattering, a dynamic range, and a low temporal resolution. In the following sections, we discuss the determinants of the quality of images in CBCT with emphasis on various methods of improving the image quality [17].

2.6.1 Scatter

Scatter radiation is the secondary radiation emitted from the patient after the initial X-ray beam interacts with the patient's tissues. In other words, the scatter is the off-axis photon fluence at the detector that is not a result of the source radiation [18]. As compared with MDCT, the scatter is more of a problem with CBCT since pre-patient collimators used in MDCT limit the z-axis coverage of X-ray, while in CBCT, the z-axis coverage is increased, and this allows for the scatter to originate from the whole volume of the scanned part. Scatter reduces "the contrast-to-noise ratio". The contribution of scatter to image may be quantified as a ratio of scatter to primary radiation, i.e. SPR. In CBCT, SPR may be as high as 3 in comparison with 0.2 in MDCT.

2.6.2 Approaches to the Reduction of Scatter in CBCT

- Reduction of FOVz

  Although the physical dimensions of the part of the body to be scanned put a constraint on the FOV along the z-axis, FOVz should be restricted to the area of interest [18].
- Air gap

  Air gap introduction between the detector and patient is a basic physical concept that may reduce the SPR. However, the CBCT systems in use in most in-office locations may not allow for sufficient air gaps to reduce scatter. Thus, the use of air gaps may not be useful in practice in most of the CBCT systems [19].
- Filters and collimators

  The use of filters at X-ray sources remains one of the most effective ways of reducing scatter radiation by eliminating the low-energy X-ray photons using aluminium filters that are primarily responsible for scatter. Collimation helps in restricting the X-Ray beam to the FOV, thus eliminating the peripheral photons contributing to scatter [19].

  Compensatory collimators are shaped in the form of a bow tie. The idea behind this configuration stems from the concept that the peripheral part of the imaged structure has a reduced X-ray path length as compared to the central part, thus leading to more scatter [20]. This forms the basis of streak and cupping artefacts. With the use of a bow-tie filter, which is thicker at the periphery and thinner in the centre, the periphery portion of the X-ray beam has higher energy and thus reduced scatter. Indeed, in an investigation by Graham et al., the authors demonstrated a $> 50\%$ reduction in the scatter by using copper bow-tie filters. However, bow-tie collimators may lead to beam hardening and thus may reduce the DQE [21].
- Reduction of KVp

  Lower KVp reduces the effect of Compton scatter and thus reduces SPR [22].
- Anti-scatter grids

  Anti-scatter grids are used between the patient and the detector to absorb the off-line scatter radiation while allowing the primary radiation to reach the detector. Multiple lead leaves are used to accomplish this. In CBCT, anti-scatter grids have a radial arrangement of the lead leaves centred at the focal point of the FPD. Even though grid anti-scatter significantly eliminates scatter, it increases noise and radiation dose, or, to overcome the increased noise with the use of the grid, the resolution can be diminished. Siewerdsen et al. evaluated the impact of anti-scatter grids in improving the image quality in CBCT and found that the use of anti-scatter grids was associated with improvement in image quality only in cases where a large volume was to be scanned or in input quantum limited states like high noise and low spatial resolution [19, 20, 23].

2.6.3 Scatter Correction Algorithms

Most clinical CBCT systems utilize one or more scatter subtraction or homogenization algorithms. Some of the most studied algorithms include beam stop or blocker-based techniques, Monte Carlo simulations, collimator shadow assessment, and analytics calculation. Monte Carlo simulations are one of the most theoretically robust scatter correction algorithms. In this algorithm, the scatter is predicted during the pre-processing of the data based on the voxel tissue densities of the entire volume of the acquired tissue. This is followed by subtraction of the predicted scatter contribution at every detector element from the whole acquired dataset. The scatter correction algorithms may not decrease the total radiation dosage due to scatter; however, they may enhance the 'contrast/noise ratio', uniformity of the image, and accuracy of CT number estimation. The algorithms are computationally challenging and require considerable computation time. At present, these algorithms may be used as an adjunct to direct scatter reduction techniques [24–26].

2.6.4 Dynamic Range

The term 'dynamic range' describes the range of incident signal intensities that a detector may successfully transform into a transmitted signal. CBCT systems with 'solid-state aSI: H FPDs' RATIO transforms from ~10^4:1 to a 14-bit digital readout than 10^6:1 dynamic range of ceramic detectors sometimes used in MDCT. Roos et al. depicted FPD with dynamic-switch mode which increased the dynamic range of CBCT FPDs sixfold. Also, the dynamic-switch FPDs increase the low contrast detectability of CBCT to 3HU, which is comparable to MDCT and better than current CBCT systems which have a low contrast detectability in the range of 5–10HU [27].

2.6.5 Temporal Resolution

Temporal resolution is the detector's capacity to distinguish between projection datasets taken sequentially and separated by brief time intervals. In comparison to ceramic-based detectors utilized in MDCT, 'solid-state aSi: H FPDs' have a lower temporal resolution. CsI is particularly slow and has a problem with 'after-glow', ghost, and streak artefacts. Due to these limitations, the CBCT system has a limit for rotation speeds. The after-glow effect is more pronounced after exposure to high-intensity incident radiation. Subtraction of a portion of the previously acquired image from the present image may mitigate the after-glow effect in post-processing and may help in improving the low contrast detectability and resolution [27, 28].

2.6.6 Spatial Resolution

The term 'spatial resolution' describes a system's capacity to discriminate between two structures of different contrasts separated by a small distance. Line pairs per centimetre (lp/cm) are used to characterize the spatial resolution of CBCT. The MTF (modulation transfer function) is a composite function that describes the relation between unsharpness, image blur, and contrast response referring to the capability of resolving line pairs per unit length. In an attempt to increase spatial resolution, a technique known as 'binning' is used. Binning means combining two or more detectors to transmit a single uniform signal. 1 × 1 binning confers the highest possible spatial resolution, however, at the cost of SNR. 2 × 2 and higher binning confers an optimum balance between SNR and spatial resolution. At KVp of 120 KV, spatial resolution of 20–22 lp/cm has been described using FPD CBCT systems at 2 × 2 binning, transforming into an isotropic voxel size of 200–250 μm^3. High spatial resolution and isotropic voxel size of as low as 150 $\mu m^3$are attractive features of CBCT [29, 30].

2.6.7 Detector Quantum Efficiency (DQE)

DQE denotes the detector's overall efficiency. DQE denotes the overall efficiency of the detector in transforming information from the incident projection data into the imaging data. Mathematically, DQE is the ratio between the square of input SNR and the square of output SNR and ranges between 0 and 1. DQE of 1 (a hypothetical situation) would mean a completely congruent output from the detector concerning the input information contained in the X-ray beam. Most CBCT systems using aSi: H solid-state detectors have a DQE of 0.6–0.7, which is higher than direct conversion amorphous selenium (aSe) detectors but lower than ceramic detectors used in CBCT. Improvements in DQE in CBCT systems remain a technical challenge [31].

2.6.8 Contrast Resolution and Low-Contrast Detectability

The capability of a system to discriminate between several grey shades is referred to as contrast resolution and is described in terms of low-contrast detectability. Modern MDCT has a low-contrast detectability of ~1 HU, while CBCT is limited to 10 HU. Although recent CBCT systems with dynamic-switch technology have made it possible to achieve a low-dose detectability of 3HU, still the contrast resolution of CBCT is lesser compared to MDCT, which limits its use in diagnostic imaging dealing with soft tissue imaging. Scatter, quantum noise, low DQE, and low temporal resolution are the factors limiting low-contrast detectability in CBCT systems as described in previous sections [29, 30].

2.7 Radiation Dose

Radiation dose is a parameter that has implications for patient safety as well as image quality. In general, higher radiation dose leads to lower quantum noise and better quality of image. In conventional CT imaging, higher KVp and mAs translate into a higher radiation dose [32]. For a given anatomical part scanned, CT protocol must ensure optimal image quality while keeping radiation dose ALARA ('As Low As Reasonable Achievable'). In conventional CT scans, the most commonly used radiation doses are parameters like DLP ("dose length product") and CTDI ("CT dose index"). These are measured using phantoms for the head and body. CTDIw (weighted CTDI) is considered to be a better indicator of dose profile in a single section FOV [32].

CBCT systems have been considered to have a lower radiation dose exposure than MDCT. However, the CT dosimetry as applied to MDCT systems does not work with CBCT since X-ray beam geometry is different, and CT phantoms do not absorb the radiation from the complete X-ray beam leading to an underestimation of the dosimetry. Also, the acquisition protocols and dose calculation methods vary between CBCT dosimetry studies published in the literature, thus limiting the generalization of protocols [33].

Presently, radiation dosimetry in CBCT for the head and neck utilizes anthropometric skull phantoms with thermoluminescent devices for point dose measurements using specific protocols for imaging a particular FOV and limiting the exposure to adjacent structures. Using 16-cm phantoms for point dose measurements for neck and head CBCT, Daly et al. obtained the effective dose to be in the range of 0.1 and 0.35 mSv based on the exposure parameters. For sinus imaging, the effective dose has been measured to be 0.2 mSv. In one study, limited CBCT of the middle ear yielded an effective dose of 13 μS, which is 60 times lower than HRCT temporal bone imaging. For comparative analysis, head MDCT has an effective dose of approximately 1–2 mSv. Commercially available dentomaxillofacial CBCT systems have a point dose measurement in the range of 13–498 μS, while most fall in the range of 30–80 μS [34].

A summary of the differences between MDCT and CBCT is provided in Table 2.1.

Table 2.1 A summary of differences between MDCT and CBCT

Parameter	MDCT	CBCT
X-ray beam geometry	Fan-beam	Cone-beam
Detector	Ceramic detectors	Solid-state amorphous silicon or selenium detectors with an array of cesium iodide crystals
Spatial resolution	Lower (10–12 lp/cm)	Higher (up to 22 lp/cm)
Temporal resolution	Good	Lower
Contrast resolution	Good	Lower
DQE	Good	Lower
Quantum noise	Low	Higher
Reconstruction algorithm	Filtered back projection, iterative reconstruction	Feldkamp algorithm, modified Feldkamp algorithm
Radiation dose	1–2 mSv	0.1–0.35 mSv

2.8 CBCT Applications in the Neck and Head

CBCT was first utilized in dentistry in the USA at 'Loma Linda University' in 2000. Since then, it has experienced rapid expansion, wide clinical use, and significant technological advancement, including increased imaging speed and resolution [35].

All areas of dentistry, like endodontics, orthodontics, pathology/oral surgery, periodontics, and implant therapy planning, use CBCT technology extensively. Different applications may be chosen depending on the features of the CBCT device, like the size of the detector and voxel size. Before getting CBCT images of a patient, the clinician needs to look at the patient's medical history, previous radiographic images, and clinical information to check the requirement for CBCT pictures. There should be a balance between risks of radiation exposure and information gained by analysis [35].

2.8.1 Applications in Implant Dentistry

The growing requirement for dental implants to substitute lost teeth necessitates a method that can evaluate the alveolar and implant site with extreme accuracy. This will help with treatment planning and prevent injury to nearby important tissues during surgery. In past, these measurements were often collected using 2D radiography and (in certain circumstances) by taking the help of traditional CT. Nevertheless, CBCT is the ideal method for implant dentistry, as it provides more accurate measurements than 2D imaging while using less radiation. The new software has decreased the likelihood of injured anatomical structures and malpositioned fixtures [36–38]. In implant planning, CBCT uses multiplanar and three-dimensional images to determine the width, height, and alveolar ridge morphology of alveolar bone and the relationship between edentulous sites and neighbouring anatomical structures. These essential structures consist of "mandibular canal, mental foramen, maxillary sinus, and nasal fossa". The CBCT datasets used can be to perform guided implant placement operations (Fig. 2.5). The doctor has assessed whether pre-prosthetic surgery, like sinus lift or bone grafting, is needed before implant implantation using the CBCT's 3D capacity. CBCT has decreased implant failures by revealing details regarding each patient's individual bone density, alveolus shape, and width and height of the intended implant location. The HU (Hounsfield Unit) numbers taken from this technology could not be recognized over CBCT individuals or machines because 'bone density numbers' from CBCT are not precise and could not be associated with HU units taking into account image acquisition techniques used in CBCT machines opposed to HU numbers taken from conventional CT [39].

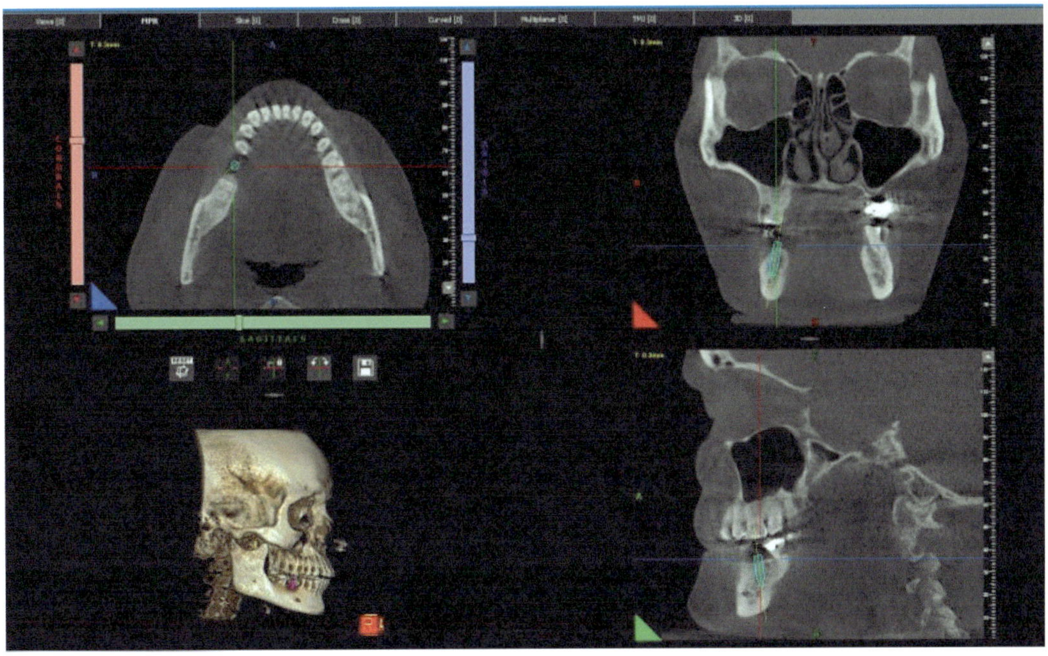

Fig. 2.5 Implant placement planning in CBCT

2.8.2 Orthodontics Application

CBCT provides superimposition-free pictures that are auto-corrected to magnify, having a measuring ratio of 1:1, for morphometric examination of structures and anatomical relations necessary for meeting a variety of orthodontic requirements. The estimation of skeletal growth patterns, palatal bone thickness, dental age, visualization of impacted teeth, measurement of 'alveolar bone width' for buccolingual teeth motion, evaluation of upper airway, and planning of facial 'orthognathic and orthomorphic' operations are some of the uses of orthodontics [40–43]. The chief method for determining facial age, growth, airway function, and abnormalities in tooth eruptive patterns is the availability of software such as dolphin as well as in vivo dental in combination with CBCT pictures for analysis of cephalometric. CBCT gives graphical instructions for the safe implantation of mini-implants, thereby preventing unintentional and permanent damage to essential structures [44, 45]. CBCT is an effective technique for evaluating the impacted teeth's proximity to critical structures that may restrict the movement of orthodontics. During mini-implant placement as a temporary anchor, CBCT provides necessary visual instructions for secure insertion, which avoids unintentional and permanent root injury. Bone density can be assessed before, during, and after therapy to see whether it is increasing, decreasing, or the same [46, 47].

2.8.2.1 CBCT in OSA (Obstructive Sleep Apnoea)

Determining the size and form of the pharynx is essential when diagnosing obstructive sleep apnoea and considering surgery, especially mandibular or maxillary setback treatments. "In cross-section, the pharynx is more elliptical compared to round"; therefore, 2D data from 'lateral cephalogram' might be misleading or insufficient for obstructive sleep apnoea detection [48].

2.8.2.2 Cleft Lip and Palate (CL/P)

Three-dimensional volumetric reconstructions of a patient having bilateral CL/P are beneficial for getting specific information on the defect's size, status, and position of teeth (Fig. 2.6).

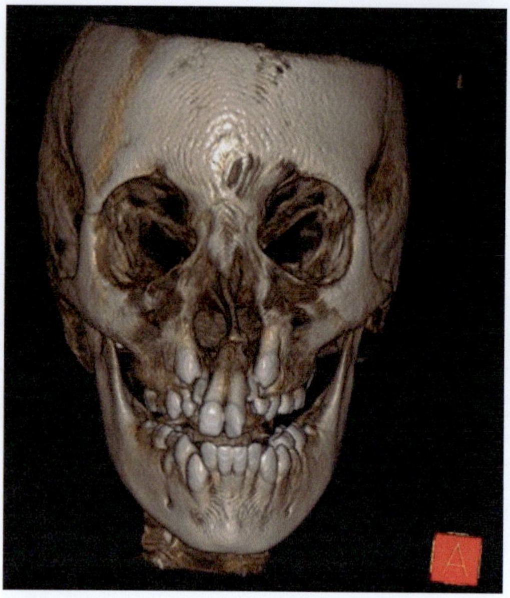

Fig. 2.6 3D volumetric reconstruction of a patient with bilateral CL/CP-frontal view

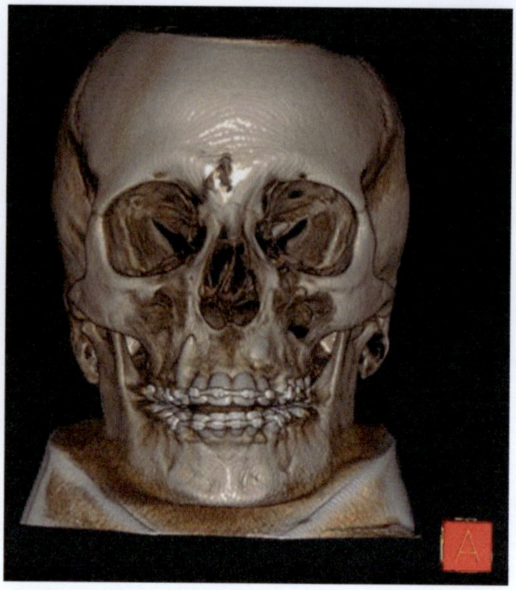

Fig. 2.7 3D volumetric reconstruction that aids in computer-aided orthognathic surgery (CAOS)

2.8.2.3 Craniofacial and Orthognathic Anomalies Surgical Planning and Implementation

Combining CBCT with CASS ('computer-aided surgical simulation') or CAOS ('computer-aided orthognathic surgery') allows for refining diagnosis and improving objectives in three-dimensional virtual treatment planning in improving surgical procedures and results (Fig. 2.7).

2.8.2.4 Asymmetry

When there are significant disparities between bilateral structures, CBCT scans make it possible to apply a technique known as 'mirroring', in which the 'normal side' is projected onto the 'discrepant side' to stimulate and see wanted outcome and to design surgical procedures to facilitate correction.

2.8.2.5 TMJ Degeneration, Functional Shifts, Progressive Bite Changes, and Responses to Therapy

The precision and superior dependability of the CBCT pictures for the diagnosis of condylar morphology and erosion were demonstrated by McCrillis MJ, et al. in their comparison of the CBCT imaging with complicated panoramic radiography and linear tomographic views [49].

2.8.2.6 Interpreting the Cone-Beam Data Volume for Occult Pathology"

Clinical examination or the patient'' medical history did not indicate or suggest sinus blockage, a calcified plaque, osteoarthritic alterations in vertebral bodies or TMJ ('temporomandibular joint') condyle, or even cysts or tumours. These results are referred to as 'occult' (Fig. 2.8).

2.8.2.7 Alveolar Boundary Conditions

The planned or projected tooth movement may be restricted or interfered with by compromised pretreatment alveolar border conditions. The condition will probably get worse during orthodontic treatment if weakened alveolar bone is not detected before starting treatment and taken into consideration in the treatment plan (Fig. 2.9). Table 2.2 summarizes the orthodontic applications of CBCT.

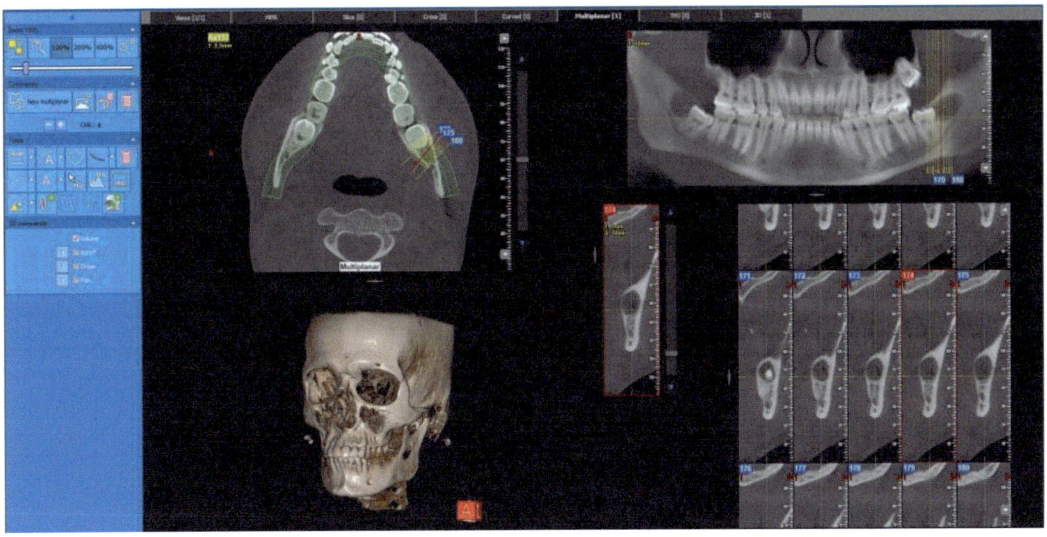

Fig. 2.8 Interpreting the cone-beam data volume for occult pathology

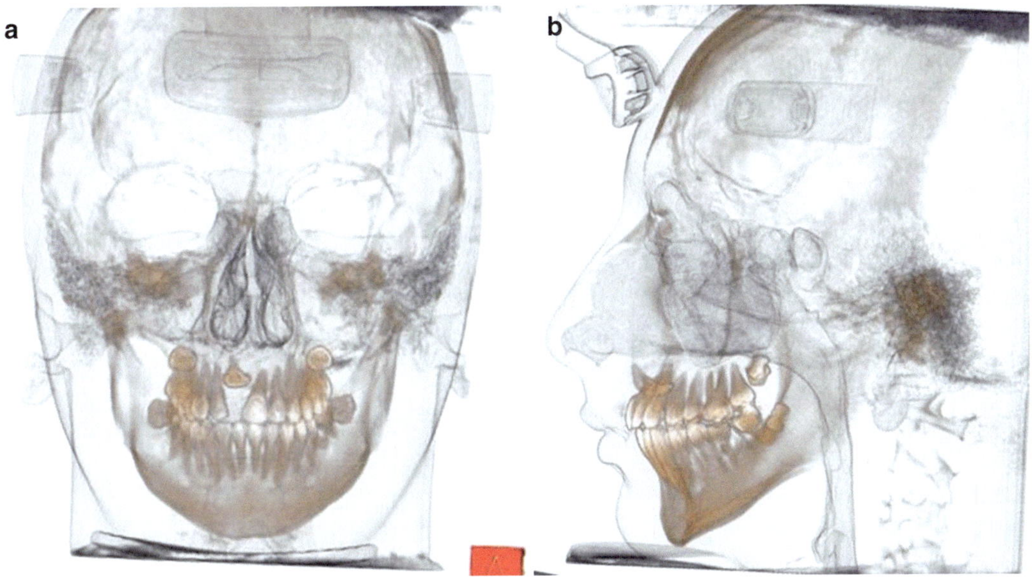

Fig. 2.9 (**a** and **b**) Alveolar boundary conditions

2.8.2.8 Treatment of Impacted Teeth

3D assessment of anomalies in dental position such as impactions and ectopic teeth becomes possible with the use of CBCT. It allows the visualization of impacted teeth in three dimensions, as well as the evaluation of the roots of the impacted and adjacent teeth. It has also become possible to assess the prognosis of tooth de-impaction using CBCT. CBCT can also be used for 3D reconstruction of tooth structure to appreciate root resorption on teeth adjacent to impacted teeth and other surface anomalies [35].

Table 2.2 Application of CBCT in orthodontics

Orthodontic situation	CBCT application
Diagnosis	Estimation of dental and skeletal structures
	Skeletal jaw relation
	Symmetry/asymmetry
	3D evaluation of the impacted tooth and evaluating the position and anatomy
	Growth assessment and the pharyngeal airway analysis
	3D assessment of the TMJ complex
	Assessment of cleft palate
	Assessment of mid-palatal suture maturation
Treatment planning	Orthognathic surgical treatment
	Planning for placement of temporary anchorage devices (TADs)
	Accurate estimation of space requirement for unerupted/impacted teeth
	Used in association with CAD/CAM technology for the fabrication of custom appliances (lingual orthodontic appliance)
Treatment progress	Estimation of dentofacial orthopaedics
	Results of alveolar bone grafts in cleft palate instances
	Superposition of orthognathic surgery
Risk assessment	Examination of orthodontic-associated paraesthesia
	Evaluation of orthodontics-related root resorption
	TMD after therapy

Machado et al (2015) [50]

2.8.2.9 Mid-Palatal Suture Evaluation

Mid-palatal sutural fusion has been classified using CBCT which allows the diagnosis of the overall anteroposterior characteristics of the mid-palatal suture, without the issue of superimposition of other anatomic structures. This provides reliable parameters for the clinical decision between conventional and surgically assisted RME for adolescent and young adult patients [35].

2.8.3 CBCT Applications in Endodontics

The CBCT use in endodontics has a wide range of potential benefits, particularly when evaluating complicated anatomical structures [51]. However, the increased effective dosage of ionizing radiation compared to conventional 2D radiographs is not always justified. CBCT should generally only be used in endodontics for the management and evaluation of the difficult endodontic problems that would be listed here.

2.8.3.1 Apical Periodontitis Detection

Inflammatory lesions of pulp and periapical regions are the pathologic disorders that affect teeth most frequently. In this aspect, CBCT is far more sensitive and accurate than conventional radiography to diagnose apical periodontitis in human patients; periapical bone loss as a sign of endodontic infection can be detected with CBCT before it is visible on conventional radiographs. Although there are numerous inconsistencies between periapical radiographs and CBCT in identifying the apical status of molar teeth, especially in the maxillary arch, CBCT detects periapical lesions in 62 per cent more cases when compared to conventional radiographs, and even the evaluation of subject teeth has been improved by parallax views in the latter method. Additionally, CBCT can show discrete cancellous and cortical bone abnormalities. Consequently, CBCT significantly outperformed periapical radiography in terms of detecting apical periodontitis [52] (Fig. 2.10).

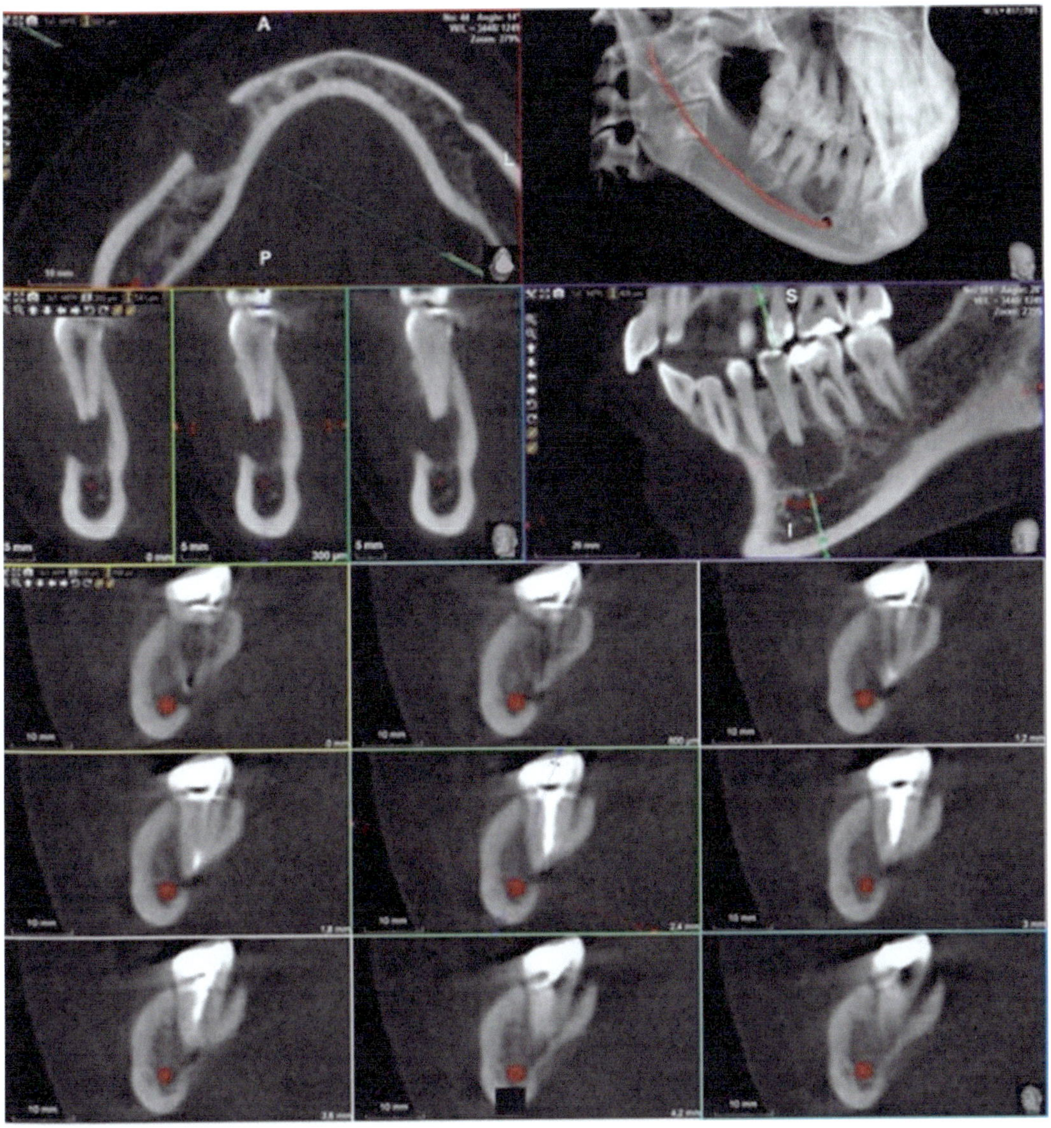

Fig. 2.10 CBCT showing periapical radiolucency in mandibular premolar

2.8.3.2 Potential Surgical Sites Assessment

A very helpful tool for planning surgical endodontic treatment is CBCT. It is possible to carefully examine the spatial relation between particular tooth roots going through surgery (and resulting bone destruction) and surrounding anatomical structures like 'maxillary sinuses, inferior oral nerve canal, and mental foramen'. "Rigolone et al. [52] determined that CBCT plays an essential role in periapical microsurgery" planning on endodontic root resorption from other conditions, determining the prognosis, classification of the lesion, and treatment. The resorptive lesion goes undiscovered till it is visible on conventional scans, by which time the tooth may have sustained substantial damage.

2.8.3.3 Root Canal Anatomy and Morphology Assessment

Identification, cleansing, obturation, and shape of all accessible parts of the root canal system are essential for endodontic treatment to be successful. Because of this, a treatment's success may be adversely impacted by failing to identify and treat all canals. For instance, depending on the research approach, it has been reported that the occurrence of second mesiobuccal canal (MB2) in maxillary first molars ranges from 69% to 93% [53]. The superimposition of anatomical components causes this diversity in the buccolingual plane. At their best, conventional radiography can only show up to 55% of these configurations. Contrarily, the detection rate of CBCT increased from 60% to 93.36% with the increase in resolution. CBCT is a reliable tool for precisely evaluating curvature degree related to the roots of teeth, and preoperative availability of this data minimizes the likelihood of the above-mentioned aberrations [54, 55]. Furthermore, when endodontic therapy for teeth with morphological and anatomical abnormalities, like tooth fusion and dens invaginatus, is necessary, CBCT was demonstrated as a valuable treatment and assessment planning tool (Fig. 2.11).

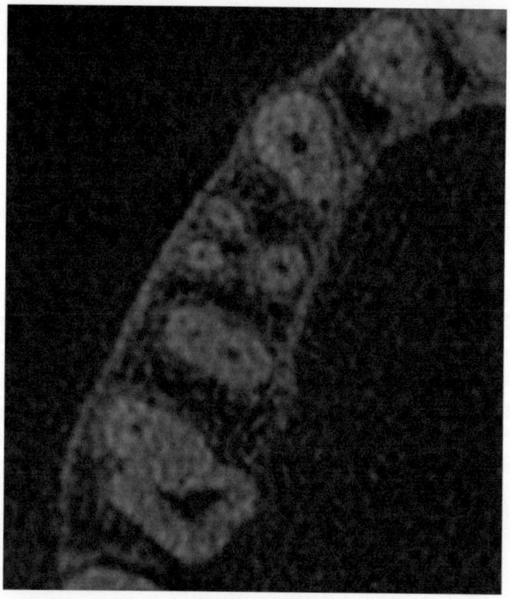

Fig. 2.11 CBCT image of maxillary first molar showing MB2 canal

2.8.3.4 Diagnosis of Various Types of Root Resorption

After avulsion injury and dental luxation, ERR ('external root resorption') is a frequent problem. Conventional radiography has a much lower sensitivity than CBCT for identifying 'ERR in the early stages before resorption can be seen on conventional radiographs'; the impacted tooth may have suffered serious hard tissue damage. Furthermore, it should be understood that "ERR superimposed on root canal could mimic internal resorption" when root resorption is diagnosed depending on conventional radiographic results and that it can be particularly challenging to distinguish between internal resorption and ECR ('external cervical resorption'). The resorptive lesion goes undetected till it is visible on conventional scans, by which time the tooth may have sustained substantial damage. Now, CBCT is frequently utilized to evaluate the severity of specific kinds of ERR and prognosis of the impacted tooth [56] (Fig. 2.12).

2.8.3.5 Vertical Root Fractures Diagnosis

Root fractures are hard to reliably detect with standard radiography, although they are less prevalent compared to crown fractures and account for 7% of dental injuries. The root fracture presence is not necessarily clinically or radiographically evident until the fracture has been for some time. It must be emphasized that radiographic signs of VRF, like halo- and J-shaped radiolucencies, do not emerge till considerable bone loss takes place. Same-shaped radiolucencies can also develop in apical periodontitis cases unrelated to VRF. Research has confirmed that CBCT is highly sensitive compared to traditional radiography in detecting VRF. VRFs of teeth with endodontic treatment should be represented by small-FOV CBCTs. However, it must be considered when evaluating 'root-filled teeth for VRF' with CBCT as scatter created by "root filling or other high-density intra-articular" materials can mistakenly propose the fracture presence [57].

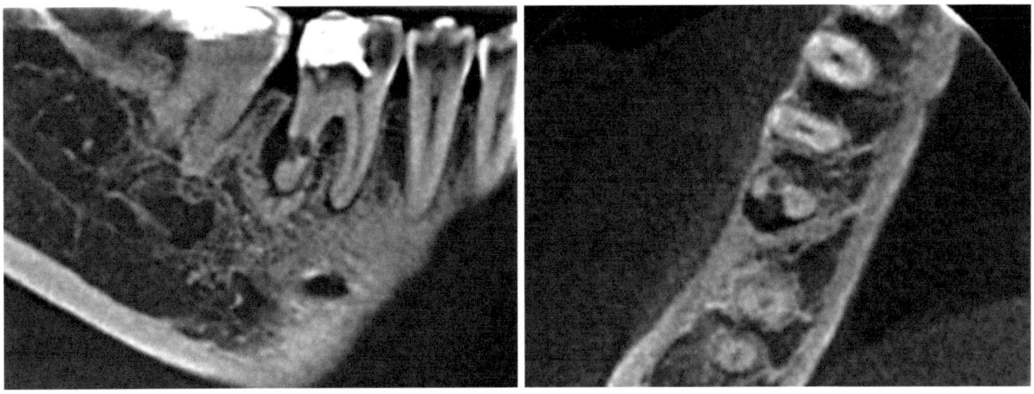

Fig. 2.12 CBCT showing external root resorption

2.9 Application in the Detection of Maxillofacial Fractures

Due to the overlap of multiple tissues, it is extremely difficult to evaluate a fracture using conventional 2D radiography, especially in the maxillary complicated region. Also, due to the clinical condition and the patients' uncooperative attitude, the examination of patients having 'maxillofacial injuries' could be very difficult. Instead, for the detection of complicated maxillary fractures, three-dimensional CBCT is a more affordable and dose-effective option than traditional two-dimensional imaging provides the physician with three-dimensional reconstructed images for the study of the injury's nature, fracture's location, and degree of fractured segments' displacement. These images aid the doctor in formulating the best clinical strategy for stabilization and reduction of fractured segments. Panoramic radiographs in most of the cases show mandibular fracture, but a few instances require confirmation through CBCT when there is the displacement of 'fracture fragments in mandibular corpus and fractures' having fracture lines not parallel to the X-ray beam [58]. To better the management of trauma patients, the CBCT must be done for patients suspected of mandibular and maxillofacial fractures. This procedure should be employed along with panoramic radiographs which are particularly advantageous as the first screening of complex fractures (Fig. 2.13).

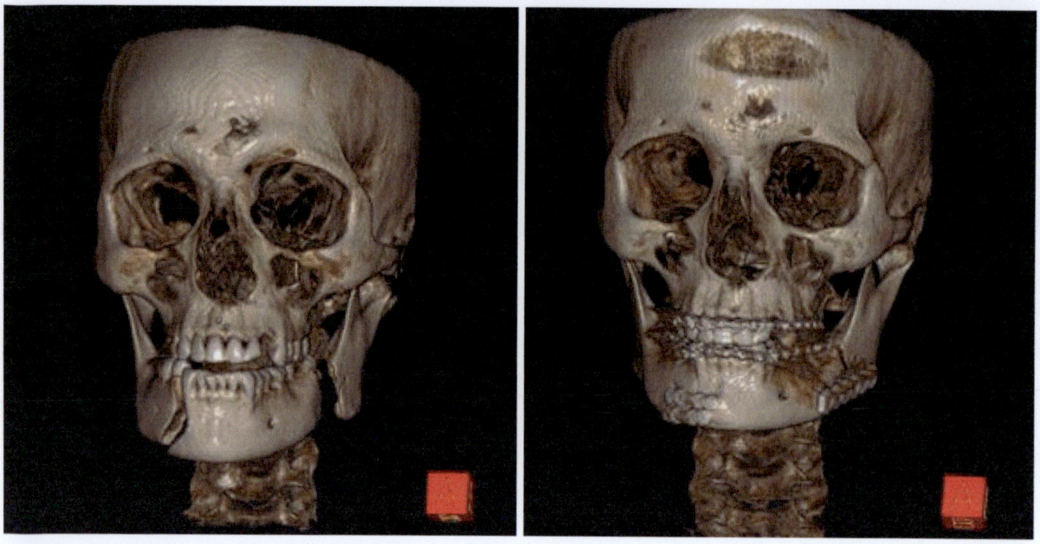

Fig. 2.13 CBCT showing Mandibular fracture

2.10 Application in Diagnosing TMDs ('Temporomandibular Joint Disorders')

TMDs are the most prevalent type of orofacial pain affecting the TMJ and its accompanying muscles. Fractures, dislocation, ankylosis, growth anomalies, and a variety of degenerative joint illnesses, such as erosions, subchondral sclerosis, osteophytes, flattening, and pseudocysts, are the TMJ conditions for which CBCT is the most beneficial [59]. To evaluate the strain the articular disc experiences while chewing, analysis of dynamic interaction between the articular surfaces of the TMJ is important; if this strain is significant, the integrity of the disc may be compromised. In the course of a CBCT scan, three-dimensional visuals of the mandibular condyle and adjacent structures are captured. These images are crucial for analysing and diagnosing the bone's morphological characteristics, joint space, and dynamic functionality. These factors significantly influence the treatment results for patients exhibiting symptoms and diagnoses of temporomandibular disorders (TMD). Research utilizing Field of Views (FOVs) of 6, 9, and 12 inches and voxel sizes of 0.2, 0.3, and 0.6 mm each has shown that the FOV can impact the diagnostic precision of CBCT in identifying erosive modifications of the condyle. A CBCT scanner, recognized for its superior resolution and smallest FOV (voxel size of 0.2 mm), has been demonstrated to detect irregularities in the condyle with a sensitivity exceeding 80% [60]. Previous research has demonstrated that MRI ("magnetic resonance imaging") is the chosen imaging modality for evaluating anterior disc displacement without declining; however, this method has less diagnostic precision for bony alterations, which must be further investigated with CBCT. Automatic registration of CBCT scans and MRI was introduced in recent times to provide complimentary images of both soft and hard tissues of TMJ in a single imaging frame. This advancement has significantly improved the accuracy of diagnoses and treatments. Al-Saleh et al. [60] discovered that fused MRI-CBCT ('magnetic resonance imaging–cone-beam computed tomography') registered pictures increased intra- as well as inter-examiner consistency and exhibited greater diagnostic value in the diagnosis of internal TMJ derangement. To establish the dependability and precision of MRI-CBCT registration for TMDs, additional clinical research is required (Fig. 2.14).

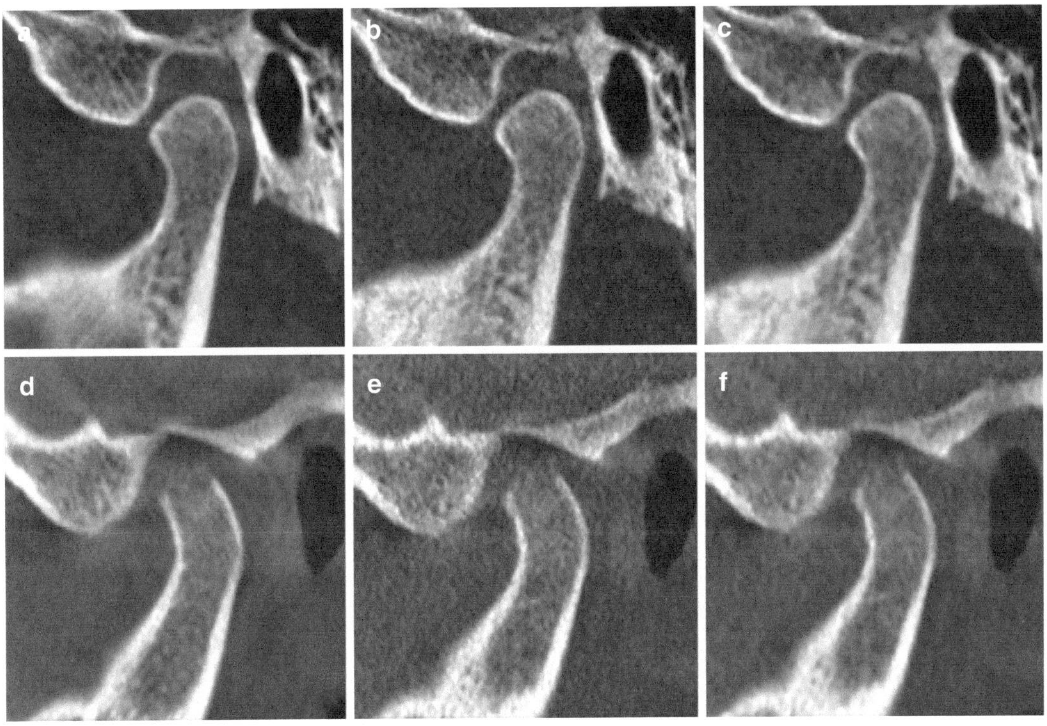

Fig. 2.14 CBCT aids in diagnosing temporomandibular joint disorders-normal vs. TMJ with joint pathology

2.11 Application in Periodontics

CBCT proved to be more reproducible and reliable than 2D radiography and defines the level of incipient furcation involvement, buccal and lingual periodontal bone, and intrabody defect [61]. Volume rendering of CBCT can facilitate the assessment of 'pre-operative alveolar bone volume and post-operative bone fill adequacy'. Additionally, CBCT makes it possible to perform a quantitative assessment of the outcome of regenerative periodontal treatment or grafts [62].

Although conventional radiography may more accurately depict bone quality, bone levels, and periodontal ligament space, it was recommended that CBCT has considerable diagnostic uses in periodontics. As a result, the choice to use CBCT imaging must be made after carefully weighing its potential advantages and disadvantages. The reproducibility, together with the reliability of CBCT used for the assessment of alveolar bone thickness and height, may be affected by variations in imaging protocol parameters. Peterson et al. [63] observed that the alveolar bone height is often underestimated by CBCT. The average facial bone height, as observed in CBCT images, ranges from 0.33–0.78 mm to 0.88–1.14 mm, which is less than the range of 0.56–0.35 mm to 1.08–0.92 mm. Mengel et al. demonstrated that CBCT images were better in the detection of periodontal defects compared with periapical radiographs and medical CT. Likewise, Noujeim et al. concluded that the CBCT technique has better diagnostic accuracy than periapical films in the detection of inter-radicular periodontal bone defects.

The effectiveness of CBCT in detecting dehiscence and fenestrations was shown to be inferior to that of traditional two-dimensional radiography, despite CBCT's superior image quality. It was hypothesized that the reduced precision of CBCT could be owing to the metallic dental fillings, the presence of teeth, or other beam-hardening artefacts. 'Full-scan CBCT' (360°) with a voxel size of 0.2 mm and a modest FOV is more successful at detecting dehiscence and fen-

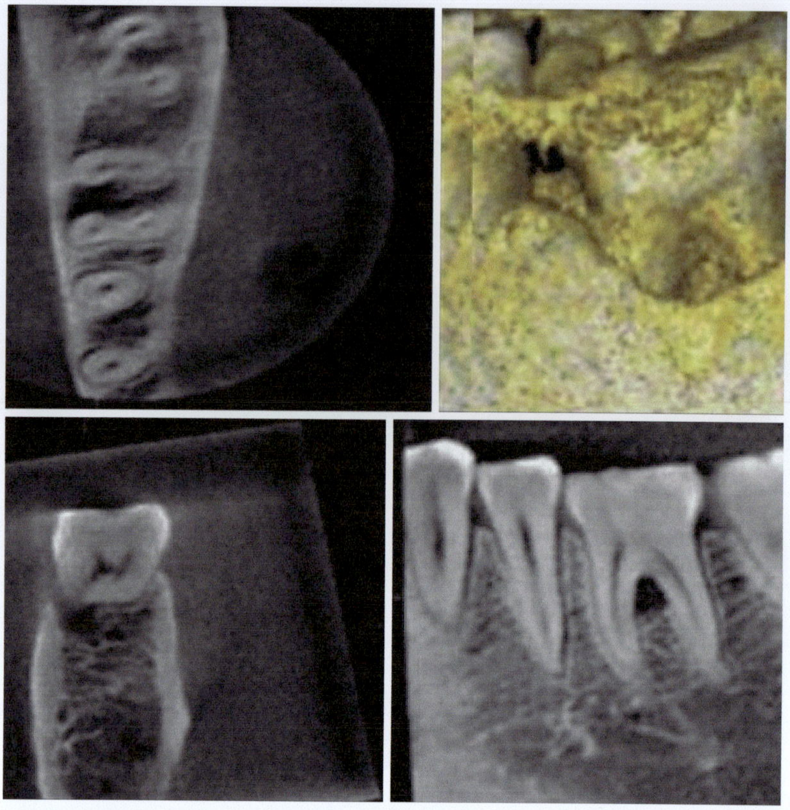

Fig. 2.15 CBCT showing periodontal bone loss

estrations, particularly in peri-implant patients. Peterson et al. observed that CBCT appeared to overrate the presence of fenestration and dehiscence defects and the inter-examiner reliability level varied from poor to moderate ('Cohen's Kappa = −0.09–0.66'). In a different research, Xu et al. [64] discovered that CBCT had limited diagnostic value in clinical practice because the method overestimated the presence of fenestrations and dehiscence in patients with "angle class III" malocclusion's maxillary anterior teeth; however, the agreement level between CBCT imaging and clinical examination was greater for dehiscence compared to fenestration. In contrast to this finding, Leung et al. [65] discovered that root fenestration detection had a greater percentage of diagnostic accuracy than dehiscence detection (Fig. 2.15).

2.12 Application in Forensic Odontology

An important part of forensic investigation is estimating the ages of living or deceased people. In the literature, several methods for determining an individual's age by analysing their teeth have been documented. Examining the pulp area is one method that presents new opportunities in dental age determination. Several techniques, such as tooth cross-sections and radiography, were established to examine pulp chamber size; however, CBCT offers a three-dimensional picture of the pulpal cavity, permitting a more precise calculation of an individual's dental age. CBCT is a reliable imaging technique that concurrently measures the mesiodistal and buccolingual dimensions of a tooth. This allows for the analysis of secondary dentin deposition as age progresses [65]. By creating facial reconstruction at reduced exposure and enhanced speed, CBCT also provides accurate and dependable measurements of the soft tissue thickness for particular landmarks on the scalp and the face. The understanding of the average thickness of the facial soft tissue, which differs in people from different racial and geographic backgrounds, is important for facial reconstruction. This technique is applied in forensic research for the identification of skeletal remains, and it aims to recreate the appearance of a person's face using the skull [66]. Currently, CBCT is applied in forensic studies for postmortem imaging and imaging of metal projectiles with high-density metal balls, e.g. in gunshot cases. It is mainly used because of its small apparatus size, low cost, portability, and metal artifact reduction functionality which it includes.

2.13 Future Perspectives of CBCT

2.13.1 CBCT Images Optimization

CBCT was shown to have greater diagnostic effectiveness in the precise detection of complicated oral as well as maxillofacial diseases when compared to other modalities. The performance of CBCT could potentially be enhanced by adjusting several factors. These include the size of the focal spot, modifications to the beam structure, boosting detector productivity, and fine-tuning both the exposure and the process of image reconstruction. Additionally, because older CBCT scanners typically have large FOV, more scattered radiation is generated and is thus supplied to the patient in higher doses. Using a "small-diameter FOV" that just encompasses the area of interest can optimize older scanners [67]. The first CBCT characteristic to be enhanced was the focused spot size, which was reduced from the 0.5 mm standard focal spot size to enhance image resolution. The creation of adaptive exposure enables the clinician to choose the ideal exposure based on the patient's size, which is another significant advancement. Most CBCT devices rely on their determination of tube voltage and current on grey values of scout images, which automatically reduce exposure levels for patients with modest mass and size. Dynamic automatic exposure control, which adjusts exposure during image acquisition, has recently been used by some machines. To improve image quality, a method called off-axis scanning has been developed. This method uses a half cone with a small overlap at the iso-centre, which effectively doubles the Field of View (FOV) compared to full-cone scanning. As a result, the radiation dose delivered to the patient is reduced. Additionally, it was shown that using a 180° rotation as opposed to a 360° rotation resulted in a dosage reduction of 60% in the posterior and 40% in the anterior. Off-axis scanning lowers the radiation exposure, although the influence on image quality is still being studied. Optimization may potentially be achieved by improving the detector's performance.

2.13.2 Optical Scanners with CBCT

The development of optical scanners recently improved the diagnostic procedure, and the use of CBCT in conjunction with these methods may improve treatment planning. CBCT may produce cross-sectional 3D pictures of the mandible and maxilla for implant surgery; however, it is unable to accurately replicate the surface details as well as the occlusal morphology of teeth. In place of traditional impression materials, we can use intraoral scanners to digitally record the occlusal surfaces of teeth, thus removing the necessity for old-fashioned impression substances. This procedure requires the insertion of a stone cast into an optical scanner, followed by a CBCT machine that mirrors the patient's scanning parameters. When planning minimally invasive surgery [68], these digital tools permit the physician to properly visualize the patient's anatomy. Software advancement has integrated optical facial scanning and CBCT to assess the impact of orthodontic procedures or orthognathic surgery on facial structures. Nevertheless, this three-dimensional illustration of facial characteristics must be validated in future clinical trials [69].

2.13.3 Non-odontogenic Pathologies

Initially, CBCT scans were primarily used for imaging the dental and maxillofacial complex. However, their use has expanded to include the visualization of non-dental-related abnormalities and pathologies in the head and neck region. This primarily includes sinus pathologies such as mucosal thickening, complete opacification, partial opacification with fluid accumulation, and polypoidal mucosal thickening. The imaging of the sinuses has traditionally been done using low-dose multidetector CT; however, this method has some drawbacks. The resulting images, for instance, typically have lesser spatial resolution and are noisier due to metal artefacts. In comparison to multidetector CT, CBCT pictures offer detailed diagnostic information about sinus diseases with superior spatial resolution. CBCT plays a significant role in the calcification process detection and circumstances requiring sinus lifting or bone augmentation treatments. However, MRI is a better tool for detecting tumours of the skull base. Additionally, CBCT can be used to perform a 3D analysis of the upper airway dimensions in patients suffering from conditions such as cleft lip and palate or obstructive sleep apnoea. In circumstances when video fluoroscopy is not available, CBCT scanning has also been performed to evaluate swallowing function. Orthopaedic surgeons are now using it more frequently to photograph the lower and upper extremities and ENT doctors to examine ear and sinus infections at a low radiation dose [70].

2.13.4 Phase Contrast Tomography

Several studies have been published in the literature examining the object's X-ray absorption during phase contrast tomography; nevertheless, more study is still required to understand the phase nature of the X-rays. A new technique known as quantitative phase-contrast cone-beam tomography has been developed by scientists. This approach reconstructs images using the phase coefficient instead of the attenuation coefficient. It utilizes unfiltered radiation from a small polychromatic source, which reduces high spatial frequency noise and enhances the contrast of soft tissues [71].

2.13.5 Advances in Head and Neck Imaging

With advancements in technology and more widespread availability of CBCT systems, its use in diagnostic and intraoperative imaging has expanded. CBCT protocols for imaging of temporal bone structures, paranasal sinuses, and skull bases were developed and are being increasingly used for imaging of these regions. CBCT, owing to low radiation dosage and high spatial resolution, appears to be an attractive imaging modality in an anatomically complex region such as the neck and head. In the below sections, we briefly discuss the applications of CBCT in temporal bone, paranasal sinus, and skull base imaging.

2.13.5.1 CBCT in Temporal Bone Imaging

Temporal bone imaging has been an area of widespread interest as far as the application of CBCT in neck and head imaging is concerned.

In a study on the CBCT of partially modified cadaveric temporal bones, Gupta et al. reported a higher observer score for CBCT as compared with MDCT for the identification of temporal bone structures. In particular, the ossicular chain, internal cochlear anatomy, bony labyrinth, and facial nerve were well visualized on CBCT. The authors also reported reduced streak artefacts in the imaging of cochlear implants and were able to identify laser-induced small changes in the ossicular chain [71]. In another study by Peltonen et al., CBCT compared to MDCT, the authors found CBCT to be at least as precise as MDCT in identifying surgically related structures of the middle ear. The effective radiation dosage reported in their analysis was 60-fold lower than MDCT; however, the authors attributed this reduced effective dose to the very low FOV and short scan time in their study [71]. Imaging middle ear and inner ear implants is one of the most well-researched uses of CBCT in temporal bone imaging. In preclinical cadaveric as well as clinical studies, CBCT has shown reduced streak artefacts and precise electrode-modius relationships. CBCT allows for a detailed evaluation of electrode array placement within the scala vestibule or scala tympani. Apart from imaging of inner and middle ear implants, CBCT has also been applied in the evaluation of hearing loss. In this regard, CBCT is accurate in its depiction of the ossicular erosions and assessment of the continuity of the ossicular chain. CBCT was used in the assessment of the middle and inner ear implants after surgery, intraoperative assessment, and identification of the ductus reuniens [72–80].

Low contrast resolution is a limitation of CBCT while imaging the temporal bone for soft tissue lesions such as vascular tumours. At present, CBCT is useful in the assessment of middle and inner ear implants, while applications in the evaluation of hearing loss continue to evolve.

2.13.5.2 CBCT in Imaging of Paranasal Sinuses

CBCT offers a high spatial resolution and definition for bone imaging with a limited FOV and is an attractive modality for paranasal sinus imaging [81, 82]. In a comparative study between CBCT and 64-slice MDCT, it was found that CBCT achieved an isotropic spatial resolution of 12-line pairs per centimetre (lp/cm) at an effective dose of 0.17 mSv. This is in contrast with MDCT, which achieved a spatial resolution of 11 lp/cm at a higher effective dose of 0.87 mSv. There is substantial evidence supporting the use of CBCT in imaging the paranasal sinuses, particularly in the context of endoscopic sinus surgery (ESS). In these cases, CBCT has proven to be effective in identifying sinus partitions, visualizing stents, facilitating sinus irrigation, and guiding surgical navigation into the frontal recess [83, 84]. Intraoperative CBCT was shown to improve surgical outcomes, help in modification of surgical techniques, and help in a better understanding of intraoperative anatomy. While useful in intraoperative imaging for endoscopic surgery, CBCT still has a long way to go as far as routine diagnostic imaging of paranasal sinuses is concerned due to its low soft-tissue resolution [85]. Also, complications of endoscopic sinus surgery such as encephalocele, meningitis, and subarachnoid haemorrhage may not be detected by CBCT and remain a limitation as compared to MDCT [86].

2.13.5.3 CBCT in Imaging of the Skull Base

The skull base offers itself as a viable ground for exploring the potential CBCT use in high-resolution 3D imaging given the complexity of the anatomy of the skull base [87]. Current imaging of the skull base is catered to by CT and MRI which not only delineate the bony anatomy but also the soft tissue anatomy, which is vital for the diagnosis and treatment in skull base pathologies. To this end, few study protocols have evaluated the function of CBCT in imaging of the skull base. One such CBCT system is the xCAT intraoperative CBCT scanner (Xoran Technologies), which has shown positive results in preliminary studies [88–90]. With advances in CBCT technology, it may be reasonable to expect more positive results on CBCT use in skull base imaging lesions.

2.14 Micro-CT

Micro-CT is a high-resolution CT technique. In the early 1980s, micro-CT was developed by Feldkamp as a tool to study ceramics [91]. Over some time, the micro-CT scanners were used in academic and industrial research and began to be considered as a potential replacement for histological sectioning of materials to determine the internal structure [92, 93].

Various components of micro-CT scanners are depicted in the schematic diagram below.

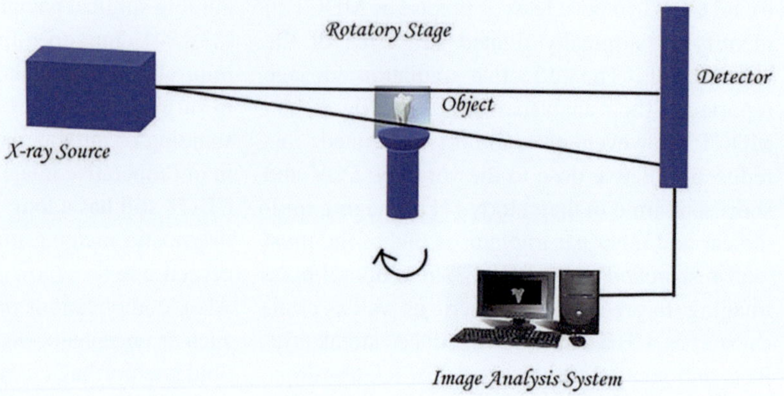

Fig. 2.16 Schematic representation of the mechanism of image acquisition in micro-CT

Essential components of micro-CT include an X-ray tube (90–150 KV), filters, collimators, a computer-controlled electric motor, a charge-coupled device, image intensifiers, a computer, and a specimen stand. Broadly, two types of image acquisition are done using micro-CT [94]. During in vivo imaging, an optical X-ray tube and detector are rotated around the structure to be imaged, while during ex vivo imaging, the object is rotated on a rotating platform, and the X-ray detector and the tube are held stationary. During ex vivo imaging, an electric motor is used to rotate the platform, and the electric motor in turn is regulated by the computer [95, 96]. Lead shielding is used during scanning to protect the operators from radiation. The data acquired during micro-CT is reconstructed into a high spatial resolution image with an isotropic voxel volume of 5–50 μm^3, which is approximately 10^6 times smaller as compared with conventional CT (Fig. 2.16).

The high spatial resolution offered by micro-CT puts it in an advantageous position as far as exploring the microstructural details of bone and tooth is concerned. This makes micro-CT a non-destructive technique for the analysis of tissues as opposed to tissue sectioning. With micro-CT, the same structure may be imaged repeatedly while maintaining the anatomical and biochemical properties of the structure. This offers the advantage that the structure can be subjected to further analysis by other methods [97].

High radiation dose, requirement for computer expertise, and limited field of view for imaging are some of the potential drawbacks of micro-CT, which have prevented a more widespread utilization of micro-CT in clinical practice. Also, the volume of data is enormous and puts a lot of demand on storage and retrieval. A single data file from micro-CT may have a size of about 3 GB [92].

Recently, micro-CT has been used in preclinical and experimental studies, mainly in dentistry. As compared with CBCT, micro-CT has a higher spatial resolution and a shorter scan time, enabling a more detailed analysis of subtle structural changes. Furthermore, the attenuation values (HU) computed using CBCT are erroneous due to cone-beam geometry, artefacts and flat panel detectors, and thus computation of HU using CBCT must be avoided. Measurements of HU using micro-CT are more reliable. Micro CT may be more suitable in the detection of periodontal disease, bone erosions, carious lesions, and intraoperative imaging as compared with CBCT [93, 94, 98, 99].

The applications of micro-CT such as bioengineering biomedical research and tissue engineering. In dentomaxillofacial imaging, micro-CT has been evaluated in endodontics, the study of dental apex resorption due to bacterial disease, surrounding bone and implants, development of the craniofacial skeleton, and tooth-restorative interfaces [100]. Moreover, micro-CT reconstructions of tooth crowns and tooth roots are considered the gold standard for volume or surface area measurements.

Micro-CT has emerged as a useful technology for the evaluation of burs used for the removal of adhesives post orthodontic treatment. This aids in deciding the appropriate bur for debonding procedures as well as assessment of enamel surface to check for cracks or micro damages. It can also be used for the assessment of microleakages following orthodontic bonding procedures.

2.15 Summary

The recent advances in CBCT technology, particularly in craniofacial imaging, have significantly expanded its range of applications. Since CBCT also allows for a limited field of view and thus reduces unnecessary radiation exposure, it has found its way as one of the necessary armamentaria for dental imaging and clinical setups. Soon, it may become an essential prerequisite for such setups, and with the future perspective in mind, it will be paired with optical scanners for optimum results intraorally as well as extra-orally.

References

1. Robb RA. The dynamic spatial reconstructor: an x-ray video-fluoroscopic CT scanner for dynamic volume imaging of moving organs. IEEE Trans Med Imaging. 1982;1(22–33):34.
2. Orth RC, Wallace MJ, Kuo MD, for the Technology Assessment Committee of the Society of Interventional Radiology. C-arm cone-beam CT: general principles and technical considerations for use in interventional radiology. J VascInterv Radiol. 2008;19:814 –20. Epub 2008 Apr 23
3. Dörfler A, Struffert T, Engelhorn T, et al. Rotational flat-panel computed tomography in diagnostic and interventional neuroradiology. Rofo. 2008;180:891–8.
4. Moore CJ, Am A, Marchant T, et al. Developments in and experience of kilovoltage x-ray cone beam image-guided radiotherapy. Br J Radiol. 2006;79 Spec No 1:S66–78.
5. Hounsfield GN. Nobel award address: computed medical imaging. Med Phys. 1980;7:283–90.
6. Seeram E. Computed tomography: physical principles, clinical applications, and quality control. Philadelphia, PA: W.B. Saunders; 2001. p. 2–3.
7. Scarfe WC, Farman AG, Sukovic P. Clinical applications of cone-beam computed tomography in dental practice. J Can Dent Assoc. 2006;72:75–80.
8. Gupta R, Grasruck M, Suess C, et al. Ultra-high resolution flat-panel volume CT: fundamental principles, design architecture, and system characterization. Eur Radiol. 2006;16:1191–205. Epub 2006 Mar 10
9. Baba R, Konno Y, Ueda K, et al. Comparison of flat-panel detector and image intensifier detector for cone-beam CT. Comput Med Imaging Graph. 2002;26:153–8.
10. Feldkamp LA, Davis LC, Kress JW. Practical cone-beam algorithm. J Opt Soc Am. 1984;A1:612–9.
11. Yan XH, Leahy RM. Derivation and analysis of a filtered back projection algorithm for cone beam projection data. IEEE Trans Med Imaging. 1991;10:462–72.
12. Kudo H, Noo F, Defrise M, et al. New super-short-scan algorithm for fan-beam and cone-beam reconstruction. IEEE NSS-MIC. 2002:902–6.
13. Gupta R, Bartling SH, Basu SK, et al. Experimental flat-panel high-spatial resolution volume CT of the temporal bone. AJNR Am J Neuroradiol. 2004;25:1417–24.
14. Siewerdsen JH, Jaffray DA. Cone-beam computed tomography with a flat panel imager: magnitude and effects of x-ray scatter. Med Phys. 2001;28:220–31.
15. Graham SA, Moseley DJ, Siewerdsen JH, et al. Compensators for dose and scatter management in cone-beam computed tomography. Med Phys. 2007;34:2691–703.
16. Siewerdsen JH, Moseley DJ, Bakhtiar B, et al. The influence of anti scatter grids on soft-tissue detectability in cone-beam computed tomography with flat panel detectors. Med Phys. 2004;31:3506–20.
17. Ning R, Chen B, Yu R, et al. Flat panel detector-based cone-beam volume CT angiography imaging: system evaluation. IEEE Trans Med Imaging. 2000;19:949–63.
18. Fahrig R, Dixon R, Payne T, et al. Dose and image quality for a cone-beam C-arm CT system. Med Phys. 2006;33:4541–50.
19. Neitzel U. Grids or air gaps for scatter reduction in digital radiography: a model calculation. Med Phys. 1992;19:475–81.
20. Nickoloff EL, Lu ZF, Dutta A, et al. Influence of flat-panel fluoroscopic equipment variables on cardiac radiation doses. Cardiovasc Intervent Radiol. 2007;30:169–76.
21. Wiegert J, Bertram M, Schafer D, et al. Soft tissue contrast resolution within the head of human cadaver by means of flat detector based cone-beam CT. Proc SPIE. 2004;5368:330–7.
22. Jarry G, Graham SA, Moseley DJ, et al. Characterization of scattered radiation in kV CBCT images using Monte Carlo simulations. Med Phys. 2006;33:4320–9.

23. Siewerdsen JH, Daly MJ, Bakhtiar B, et al. A simple, direct method for x-ray scatter estimation and correction in digital radiography and cone-beam CT. Med Phys. 2006;33:187–97.
24. Ning R, Tang X, Conover D. X-ray scatter correction algorithm for cone beam CT imaging. Med Phys. 2004;31:1195–202.
25. Malusek A, Sandborg M, Carlsson GA. Simulation of scatter in cone beam CT: effect on projection image quality. Proc SPIE. 2003;5030:740–51.
26. Cowen AR, Kengyelics SM, Davies AG. Solid-state, flat-panel, digital radiography detectors and their physical imaging characteristics. Clin Radiol. 2008;63:487–98. Epub 2008 Jan 31
27. Roos PG, Colbeth RE, Mollov I, et al. Multiple gain ranging readout method to extend the dynamic range of amorphous silicon flat panel imagers. Proc SPIE. 2004;5368:139–49.
28. Bacher K, Smeets P, Vereecken L, et al. Image quality and radiation dose on digital chest imaging: comparison of amorphous silicon and amorphous selenium flat-panel systems. AJR Am J Roentgenol. 2006;187:630–7.
29. Bacher K, Smeets P, Bonnarens K, et al. Dose reduction in patients undergoing chest imaging: digital amorphous silicon flat-panel detector radiography versus conventional film-screen radiography and phosphor-based computed radiography. AJR Am J Roentgenol. 2003;181:923–39.
30. Völk M, Paetzel C, Angele P, et al. Routine skeleton radiography using a flatpanel detector: image quality and clinical acceptance at 50% dose reduction. Investig Radiol. 2003;38:230–5.
31. Farman TT, Vandre RH, Pajak JC, et al. Effects of scintillator on the detective quantum efficiency (DQE) of a digital imaging system. Oral Surg Oral Med Oral Pathol Oral Radiol Endod. 2006;101:219–23. Epub 2005 Nov 11
32. Bauhs JA, Vrieze TJ, Primak AN, et al. CT dosimetry: comparison of measurement techniques and devices. Radiographics. 2008;28:245–53.
33. Mori S, Endo M, Nishizawa K, et al. Enlarged longitudinal dose profiles in cone-beam CT and the need for modified dosimetry. Med Phys. 2005;32:1061–9.
34. Kyriakou Y, Deak P, Langner O, et al. Concepts for dose determination in flat-detector CT. Phys Med Biol. 2008;53:3551–66. Epub 2008 Jun 13
35. Mah J, Hatcher D. Three-dimensional craniofacial imaging. Am J Orthod Dentofacial Orthop. 2004;126(3):308–9. https://doi.org/10.1016/j.ajodo.2004.06.024.
36. Pauwels R. Cone beam CT for dental and maxillofacial imaging: dose matters. Radiat Prot Dosim. 2015;165(1–4):156–61. https://doi.org/10.1093/rpd/ncv057. Epub 2015 Mar 23
37. Yajima A, Otonari-Yamamoto M, Sano T, Hayakawa Y, Otonari T, Tanabe K, Wakoh M, Mizuta S, Yonezu H, Nakagawa K, Yajima Y. Cone beam CT (CB Throne) applied to dentomaxillofacial region. Bull Tokyo Dent Coll. 2006;47(3):133–41.
38. Almog DM, LaMar J, LaMar FR, LaMar F. Cone beam computerized tomography-based dental imaging for implant planning and surgical guidance, part 1: single implant in the mandibular molar region. J Oral Implantol. 2006;32(2):77–81.
39. Tyndall DA, Price JB, Tetradis S, Ganz SD, Hildebolt C, Scarfe WC, American Academy of O, Maxillofacial R. Position statement of the American academy of oral and maxillofacial radiology on selection criteria for the use of radiology in dental implantology with emphasis on cone beam computed tomography. Oral Surg Oral Med Oral Pathol Oral Radiol. 2012;113(6):817–26.
40. Tischler M. In-office cone beam computerized tomography: technology review and clinical examples. Dent Today. 2008;27(6):102. 104, 106
41. Aboudara CA, Hatcher D, Nielsen IL, Miller A. A three-dimensional evaluation of the upper airway in adolescents. Orthod Craniofac Res. 2003;6(Suppl 1):173–5.
42. Harrell WE Jr. Three-dimensional diagnosis and treatment planning: the use of 3d facial imaging and 3d cone beam CT in orthodontics and dentistry. Austral Dent Pract. 2007;18(4):102–13.
43. Kapila S, Conley RS, Harrell WE Jr. The current status of cone beam computed tomography imaging in orthodontics. Dentomaxillofac Radiol. 2011;40(1):24–34.
44. Peck JL, Sameshima GT, Miller A, Worth P, Hatcher DC. Mesiodistal root angulation using panoramic and cone beam CT. Angle Orthod. 2007;77(2):206–13.
45. Kim SH, Choi YS, Hwang EH, Chung KR, Kook YA, Nelson G. Surgical positioning of orthodontic mini-implants with guides fabricated on models replicated with cone-beam computed tomography. Am J Orthod Dentofacial Orthop. 2007;131(4 Suppl):S82–9.
46. Kim SH, Kang JM, Choi B, Nelson G. Clinical application of a stereolithographic surgical guide for simple positioning of orthodontic mini-implants. World J Orthod. 2008;9(4):371–82.
47. Gracco A, Lombardo L, Cozzani M, Siciliani G. Quantitative evaluation with CBCT of palatal done thickness in growing patients. Prog Orthod. 2006;7(2):164–74.
48. Hungcharassaeng K, Caruso PM, Kan BY, Kim TG. Factors affecting bu al bone changes of maxillary posterior teeth after rapid maxillary expansion. Am J Orthod Dentofacial Orthop. 2007;132(4):428. e1 e8.
49. McCrillis MJ, et al. Obstructive sleep apnea and the use of cone beam computed tomography in airway imaging: a review. Semin Orthod. 2009;15(1):63–9.
50. Machado GL. CBCT imaging–A boon to orthodontics. Saudi Dent J. 2015;27(1):12–21.
51. Lofthag-Hansen S, Huumonen S, Grondahl K, Grondahl HG. Limited cone-beam CT and intraoral radiography for the diagnosis of periapical pathology. Oral Surg Oral Med Oral Pathol Oral Radiol Endod. 2007;103(1):114–9.

52. Rigolone M, Pasqualini D, Bianchi L, Berutti E, Bianchi SD. Vestibular surgical access to the palatine root of the superior first molar: "low-dose cone-beam" CT analysis of the pathway and its anatomic variations. J Endod. 2003;29(11):773–5.
53. Wolcott J, Ishley D, Kennedy W, Johnson S, Minnich S, Meyers J. A 5 yr clinical investigation of second mesiobuccal canals in endodontically treated and retreated maxillary molars. J Endod. 2005;31(4):262–4.
54. Estrela C, Bueno MR, Azevedo BC, Azevedo JR, Pecora JD. A new periapical index based on cone beam computed tomography. J Endod. 2008;34(11):1325–31.
55. D'Addazio PS, Campos CN, Ozcan M, Teixeira HG, Passoni RM, Carvalho AC. A comparative study between cone-beam computed tomography and periapical radiographs in the diagnosis of simulated endodontic complications. Int Endod J. 2011;44(3):218–24.
56. Hassan B, Metska ME, Ozok AR, van der Stelt P, Wesselink PR. Detection of vertical root fractures in endodontically treated teeth by a cone beam computed tomography scan. J Endod. 2009;35(5):719–22.
57. Ersan N, Ilguy M. Diagnosis of unusual mandibular split fracture with cone-beam computed tomography. J Oral Maxillofac Radiol. 2015;3:67–9.
58. Lewis EL, Dolwick MF, Abramowicz S, Reeder SL. Contemporary imaging of the temporomandibular joint. Dent Clin N Am. 2008;52:875–90.
59. Librizzi ZT, Tadinada AS, Valiyaparambil JV, Lurie AG, Mallya SM. Cone-beam computed tomography to detect erosions of the temporomandibular joint: effect of field of view and voxel size on diagnostic efficacy and effective dose. Am J Orthod Dentofacial Orthop. 2011;140:e25–30.
60. Al-Saleh MA, Alsufyani NA, Lagravere M, Nebbe B, Lai H, Jaremko JL, et al. MRI alone versus MRI-CBCT registered images to evaluate temporomandibular joint internal derangement. Oral Surg Oral Med Oral Pathol Oral Radiol. 2016;122:638–45.
61. Oberoi S, Chigurupati R, Gill P, Hoffman WY, Vargervik K. Volumetric assessment of secondary alveolar bone grafting using cone beam computed tomography. Cleft Palate Craniofac J. 2009;46:503–11.
62. Takane M, Sato S, Suzuki K, Fukuda T, Asano Y, Honda K, et al. Clinical application of cone beam computed tomography for ideal absorbable membrane placement in inter-proximal bone defects. J Oral Sci. 2010;52:63–9.
63. Peterson AG, Wang M, Gonzalez S, Covell Jr DA, Katancik J, Sehgal HS. An in vivo and cone beam computed tomography investigation of the accuracy in measuring alveolar bone height and detecting dehiscence and fenestration defects. Int J Oral Maxillofac Implants. 2018;33(6):1296–304.
64. Xu X, Xu L, Jiang JH, Wu JQ, Li XT, Jing WD. Accuracy analysis of alveolar dehiscence and fenestration of maxillary anterior teeth of angle class III by cone-beam CT. Beijing Da Xue Xue Bao. 2018;50:104–9.
65. Leung CC, Palomo L, Griffith R, Hans MG. Accuracy and reliability of cone-beam computed tomography for measuring alveolar bone height and detecting bony dehiscences and fenestrations. Am J Orthod Dentofacial Orthop. 2010;137(4):S109–19.
66. Hwang HS, Choe SY, Hwang JS, Moon DN, Hou Y, Lee WJ, et al. Reproducibility of facial soft tissue thickness measurements using cone-beam CT images according to the measurement methods. J Forensic Sci. 2015;60:957–65.
67. Pauwels R, Jacobs R, Bosmans H, Schulze R. Future prospects for dental cone beam CT imaging. Imaging Med. 2012;4:551–63.
68. Hiraiwa T, Ariji Y, Fukuda M, Kise Y, Nakata K, Katsumata A, et al. A deep-learning artificial intelligence system for assessment of root morphology of the mandibular first molar on panoramic radiography. Dentomaxillofac Radiol. 2019;48:2018.
69. Lata S, Mohanty SK, Vinay S, Das AC, Das S, Choudhury P. Is cone beam computed tomography (CBCT) a potential imaging tool in ENT practice? A cross-sectional survey among ENT surgeons in the State of Odisha, India. Indian J Otolaryngol Head Neck Surg. 2018;70:130–6.
70. Liu J, Cai W, Ning R. Evaluation of differential phase contrast cone beam CT imaging system. J Xray Sci Technol. 2017;25:357–72.
71. Peltonen LI, Aarnisalo AA, Kortesniemi MK, et al. Limited cone-beam computed tomography imaging of the middle ear: a comparison with multislice helical computed tomography. Acta Radiol. 2007;48:207–12.
72. Cerini R, Faccioli N, Barillari M, et al. Bionic ear imaging. Radiol Med. 2008;113:265–77. Epub 2008 Apr 2
73. Yamane H, Takayama M, Sunami K, et al. Three-dimensional images of the reuniting duct using cone beam CT. Acta Otolaryngol. 2009;129:493–6.
74. Husstedt HW, Aschendorff A, Richter B, et al. Nondestructive three-dimensional analysis of electrode to modiolus proximity. Otol Neurotol. 2002;23:49–52.
75. Richter B, Aschendorff A, Lohnstein P, et al. The nucleus contour electrode array: a radiological and histological study. Laryngoscope. 2001;111:508–14.
76. Aschendorff A, Kubalek R, Hochmuth A, et al. Imaging procedures in cochlear implant patients: evaluation of different radiological techniques. Acta Otolaryngol Suppl. 2004;552:46–9.
77. Offergeld C, Kromeier J, Aschendorff A, et al. Rotational tomography of the normal and reconstructed middle ear in temporal bones: an experimental study. Eur Arch Otorrinolaringol. 2007;264:345–51. Epub 2006 Oct 18

78. Aschendorff A, Kubalek R, Turowski B, et al. Quality control after cochlear implant surgery by means of rotational tomography. Otol Neurotol. 2005;26:34–47.
79. Dalchow CV, Weber AL, Bien S, et al. Value of digital volume tomography in patients with conductive hearing loss. Eur Arch Otorrinolaringol. 2006;263:92–9. Epub 2005 Sep 15
80. Jackman AH, Palmer JN, Chiu AG, et al. Use of intraoperative CT scanning in endoscopic sinus surgery: a preliminary report. Am J Rhinol. 2008;22:170–4.
81. Rafferty MA, Siewerdsen JH, Chan Y, et al. Investigation of C-arm cone-beam CT-guided surgery of the frontal recess. Laryngoscope. 2005;115:2138–43.
82. Chennupati SK, Woodworth BA, Palmer JN, et al. Intraoperative IGS/CT updates for complex endoscopic frontal sinus surgery. ORL J Otorhinolaryngol Relat Spec. 2008;70:268–70. Epub 2008 May 19
83. Batra PS, Kanowitz SJ, Citardi MJ. Clinical utility of intraoperative volume computed tomography scanner for endoscopic sinonasal and skull base procedures. Am J Rhinol. 2008;22:511–5.
84. Harvey RJ, Goddard JC, Wise SK, et al. Effects of endoscopic sinus surgery and delivery device on cadaver sinus irrigation. Otolaryngol Head Neck Surg. 2008;139:137–42.
85. Hudgins PA, Browning DG, Gallups J, et al. Endoscopic paranasal sinus surgery: radio-graphic evaluation of severe complications. AJNR Am J Neuroradiol. 1992;13:1161–7.
86. Chong V. The skull base in oncologic imaging. Cancer Imaging. 2004;4:5–6.
87. Bachar G, Siewerdsen JH, Daly MJ, et al. Image quality and localization accuracy in C-arm tomosynthesis-guided head and neck surgery. Med Phys. 2007;34:4664–77.
88. Bartling SH, Leinung M, Graute J, et al. Increase of accuracy in intraoperative navigation through high-resolution flat-panel volume computed tomography: experimental comparison with multislice computed tomography-based navigation. Otol Neurotol. 2007;28:129–34.
89. Woodworth BA, Chiu AG, Cohen NA, et al. Real-time computed tomography image up-date for endoscopic skull base surgery. J Laryngol Otol. 2008;122:361–5. Epub 2007 Aug 16
90. Erpaçal B, Adıgüzel Ö, Cangül S. The use of micro-computed tomography in dental applications. Int J Dent Res. 2019;9:78–91.
91. Howell JD. Early clinical use of the x-ray. Trans Am Clin Climatol Assoc. 2016;127:341–9.
92. Boerckel JD, Mason DE, McDermott AM, Alsberg E. Microcomputed tomography: approaches and applications in bioengineering. Stem Cell Res Ther. 2014;5:144.
93. Ritman EL. Current status of developments and applications of micro-CT. Annu Rev Biomed Eng. 2011;13:531–52.
94. Swain MV, Xue J. State of the art of micro-CT applications in dental research. Int J Oral Sci. 2009;1:177–88.
95. Boca C, Truyen B, Henin L, Schulte AG, Stachniss V, De Clerck N, et al. Comparison of micro-CT imaging and histology for approximal caries detection. Sci Rep. 2017;7:6680.
96. Liao CW, Fuh LJ, Shen YW, Huang HL, Kuo CW, Tsai MT, et al. Self-assembled micro-computed tomography for dental education. PLoS One. 2018;13:e0209698.
97. Fouladi M, Gholami K, Ghadiri H. LOTUS-in vivo micro computed tomography system for imaging of small animals and ex vivo biological samples. Front Biomed Technol. 2020;7:134–7.
98. Cengiz IF, Oliveira JM, Reis RL. Micro-CT—a digital 3D microstructural voyage into scaffolds: a systematic review of the reported methods and results. Biomater Res. 2018;22:26.
99. Campioni I, Pecci R, Bedini R. Ten years of micro-CT in dentistry and maxillofacial surgery: a literature overview. Appl Sci. 2020;10:4328.
100. Paterson GL, Sykes D, Faulwetter S, Merk R, Ahmed F, Hawkins LE, et al. The pros and cons of using micro-computed tomography in gross and micro-anatomical assessments of polychaetous annelids. Mem Mus Vic. 2014;71:237–46.

3 Magnetic Resonance Imaging for Craniofacial Applications

Harmeet Kaur, Ramandeep Singh, Hariram Sankar, and Sharvari Vichare

3.1 Introduction

There is a paradigm shift in orthodontic imaging from conventional radiography to three-dimensional (3D) imaging modalities. Currently, MRI, CBCT, and CT are used to acquire three-dimensional pictures of the craniofacial region. The superiority of CBCT/CT over traditional radiography for treatment planning is notable. However, an important limitation is the higher radiation exposure for patients, which raises concerns about its repeatability [1]. With the increasing popularity of MRI, the use of three-dimensional imaging has significantly increased in dentistry and its sub-specialities, including orthodontics, periodontology, implantology, and endodontics.

MRI is a minimally invasive, non-radiation tool in the field of diagnostic imaging that offers excellent image quality. The absence of radiation from this system makes it non-harmful and poses minimal risk [2]. MRI may assess intra-cranial and extra-cranial pathologies ranging from infections to neoplastic causes. It is helpful in cases of soft tissue trauma, temporomandibular joint pathologies, tumour of salivary glands, and facial muscle pathologies. Despite this wide range of applications, there are a some limitations. This technique is comparatively costly and not suitable for claustrophobic patients [3].

3.2 History of MRI

Dutch scientist CJ Gorter [4] first proposed the concept called nuclear magnetic resonance (NMR) in 1936, which was promoted by the work of Bloch and Purcell. In the year 1946, they submitted a paper that the charged particle, like a proton, rotating around the axis has a magnetic field known as a magnetic moment. These theories were experimentally verified in 1950 and were awarded the Nobel Prize for this work in 1952.

In the late 1960s, Raymond Damadian found that the NMR parameters of malignant tissue differ from those of normal tissue, making tissue characterisation based on these differences possible. In the year 1977, Damadian and his co-workers created the pioneer superconducting NMR scanner, and the first human body imaging was conducted, which took almost five hours.

The idea of using an operator-controlled magnetic field to encode position-dependent information in an NMR signal was proposed by Paul

H. Kaur (✉) · R. Singh
Department of Radiodiagnosis, All India Institute of Medical Sciences, Bathinda, Punjab, India

H. Sankar · S. Vichare
Department of Dentistry, All India Institute of Medical Sciences, Bathinda, Punjab, India

S. S. Rana et al. (eds.), *Applications of Three-dimensional Imaging for Craniofacial Region*, https://doi.org/10.1007/978-981-97-4608-8_3

Lauterbur in 1973 [5]. This concept eventually contributed to the development modern MRI. Paul Lauterbur and Sir Peter Mansfield received the 2003 Nobel Prize in Medicine for their work on MRI.

Since the word 'nuclear' was not likely to be well received by the public, nuclear magnetic resonance (NMR) was subsequently modified into magnetic resonance imaging (MRI).

3.3 Basic MR Scanner Components

The MR system is made up of four important parts (Figs. 3.1 and 3.2), which are the following:

1. A magnet, to create an external magnetic field.
2. Gradients for signal localisation.

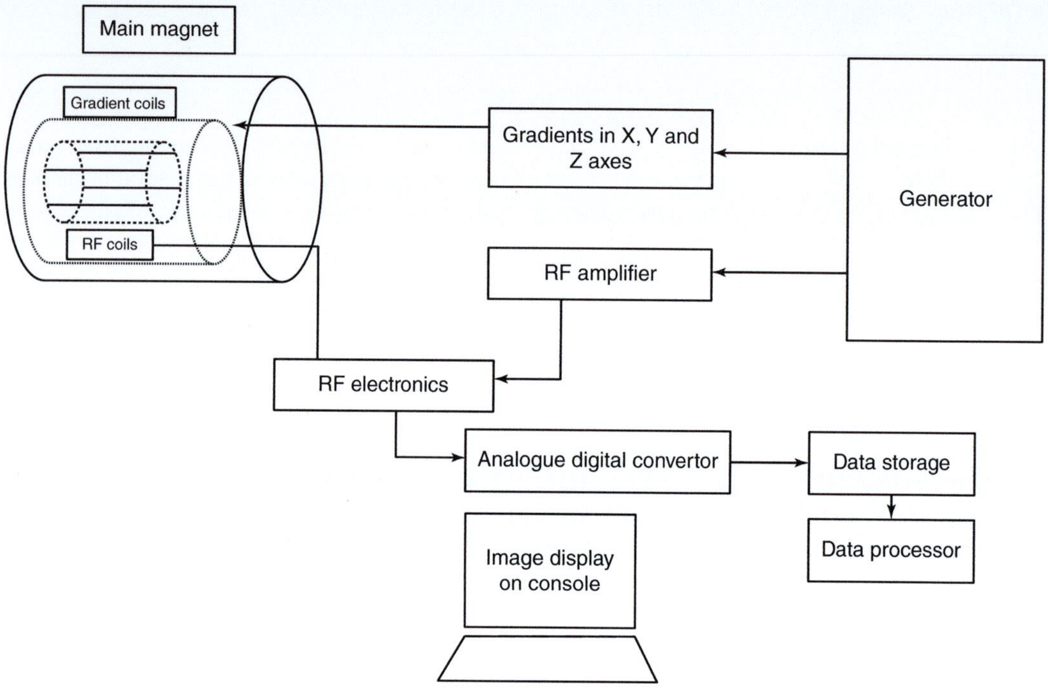

Fig. 3.1 Flowchart depicting various hardware components of MRI machine

Fig. 3.2 MRI machine with the permanent magnet (3.0 Tesla) and the patient's table

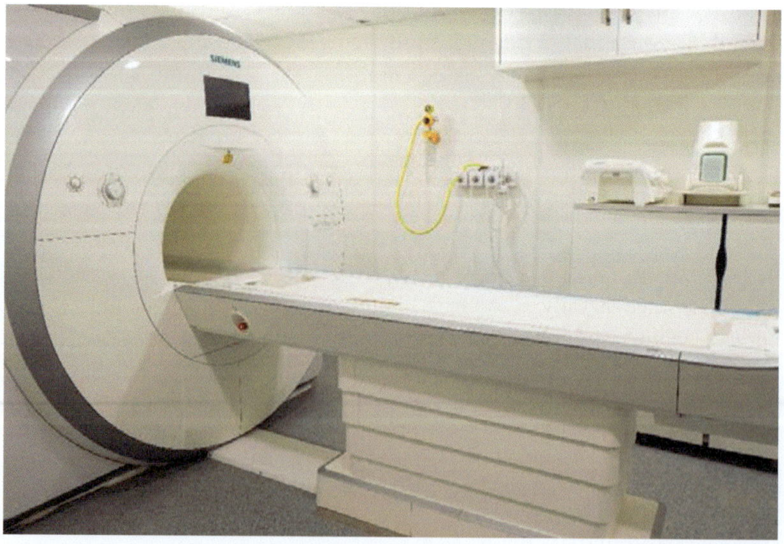

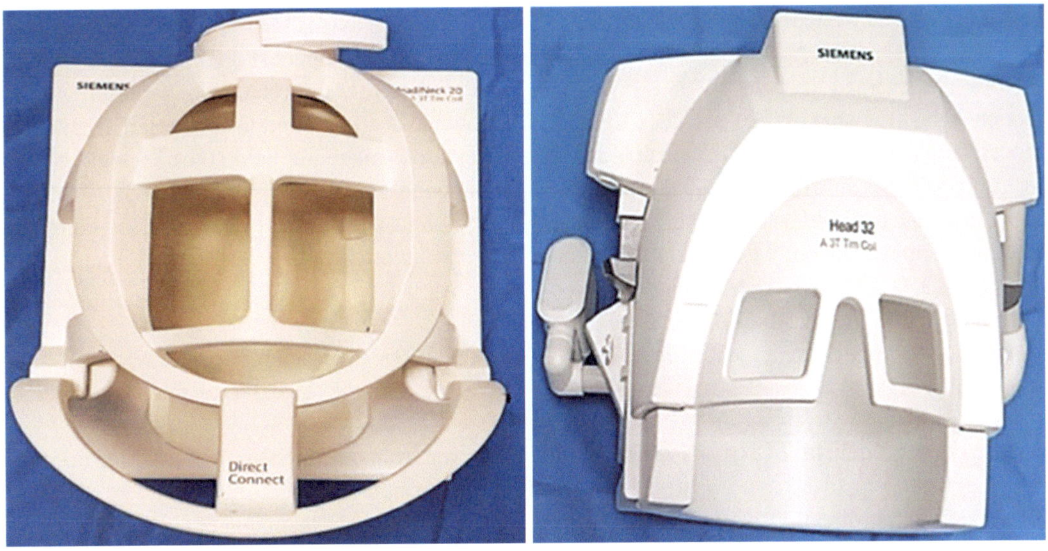

Fig. 3.3 Dedicated Head coil (both transmitter and receiver type)

3. Radiofrequency (RF) transmitter and receiver coils (Fig. 3.3).
4. System computer.

Similarly, there are four basic steps [6] for MRI, which are the following:

1. The patient is first inserted into the magnet.
2. Using the coil to provide an RF pulse to the patient.
3. Using the coil to pick up signals from the patient.
4. Signals are transformed into images using sophisticated computer processing.

3.4 MR Physics

Proton imaging refers to MR imaging. Each atom's nucleus contains a positively charged particle called a proton. The hydrogen nucleus is the most commonly used MR active nucleus in clinical MRI since it only has one proton (atomic number and mass number 1).

3.4.1 Why Are the Protons Used in MRI?

- Since it makes up the majority of the human body's nuclei, its solitary proton gives it a strong magnetic moment.
- Because of these properties, the signal produced by hydrogen is stronger than that of any other element.
- Furthermore, differences in the water (and thus hydrogen) content between normal and diseased tissues make MRI desirable for detecting pathologies.

Besides hydrogen, additional MR active nuclei include potassium (39), sodium (23), and phosphorus (15 protons, 16 neutrons) (19 protons, 20 neutrons). They are present in very small quantitities in the body, and the adequate magnetic moment for imaging does not exist; therefore, they are not used in clinical imaging. Thus, in the rest of the chapter, the term hydrogen nucleus and protons will be used interchangeably.

3.4.2 Role of Protons in MR Imaging

Protons are charged particles with a rotational motion known as spin. When a charged particle moves, current is produced, and the result is a weak magnetic field. Because of this, every proton creates a tiny magnetic field and behaves like a small magnet. Protons move randomly throughout the human body (Fig. 3.4a). These randomly aligned protons align and spin in the direction of the B0 external magnetic field while doing an MRI (Fig. 3.4b).

3.4.3 Longitudinal Magnetisation

The *z*-axis is the direction of the external magnetic field. Some of these protons align parallel to the *z*-axis under the action of B0, while others align anti-parallel. The protons' net magnetisation vector (M0), however, is aligned parallel to B0 because there are more protons spinning parallel to the *z*-axis than any other direction. M0 is also referred to as longitudinal magnetisation because the *z*-axis is the long axis to patients and the bore of the magnet (Fig. 3.5a–c).

Precession is the rotation of a proton around its own axis and around itself when it aligns with an external magnetic field (Fig. 3.6a and b) [7]. Precession frequency is the number of proton precessions per second [5]. It is expressed by the *Larmor equation*:

$$W0 = \gamma \, B0$$

where, **W0** = precession frequency (in Hz).

B0 = strength of external magnetic field in Tesla (T).

γ = gyromagnetic ratio, which is specific to a particular nucleus.

The external magnetic field's strength is directly correlated with the precession frequency. The precession frequency increases with the strength of the external magnetic field. Hydrogen has a gyromagnetic ratio of 42.57 MHz/T. In light of this, the hydrogen precession/resonant frequency is 63.9 MHz at 1.5 T and 127.7 MHz at 3 T [8].

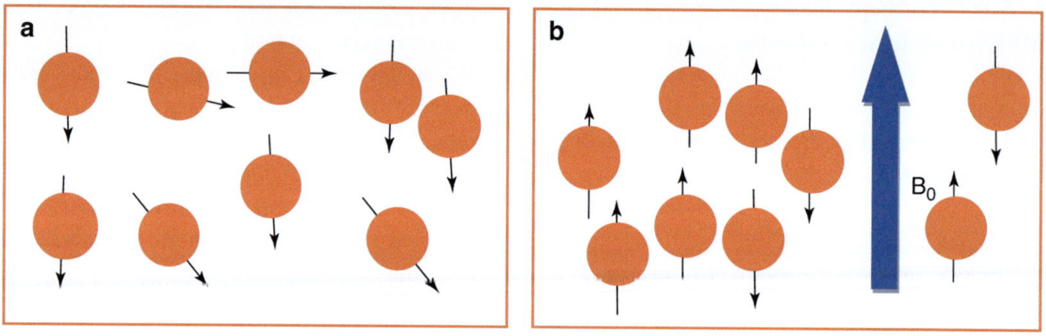

Fig. 3.4 (**a**) Random alignment of protons in the human body with no external magnetic field (B_0), (**b**) protons align in the direction of external magnetic field (B_0)

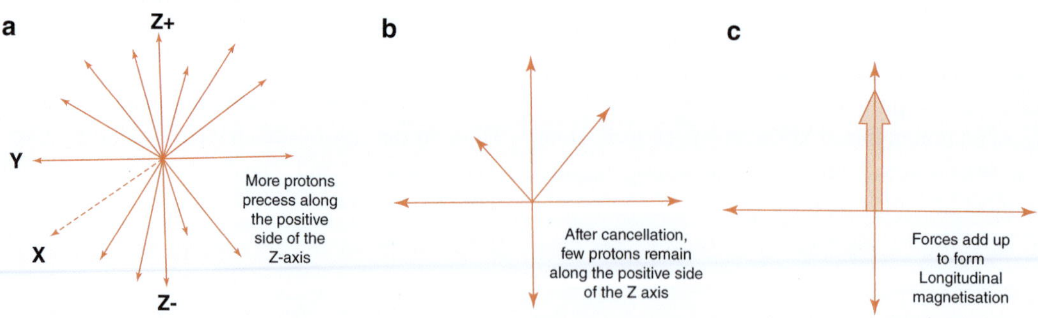

Fig. 3.5 (**a–c**) Longitudinal magnetisation

3.4.4 Transverse Magnetisation

Due to the existence of the greater external magnetic field, B0, as long as M0 and B0 are parallel, it is challenging to measure the weak magnetic field produced by M0. An Radiofrequency (RF) pulse is used to measure this weak magnetism. An RF pulse provides energy to precess protons, allowing them to gain energy and precess in phase with one another. Due to this, transverse magnetisation appears in the X-Y plane and the longitudinal magnetisation decreases (Fig. 3.7a–c). Only when an RF pulse with the same precession frequency as the proton's spinning rate is applied does this occur. The 'resonance' in an MRI stands for this phenomenon.

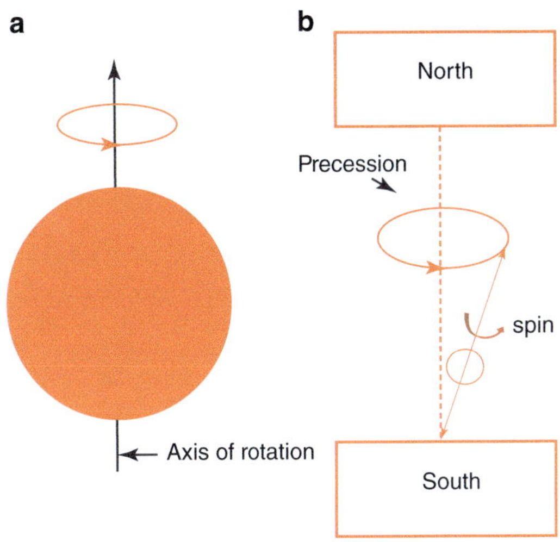

Fig. 3.6 (**a**) Spin, rotation of a proton around its own axis; (**b**) precession, rotation of the axis itself under the effect of B0

3.4.5 MR Signal

The transverse magnetisation vector constantly rotates at Larmor frequency in the transverse plane and leads to induction of electric current. The receiver RF coil receives this current as MR signal whose strength is proportional to the magnitude of the transverse magnetisation (Fig. 3.8a and b). Using various mathematical methods like

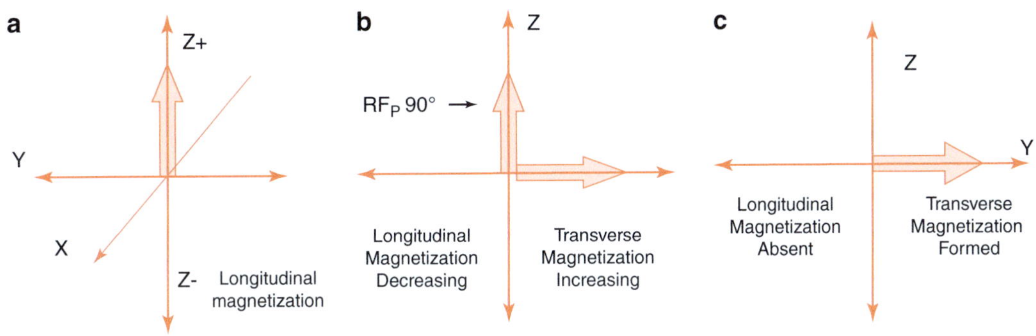

Fig. 3.7 (**a–c**) Transverse magnetisation

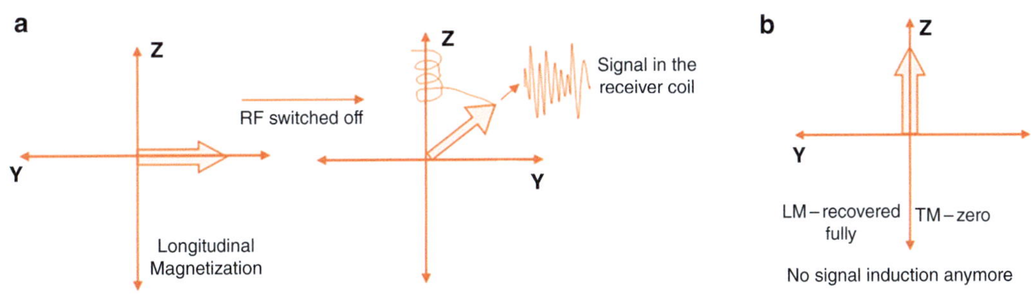

Fig. 3.8 (**a** and **b**) Magnetic signal: produced by the current that is generated by the constant precession of the transverse magnetisation vector in the transverse plane

Fourier transformation, the computer transforms MR signals into MR images.

3.4.6 Localisation of the Signal

Three gradient magnetic fields are superimposed on main magnetic field along the Z, Y, and X axes to locate the body signals. The gradient fields produced by coils are referred to as 'gradient coils'.

The three gradients are the following:

1. Slice selection gradient on the *z*-axis, which establishes slice position. The RF pulse's bandwidth affects slice thickness.
2. Frequency encoding (read out) gradient on the *y*-axis.
3. *X*-axis: Gradient of phase encoding.

Frequency encoding and phase encoding Gradients can be used to pinpoint where in the slice the signal is coming from. Both to the gradient of the slice selection and to one another, they are applied perpendicularly.

The point of the signal is located using data from all three axes.

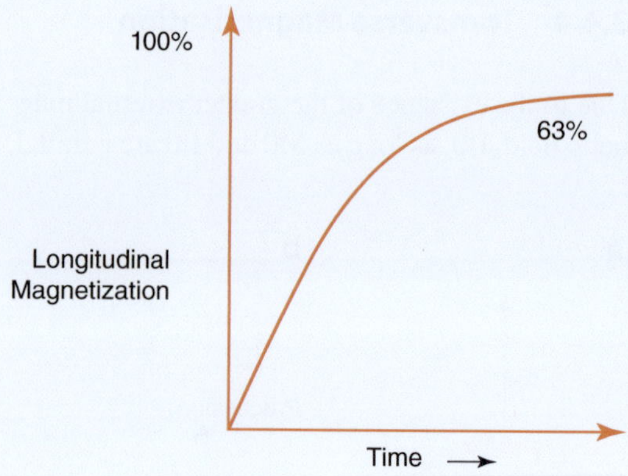

Fig. 3.9 T1 recovery curve

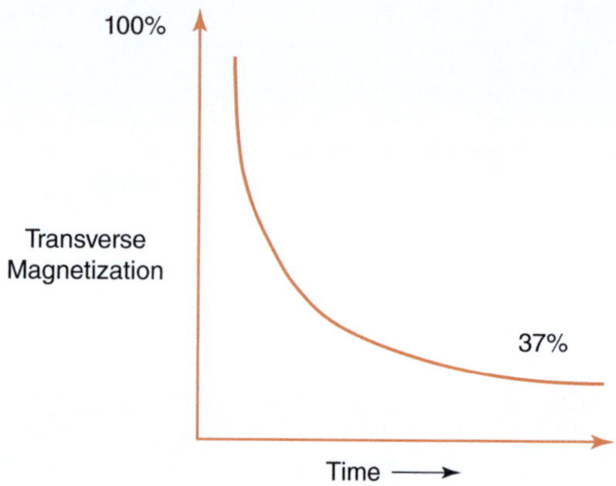

Fig. 3.10 T2 decay curve

3.4.7 Relaxation

When the RF pulse is switched off, the net magnetisation vector (M0) again starts shifting from the transverse plane (XY plane) to the longitudinal plane (along *z*-axis) under the influence of B0. The process is called 'relaxation' [9], and in this process, the hydrogen nuclei release absorbed RF energy, and M0 returns to B0.

T1 recovery: The T1 recovery mechanism is what causes the recovery of longitudinal magnetisation. The spin-lattice relaxation method for T1 recovery involves nuclei releasing energy to the lattice or environment around them. Recovery happens at an exponential rate. The T1 relaxation time is the recovery time constant. The amount of time needed for the tissue's longitudinal magnetisation to recover is 63% (Fig. 3.9). T1 depends on the surrounding matter. If the magnetic field of the surrounding matter fluctuates at Larmor frequency, the energy transfer of protons to the surroundings is faster. Fat has short T1 because the protons in fat have a frequency near the Larmor frequency, which helps quickly transfer energy from fat to the surroundings. Water has long T1 since their molecules move rapidly, and protons in water takes longer duration for their energy transfer.

T2 decay: Transverse magnetisation degrades through a process known as T2 decay. Spin-spin relaxation, which causes T2 decay, results from the magnetic fields of nearby nuclei interacting with one another. The T2 relaxation time acts as the decay time constant, and the decay rate is an exponential process. It is the amount of time needed for 37% of the transverse magnetism to remain (Fig. 3.10). Local magnetic field inhomogeneity inside the tissues is necessary for T2 decay. Liquids, whose molecules are mobile, produce local field strengths that are weak and have prolonged T2 relaxation time. Solid masses like the muscles tend to have a rigid molecular structure resulting in a strong magnetic field. This leads to rapid dephasing of dipole movements, hence short T2 relaxation times [10]. Fat has short T2, and water has long T2.

3.4.8 Image Weighting

All the intrinsic contrast parameters (these are inherent to the body's tissues and cannot be changed) simultaneously affect image contrast and would therefore produce images of mixed contrast. So, it is necessary to weight image contrast towards one of the parameters and away from the others. This can be done by knowing how extrinsic contrast parameters control the contribution of each intrinsic contrast parameter depicted in Table 3.1.

For a given pulse sequence, particular values of TR and TE are chosen to show either Tl or T2 contrast.

The repetition time (TR): Time from the application of one RF pulse to the application of the next RF pulse.

Table 3.1 Various factors affect MR image contrast

Sr. no	Intrinsic parameters	Extrinsic factors
1.	T1 recovery time	TR (repetition time)
2.	T2 decay time	TE (echo time)
3.	Proton density	Flip angle
4.	Apparent diffusion coefficient	

The echo time (TE): Time from the application of the RF pulse to the peak of signal induced in the coil.

T1 weighting: When the contrast in a picture is mostly driven by the differences between the T1 timings of fat and water, the image is said to be T1 weighted (and all the tissues with intermediate signal). The quantity of T1 weighting is controlled by TR. Tissues with short T1-like fat have a strong signal in T1-weighted pictures.

T2 weighting: A T2-weighted image is one in which the contrast is mostly determined by the variations in the T2 timings between fat and water (and all the tissues with intermediate signal). T2 weighting is regulated by TE. T2 weighted images show a strong signal in tissues containing lengthy, T2-like CSF, water, and cysts (Table 3.2).

3.4.9 MR Sequences

Routine sequences are the pulse sequences in which a series of RF pulse and gradient applications are used to get the MR signal. Pulse sequences are broadly divided into two categories:

(a) Spin echo sequence (Fig. 3.11).
(b) Gradient echo sequence.

Table 3.2 Relation of TE & TR in T1- and T2-weighted image

	T1-weighted image	T2-weighted image
TR	Short	Long
TE	Short	Long

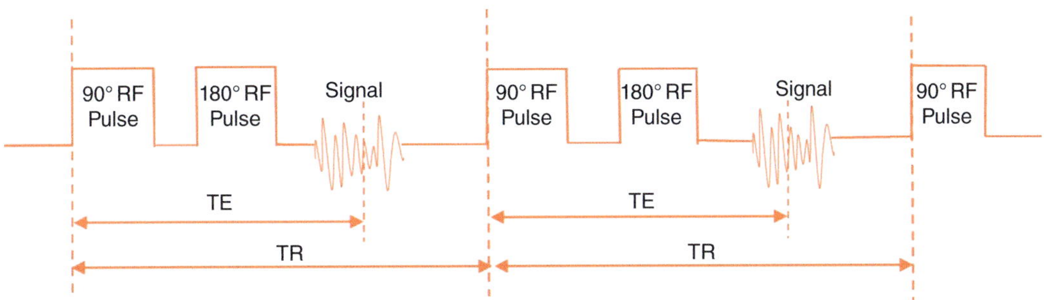

Fig. 3.11 MR basic pulse (spin echo) sequence. *TE* time to echo, *TR* time to repeat

Table 3.3 Various MR pulse sequences trademarked by different vendors

Sequences	Siemens	Philips	GE Healthcare
1. Spin echo (SE) sequences			
A. Conventional SE (90°–180° RF pulses)	SE	SE	SE
B. Double SE (90° followed by two 180° RF pulses)	PD/T2	PD	PD
C. Multi-SE (90° followed by multiple 180° RF pulses)	Turbo SE	Turbo SE	Fast SE
D. Single-shot multi-SE (multi-SE with half K-space filling)	HASTE	UFSE	SS-FSE
2. Gradient echo sequences			
A. Incoherent spoiled B. Coherent/rephased TM	FLASH (3D version-3D) FLASH VIBE FISP True FISP	T_1-FFE THRIVE FFE Balanced FFE	SPGRMPSPGR LAVA MPGR FIESTA

SE spin echo, *RF* radio frequency, *TM* transverse magnetisation, *PD* proton density, *HASTE* half Fourier single-shot turbo spin echo, *turbo SE* turbo spin echo, *SS-FSE* single-shot fast spin echo; *FLASH* fast low angle shot, *FFE* fast field echo, *SPGR* spoiled gradient recalled acquisition in the steady state, *VIBE* volume interpolated breath-hold examination, *THRIVE* T1-weighted high-resolution isotropic volume examination, *LAVA* liver acquisition with volume acceleration, *FISP* fast imaging with steady-state free precession, *FIESTA* fast imaging employing steady-state acquisition

With advancements in technology, there occurred many modifications in the basic pulse sequence that have immensely helped in improving the image quality and reducing the acquisition time. Details of these sequences are beyond the scope of this chapter; however, the names of the relevant sequences used are tabulated in Table 3.3.

3.5 Image Quality Determinants [11]

1. **Signal-to-noise ratio (SNR):** The ratio of useful signal to unwanted signal (noise) in the image. It is one of the most significant factors in determining image clarity [11].
2. **Spatial resolution:** The capacity to distinguish two points as distinct and separate is known as spatial resolution. The resolution is greater if the points can be seen separately at a smaller size. A higher matrix scale improves the spatial resolution.
3. **Contrast:** In an image, contrast is the difference in signal intensities between adjacent structures.
4. Imaging time.

$$aT = TR \times N^{*} \times NEX$$

where aT = acquisition time.
TR = time to repeat.
N^* = number of pixels (matrix).
NEX = number of excitations.

The effects of the imaging parameters on the image quality determinants are as follows:

(a) Scanning time: It increases with increasing the image matrix and the number of signal averages per excitation (NSA), whereas it decreases when increasing the receiver bandwidth.
(b) SNR: It is directly proportional to the increase in the FOV, slice thickness, and NSA, whereas it decreases with increase in matrix and receiver bandwidth.
(c) Spatial resolution: It decreases with increase in FOV and slice thickness; however, it increases with an increase in matrix.

3.6 MR Bioeffects and Safety [12]

During MR examination, the patient is exposed to three forms of electromagnetic fields:

1. **Static magnetic field:** Metal projectile damage is a significant risk that is associated with MR imaging. That happens when ferromag-

netic objects unintentionally come into contact with the MR imaging unit's powerful magnetic field. Due to the fact that accidents can occur at any time, screening patients and personnel is of utmost importance.

The external magnetic field can also cause electrical induction, cardiac effects, headaches, nausea, tinnitus, and numbness, among other negative side effects.

2. **Gradient magnetic field:** Ventricular fibrillation, epileptogenic potentials, auditory noise, and visual flashes are all potential side effects.
3. **RF electromagnetic field:** Can result in energy deposition and burns.

   In the present clinical MR system, all these effects are not that significant.

   Acoustic noise: It is caused by gradient coil vibrations. Earplugs and earphones should be made available to patients to avoid any bioeffects.

3.7 Absolute Contraindications of MRI

1. A cardiac pacemaker inside the body.
2. Implants for cardiac defibrillators.
3. Cochlear implants.
4. Neurostimulants.
5. Drugs to promote bone growth.
6. Vascular access ports and electrically programmable medication infusion pumps.
7. An inside foreign substance.
8. Non-titanium aneurysm clamps [13].

3.8 MRI and Dental Implants

Studies indicate that patients with dental implants can safely undergo MRI [11]. They are not contraindicated since they have minimal chance of displacement. Still, they can cause artifacts that are problematic.

3.9 MRI and Pregnancy

According to the latest American College of Radiology (ACR) MRI safety guidelines, if there is more benefit compared to the risks, then pregnant patients can undergo MRI. Injection of MR contrast agents like gadolinium (MR contrast agent) in pregnant patients should be avoided since they tend to cross the placenta.

3.10 MRI Contrast

MRI contrast agents play a crucial role in identifying, defining, and characterizing the illness process. Dynamic studies can evaluate perfusion and enhancement patterns utilizing the use of novel rapid sequences and contrast media. Contrast enhancement in MRI results from the interaction of the contrast agents with nearby water protons, as opposed to CT contrast agents, which create direct contrast effects on their placements based on the electron-density differential. By changing the T1 or T2 relaxation durations, these substances modify the signal intensity of tissues. The three types of MR contrast materials are ferromagnetic, paramagnetic, and super magnetic, with paramagnetic being the most well-liked and practical. The greatest notable relaxation is experienced by paramagnetic contrast agents when there are water molecule protons. Gadolinium diethylene thiamine pantothenic acid (Gd-DTPA) is the most commonly used MRI contrast media. Gadolinium predominantly affects the T1 relaxation of the tissues, reducing T1 of the tissue where the contrast medium accumulates. Reduction in T1 results in an increase in the signal intensity on T1-W images. At higher doses, it also causes a shortening of T2 relaxation time. Post-contrast T2 MR studies are commonly used for cerebral perfusion studies and currently have limited applications in dentistry.

3.11 Functional MRI (f-MRI)

In recent years, our understanding of the functional and structural neuroanatomy of the craniofacial region has undergone a revolutionary change as a result of the development of functional neuroimaging. Functional MRI (f-MRI) is based on blood-oxygen level-dependent (BOLD) changes in the cerebral cortex that occur during specific tasks. During activation of a particular brain region, an excess of oxygenated (arterial) blood is supplied. Because of this, there is more oxy-haemoglobin in the venous outflow from the active areas, which alters the tissue's paramagnetic characteristics and makes it easier to detect during a T2* acquisition. It can be used to investigate the functional anatomy of the brain, identify the areas of the brain accountable for vital functions, and examine the physiology and pathophysiology of dental problems including TM joint disorders. The key advantages of f-MRI include its lack of invasiveness, superior spatiotemporal resolution, and capacity to pinpoint the complete network of brain regions involved in a given task. In dentistry and craniomaxillofacial research, the patterns of brain activity linked to oral processes, such as chewing, swallowing, digesting, and speaking, as well as the somatotopic representation of the lips, teeth, and tongue, have been effectively assessed using f-MRI [14, 15].

Advantages of MRI

- No ionizing radiation hazard.
- Good contrast of soft tissue.
- Multiplanar anatomical display.
- Non-contrast angiography.

Relative Disadvantages

- High cost and limited availability.
- Longer examination time.
- Lower spatial resolution.
- Patients with pacemakers/non-compatible metallic implants can be excluded.
- It is not easy to perform MRI in ill patients with ventilator support or while under the influence of GA.

3.12 Applications of MRI in Craniomaxillofacial Region

In dentistry, the role of MRI as a diagnostic tool has been increasingly recognized. Various subspecialties of dentistry like orthodontics, prosthodontics, endodontics, and oral and maxillofacial surgery have been utilizing MRI for a range of purposes such as diagnosing temporomandibular disc disorders, inflammatory and infectious lesions of the maxillofacial region, diagnosing the disorders of salivary gland and paranasal sinuses. MRI is also valuable for the detection of early bone changes such as tumours, inflammatory conditions, fractures, and hematoma. In this discussion we will explore the applications of MRI in various maxillofacial conditions.

3.12.1 Orthodontics

Orthodontics is one branch of dentistry that has a significant association with radiographic examination. For routine orthodontic treatment planning, OPG, lateral and PA cephalogram, and CBCT are done before the treatment planning for the patient. Even though all these scans were used regularly, MRI in orthodontics is quite rare. With more advent MRI, the radiation exposure hazard can be reduced in these patients. The uses are listed below [16]:

- MRI may be used to provide the volume of the tongue.
- MRI also has its role in the diagnosis of TMD [17].
- To assess growth status and estimate sizes of the oropharynx and hypopharynx.

Since orthodontic procedures and orthognathic surgeries can impact the pharyngeal airway space, this estimation of their volume can be proven vital.

3.12.2 Endodontics

The role of MRI in endodontics is limited. MRI can help in assessing periapical lesions and planning periapical surgeries. MRI is unaffected by the artifacts due to metallic restorations like amalgam or metallic extra-coronal restoration, which is an issue while using CT scan [18]. Despite its advantages, MRI has several setbacks in endodontics. It has a lower resolution than normal radiographs and a prolonged scanning time. The other significant setbacks for using MRI in regular dental procedures are the higher cost and the need for a separate dedicated unit setup [19, 20].

3.12.3 Prosthodontics and Implantology

In the field of prosthodontics, the role of MRI is minimal. The prosthetic models can be constructed from 3D ear models. Coward and coworkers performed a study comparing the ear prosthesis from data obtained by various techniques like CT, MRI, and laser scanning [21]. However, the study results show significantly less difference between those groups. In the future, more studies with a large sample size as well as study design will be required to comment on this. Also, another facial prosthesis can be constructed similarly.

3.12.4 Oral and Maxillofacial Surgery

MRI is widely used in the diagnosis of various maxillofacial pathologies. This chapter will discuss some of the most frequently encountered maxillofacial pathologies and their MRI findings in detail (Table 3.4) [22–71].

The MRI images of few maxillofacial conditions like chronic fungal sinusitis and pleomorphic adenoma were given below in this chapter (Figs. 3.12 and 3.13).

Table 3.4 List of various maxillofacial pathologies

Sr. no	Clinical condition	MRI findings
Head and neck infections		
1.	Orbital and periorbital infection	MRI findings of orbital cellulitis include fat stranding and rim-enhancing abscess formation, which can be intra-coronal or extra-coronal, and oedema and abnormal enhancement of the extraocular muscles
2.	Bacterial paranasal sinusitis	MR imaging is sensitive in identifying inflammation of the paranasal sinus mucosa. Although the diagnosis of sinusitis should not be based solely on imaging findings, greater than 4 mm of sinus mucosal thickening suggests a greater likelihood of sinusitis
3.	Sialadenitis	1. Oedema and abnormal enhancement within the affected salivary gland(s) are sometimes associated with a rim-enhancing abscess 2. Inflammation of the peri-glandular fat and soft tissues 3. Associated sialolithiasis which demonstrates signal void within the obstructed ducts, most commonly Wharton's duct
4.	Facial neuritis (Bell's palsy)	MR imaging is useful in atypical clinical presentations or the setting of persistent palsy even after treatment. Abnormal enhancement of the facial nerve, typically affecting the canalicular, labyrinthine, and tympanic segment, can be seen on MR imaging
5.	Retropharyngeal abscess	1. Bow-tie-shaped distention of the retropharyngeal space causing displacement of the posterior pharyngeal wall anteriorly 2. Retropharyngeal T2 hyperintensity and T1 hypointensity indicating oedema/cellulitis 3. Loculated rim-enhancing fluid collection on post-contrast imaging indicating an abscess 4. Restricted diffusion in the area of the collection

(continued)

Table 3.4 (continued)

Sr. no	Clinical condition	MRI findings
6.	Odontogenic infection	MR imaging is more sensitive for the evaluation of complications such as osteomyelitis and extraosseous abscesses. Ludwig's angina can be a complication of periodontal disease, characterised as a necrotizing soft tissue infection of the floor of the mouth, with MR imaging demonstrating oedema and swelling, and the presence of a rim-enhancing abscess
Soft tissue tumours		
1.	Lipoma	On MRI, lipomas are well-defined T1 and T2 hyperintense lesions that show suppression on the STIR and the fat-saturated images
2.	Liposarcoma	They classically demonstrate density and signal characteristics matching that of subcutaneous fat, including high signal intensity on both T1-weighted and T2-weighted images. With fat suppression techniques, the signal within a lipoma drops out completely
3.	Fibrosarcoma	On MR imaging, fibrosarcomas are heterogeneous masses that may have well-defined or infiltrative margins. They are predominantly isointense to the muscle on T1-weighted imaging and hyperintense on T2-weighted imaging, although they may demonstrate hypointense regions related to fibrous components
4.	Leiomyosarcoma	On MR imaging, Leiomyosarcomas typically are isointense to hypointense relative to muscle on T1-weighted images and variably hyperintense on T2-weighted images, with prominent contrast enhancement. Large lesions usually are more heterogeneous due to the presence of haemorrhage, necrosis, and cystic change
5.	Leiomyoma	On MR imaging, leiomyomas appear as homogeneous masses demonstrating signal intensity hypointense or isointense to the muscle on T1-weighted images and isointense to mildly hyperintense on T2-weighted images with marked postcontrast enhancement. These tumours can demonstrate calcification or ossification
Vascular lesion		
1.	High flow lesions	High-flow vascular lesions in MRI show rapid contrast enhancement during the early arterial phase. Also enlarged vessels and pathologic arteriovenous shunting with early venous filling will be shown in MRI
2.	Low flow lesions	In conventional MRIs, low-flow lesions, such as venous malformations, show minimal contrast enhancement. It is important that the low-flow lesion has no early opacification on MR digital subtraction angiograms. Such lesions show either no vascularity on MR digital subtraction angiograms or appear during the venous phase
Salivary gland disorders		
1.	Branchial cleft cyst	On MRI, branchial cleft cyst demonstrates low T1 signals and high T2 signals. They appear as a single fluid-filled mass. Usually, there will not be any thickening or rim enhancement in MR imaging unless there is any secondary infection associated with it
2.	Lymphatic malformation	On MRI, lymphatic malformation demonstrates high T2 and low T1 signals. Sometimes, T1 signals may be raised because of the presence of blood clots. Fluid-filled cavity will also be seen
3.	Ranula	On MRI appears as T1-hypointense and T2-hyperintense with no obvious post-contrast enhancement
4.	Pleomorphic adenoma	On MRI, they have a homogenous appearance. They show a well-defined capsule. They demonstrate a moderate to low T1 signal. High T2 signals will be present. Because of fibrosis or calcification, low signals in small areas are visualised. It is difficult to differentiate pleomorphic adenoma from warthin tumour. The intense and patchy postcontrast enhancement are the major distinguishing feature
5.	Warthin tumour	On MRI, they appear as well-circumscribed mass. They show high signals for T2-weighted and intermediate signals for T1-weighted images. Peri-parotid lymph node involvement may be seen. On MRI, only minimal contrast enhancement is present. On T2-weighted imaging and proton density weighted imaging, the tumour extend appears different

Table 3.4 (continued)

Sr. no	Clinical condition	MRI findings
6.	Mucoepidermoid tumour	On MRI, well-differentiated mucoepidermoid tumour shows well-circumscribed lesion and high T2 signal. However, poorly differentiated variety shows high infiltration and irregular margins. It also has low T2 signals
7.	Adenoid cystic tumour	If the tumour involves the parotid gland, on MRI, it looks well-defined and also has high T2 content. If arising from minor salivary glands, then it has poorly defined irregular margins. In case of perineural involvement, there will be thickening of nerve structure or postcontrast enhancement seen on fat-saturated T1 imaging

3.12.5 Temporomandibular Disorder

Gross anatomy of TMJ: The TMJ is a unique synovial joint. It forms the joint between the condyle and the mandibular fossa and thus helps in jaw motion. The articulating surfaces of this joint are fibrocartilaginous unlike other body joints, which are made of hyaline cartilage. Between the mandibular condyle and mandibular fossa of the temporal bone is this fragile articular disc. The articular disc divides the synovial cavity into two compartments which are superior and inferior, respectively. The articular disc is a connective tissue which is avascular in nature and biconcave in shape. The anterior zone, intermediate zone, and posterior zone are its 3 segments. The intermediate zone, which is relatively thin, connects the anterior and posterior bands, both of which are relatively thicker [72, 73].

MR anatomy of TM joint: On sagittal view of MRI, the articular disc appears as a biconcave structure. On T2-weighted imaging, it presents as a homologous low signal. In T2-weighted imaging, the intermediate zone rarely shows as a bright signal similar to a centrally hydrated disc. On T1-weighted imaging, the retro-discal tissue or bilaminar zone appears in a higher signal intensity compared to muscles. The posterior band shows intermediate signal intensity [74–77].

Internal derangement: One of the frequent TMJ disorders is internal derangement. The mandibular condyle, glenoid fossa, and articular eminence are in an improper relationship with the articular disc. Patients with this disorder have the following presentations: tenderness on palpation over the preauricular TMJ region, tenderness on palpation over the masseteric muscle region, pain on mouth opening and closing, pain during chewing, clicking sound during jaw opening and closing, and restricted mouth opening. In some cases, headaches can also occur, which can be secondary or unrelated to this condition. Gross bony changes are rare in most internal derangement conditions. Hence, investigation in MRI is vital in assessing the severity of the condition [72, 78].

MRI findings of internal derangement: Oblique sagittal PD or T2-weighted sequences are the best suited for the diagnosis of anterior disc displacement [79]. The important findings to look out TMD in MRI imaging are the following:

- Disc position.
- Disc morphology.
- Disc signal.
- Condylar translation.
- The masticator space.
- Any joint effusion.
- Presence of osteoarthritis.

The anterior disc displacement is the most typical type of internal derangement. The posterior attachment is stretched during anterior disc

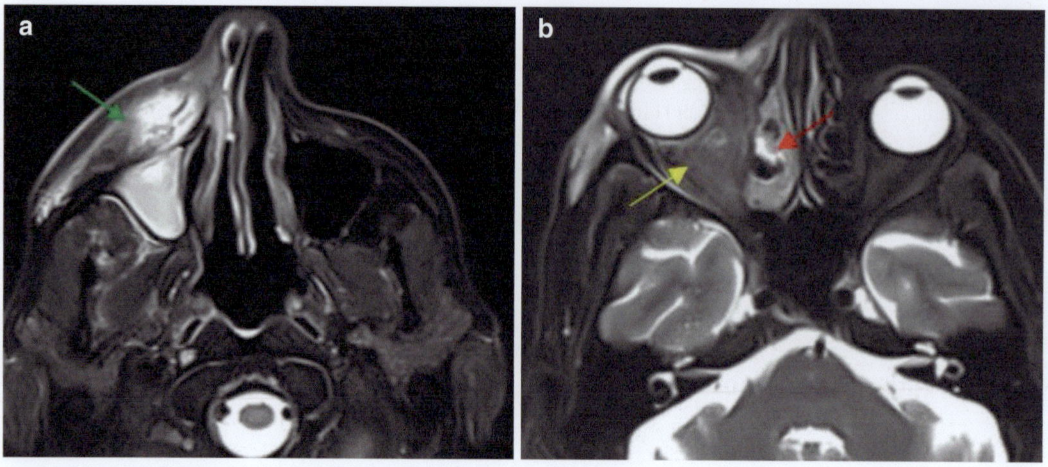

Fig. 3.12 Chronic fungal sinusitis. (**a**) Axial T2 W FS MR images of the face at the level of the maxillary sinuses, and (**b**) orbits show an ill-defined hypointensity in right ethmoid air cells (red arrow) with extension to the premaxillary region (green arrow) and orbit on the right side (yellow arrow) and resultant proptosis

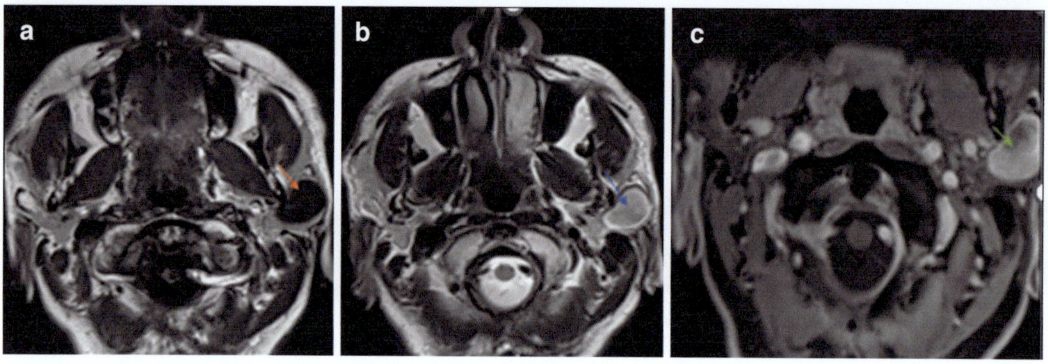

Fig. 3.13 Pleomorphic adenoma. Axial (**a**) T1, (**b**) T2, and (**c**) T1 FS post-contrast MR images of the neck at the level of the parotid gland reveal a well-defined T1 hypointense, T2 hyperintense, and homogenously enhancing lesion in the superficial lobe of the parotid gland (coloured arrows)

displacement. As a result of this stretching, there will be thickening of this posterior attachment. Normally, it is not necessary to examine the disc position in the open mouth position if the disc position is normal during the closed mouth position. When the mouth is open, the disc position is assessed if there is anterior disc displacement in the closed mouth position.

The condylar translation is the term used for the forward and downward motion of condyle while opening the mouth. It is important to assess whether the mouth opening is sufficient. If there is enough opening, then the anterior translation of the condyle is just below the articular eminence. The restriction in translation of condyle may be due to various pathologies such as a motion restriction, stuck disc, or patient cooperation. A fixed disc may be a result of intracapsular adhesions. Adhesions cannot be directly visualised by MRI. If the disc position is fixed in MRI, it could be suggestive of adhesion. In normal TMJ, a mild effusion is seen usually. Moderate to large effusions are seen in TMJ abnormalities which appear as T2 bright signal fluid. Like other synovial joints, osteoarthritis in the TMJ presents as the narrowing of the joint space, eburnation, articular erosion, and osteophytosis. Sclerosis of the condyle is seen as a decreased signal on both PD and T2-weighted images [79–81] (Fig. 3.14).

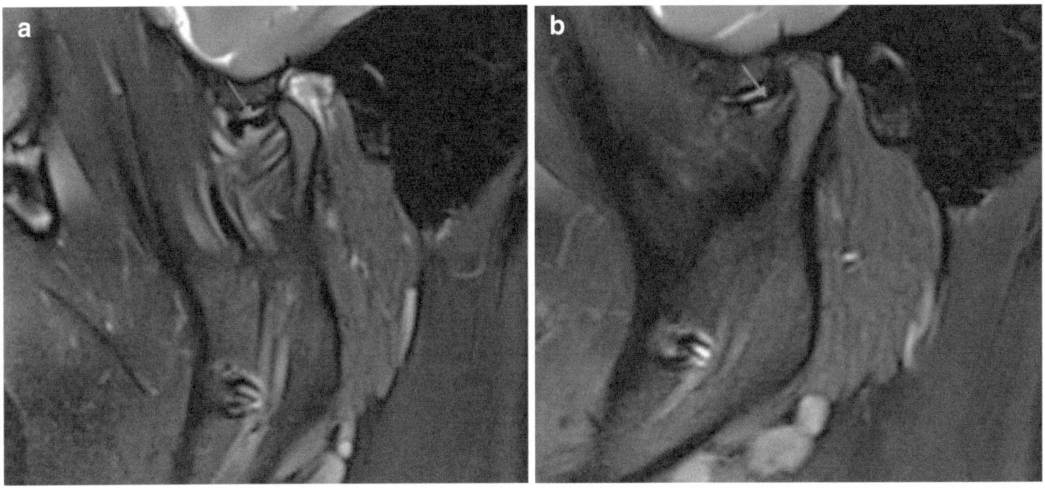

Fig. 3.14 TM joint disorder. T2FS MR (**a**) Sagittal open and (**b**) closed mouth view of the left TMJ shows irreducible internal disc derangement. The blue arrow shows the anterior displacement of the disc in the open-mouth view, which remains displaced in the closed-mouth view (shown by the orange-coloured arrow) indicating irreducible displacement

MRI of other TMJ arthropathies: Rheumatoid arthritis, pigmented villonodular synovitis (PVNS), calcium pyrophosphate dihydrate crystal deposition syndrome, gout, and infections are a few examples of the several inflammatory arthropathies that can affect TMJ. Rheumatoid arthritis is distinguished by the involvement of both soft tissues and bones. Contrast-enhanced MR imaging is most sensitive to evaluate bone abnormalities like condylar head flattening, narrowing of joint space, articular erosion, and also soft tissue abnormalities of synovial proliferation. They also play an important role in evaluating juvenile arthritis in children since a delayed diagnosis of the disorder may affect the growth of facial structures. Radiographically, it might be challenging to identify rheumatoid arthritis from other inflammatory disorders that affect the joints, like ankylosing spondylitis, psoriatic arthritis, and systemic lupus erythematosus [80, 81].

3.13 Summary

MR is a well-established and commonly used modality in the field of dentistry. Intense technological advancement is rapidly increasing its applications in the craniofacial region, not just in terms of structural details but also functional assessment of TMJ and cerebral activity in dental disorders. Nevertheless, understanding fundamental MR physics is important for clinical imaging because it allows us to modify scanning protocols to obtain optimum image quality. Proper attention to MR scanning parameters, proper use of conventional and advanced pulse sequences, and diligence of examination technique help avoid various drawbacks and attain better accuracy.

Acknowledgement The authors sincerely acknowledge the contribution of Ms. Namrata Shikhawat, our nursing officer, for her assistance with the diagrams and graphical representation of the images related to MR physics.

References

1. Smith-Bindman R, Lipson J, Marcus R, et al. Radiation dose associated with common computed tomography examinations and the associated lifetime attributable risk of cancer. Arch Intern Med. 2009;169(22):2078–86.
2. Hartwig V, Giovannetti G, Vanello N, Lombardi M, Landini L, Simi S. Biological effects and safety in magnetic resonance imaging: a review. Int J Environ Res Public Health. 2009;6(6):1778–98.
3. Okano Y, Yamashiro M, Kaneda T, Kasai K. Magnetic resonance imaging diagnosis of the temporomandibular joint in patients with orthodontic appliances. Oral Surg Oral Med Oral Pathol Oral Radiol Endod. 2003;95:255–63.
4. Gorter CJ. Negative result of an attempt to detect nuclear spins. Physica. 1936;3:995–8.
5. Lauterbur PC. Image formation by induced local interactions: examples employing nuclear magnetic resonance. Nature. 1973;242:190–1.
6. Fullerton GD. Magnetic Resonance Imaging Signal concept. Radiographics. 1978;7:579–96.
7. Chavhan GB. MRI made easy. JP Medical Ltd; 2013 Jan 30.
8. Westbrook C, Roth CK, Talbot J. MRI in practice. 4th ed, Wiley, 2011.
9. Hashemi RH, Bradley WG Jr, Lisanti CJMRI. The basics, 3, 40. Philadelphia, PA: Lippincott Williams and Wilkins; 2010.
10. Dale BM, Brown MA, Semelka RC. MRI: basic principles and applications, 5, 21. Wiley; 2015.
11. DiNardo D, Gambarini G, Capuani S, Testarelli L. Nuclear magnetic resonance imaging in endodontics: a review. J Endod. 2018;44:536–42.
12. Teitelbaum GP, Yee CA, Van Horn DD, Kim HS, Colletti PM. Metallic ballistic fragments: MR imaging safety and artifacts. Radiology. 1990;175:855–9.
13. ACR Manual on MR Safety Version 1.0 2020. ACR Committee on MR Safety.
14. Orringer DA, Vago DR, Golby AJ. Clinical applications and future directions of functional MRI. Semin Neurol. 2012;32(4):466–75.
15. Sahara Y, Kobayashi T, Toya H, Suzuki T. Applications of functional magnetic resonance imaging for analysis of oral functions. J Oral Biosci. 2012;54:101–6.
16. Tekale PD, Mhaske AR, Chitko SS, Parhad SM, Bhandari AP, Patil HA. MRI and dentistry-a contemporary review. Resonance. 2014;1:4.
17. Okano Y, Yamashiro M, Kaneda T, Kasai K. Magnetic resonance imaging diagnosis of the temporomandibular joint in patients with orthodontic appliances. Oral Surg Oral Med Oral Pathol Oral Radiol Endod. 2003;95(2):255–63.
18. Lloyd CH, Scrimgeour SN, Chudek JA, Hunter G, MacKay RL. Magnetic resonance microimaging of carious teeth. Quintessence Int. 1997;28:349–55.
19. Ploder O, Partik B, Rand T, Fock N, Voracek M, Undt G, Baumann A. Reperfusion of autotransplanted teeth—comparison of clinical measurements by means of dental magnetic resonance imaging. Oral Surg Oral Med Oral Pathol Oral Radiol Endod. 2001;92:335–40.
20. Appel TR, Baumann MA. Solid-state nuclear magnetic resonance microscopy demonstrating human dental anatomy. Oral Surg Oral Med Oral Pathol Oral Radiol Endod. 2002;94:256–61.
21. Coward TJ, Scott BJ, Watson RM, Richards R. A comparison between computerized tomography, magnetic resonance imaging, and laser scanning for capturing 3-dimensional data from an object of standard form. Int J Prosthodont. 2005;18(5):405–13.
22. Meyer DR, Linberg JV, Wobig JL, et al. Anatomy of the orbital septum and associated eyelid connective tissues. Ophthalmic Plast Reconstr Surg. 1991;7:104–13.
23. Cunnane ME, Sepahadari AR, Gardiner M, et al. Pathology of the eye and orbit. In: Som PM, Curtin HD, editors. Head and neck imaging. 5th ed. St Louis, MO: Mosby Inc.; 2011. p. 591–756.
24. LeBedis CA, Sakai O. Nontraumatic orbital conditions: diagnosis with CT and MR imaging in the emergent setting. Radiographics. 2008;28:1741–53.
25. Eustis HS, Mafee MF, Walton C, et al. MR imaging and CT of orbital infections and complications in acute rhinosinusitis. Radiol Clin North Am. 1998;36(6):1165–83.
26. Sepahdari AR, Aakalu VK, Kapur R, et al. MRI of orbital cellulitis and orbital abscess: the role of diffusion-weighted imaging. AJR Am J Roentgenol. 2009;193:W244–50.
27. Kassel EE, Schatz CJ. Anatomy, imaging, and pathology of the lacrimal apparatus. In: Som PM, Curtin HD, editors. Head and neck imaging. 5th ed. St Louis, MO: Mosby Inc.; 2011. p. 757–854.
28. Eggesbø HB. Radiological imaging of inflammatory lesions in the nasal cavity and paranasal sinuses. Eur Radiol. 2006;16:872–88.
29. Rak KM, Newell JD, Yakes WF, et al. Paranasal sinuses on MR images of the brain: significance of mucosal thickening. Am J Roentgenol. 1991;156:381–4.
30. Som PM, Brandwein MS, Wang BY. Inflammatory diseases of the sinonasal cavities. In: Som PM, Curtin HD, editors. Head and neck imaging. 5th ed. St. Louis, MO: Mosby Inc.; 2011. p. 167–252.
31. Epstein VA, Kern RC. Invasive fungal sinusitis and complications of rhinosinusitis. Otolaryngol Clin N Am. 2008;41(3):497–524.
32. De Shazo RD, Chapin K, Swain RE. Fungal sinusitis. N Engl J Med. 1997;337(4):254–9.
33. Capps EF, Kinsella JJ, Gupta M, et al. Emergency imaging assessment of acute, nontraumatic conditions of the head and neck. Radiographics. 2010;30:1335–52.
34. Som PM, Brandwein-Gensler MS. Anatomy and pathology of the salivary glands. In: Som PM, Curtin

HD, editors. Head and neck imaging. 5th ed. St Louis, MO: Mosby Elsevier; 2011. p. 2449–610.
35. Kanerva M, Nissinen J, Moilanen K, et al. Microbiologic findings in acute facial palsy in children. Otol Neurotol. 2013;34(7):e82–7.
36. Engstrom M, Abdsaleh S, Ahlstrom H, et al. Serial GD-enhanced MRI and assessment of facial nerve involvement in Bell's palsy. Otolaryngol Head Neck Surg. 1997;117:559–66.
37. Chong VF, Fan YF. Radiology of the retropharyngeal space. Clin Radiol. 2000;55(10):740.
38. Chapman MN, Nadgir RN, Akman AS, et al. Periapical lucency around the tooth: radiologic evaluation and differential diagnosis. Radiographics. 2013;33(1):E15–32.
39. Aribandi M, McCoy VA, Bazan C III. Imaging features of invasive and noninvasive fungal sinusitis: a review. Radiographics. 2007;27:1283–96.
40. The WHO Classification of Tumours of Soft Tissue and Bone Board. The WHO classification of Tumours of soft tissue and bone. 5th ed. Lyon: IARC Press; 2020.
41. Bancroft LW, Kransdorf MJ, Peterson JJ, et al. Benign fatty tumors: classification, clinical course, imaging appearance, and treatment. Skeletal Radiol. 2006;35(10):719–33.
42. Cappabianca S, Colella G, Pezzullo MG, et al. Lipomatous lesions of the head and neck region: imaging findings in comparison with histological type. Radiol Med. 2008;113(5):758–70.
43. Murphey MD, Carroll JF, Flemming DJ, et al. From the archives of the AFIP: benign musculoskeletal lipomatous lesions. Radiographics. 2004;24(5):1433–66.
44. Razek AA, Huang BY. Soft tissue tumors of the head and neck: imaging-based review of the WHO classification. Radiographics. 2011;31(7):1923–54.
45. Rydholm A, Berg NO. Size, site and clinical incidence of lipoma. Factors in the differential diagnosis of lipoma and sarcoma. Acta Orthop Scand. 1983;54(6):929–34.
46. Francom CR, Leoniak SM, Lovell MA, et al. Head and neck pleomorphic myxoid liposarcoma in a child with Li-Fraumeni syndrome. Int J Pediatr Otorhinolaryngol. 2019;123:191–4.
47. Baranov E, Hornick JL. Soft tissue special issue: fibroblastic and myofibroblastic neoplasms of the head and neck. Head Neck Pathol. 2020;14(1):43–58.
48. Sargar KM, Sheybani EF, Shenoy A, et al. Pediatric fibroblastic and myofibroblastic tumors: a pictorial review. Radiographics. 2016;36(4):1195–214.
49. Dell'Aversana Orabona G, Iaconetta G, Abbate V, et al. Head and neck myxofibrosarcoma: a case report and review of the literature. J Med Case Rep. 2014;8:468.
50. Waters B, Panicek DM, Lefkowitz RA, et al. Lowgrade myxofibrosarcoma: CT and MRI patterns in recurrent disease. AJR Am J Roentgenol. 2007;188(2):W193–8.
51. Hollinshead H. Anatomy for surgeons: the head and neck. 3rd ed. Philadelphia, PA: Lippincott; 1982.
52. Chooi WK, Woodhouse N, Coley SC, et al. Pediatric head and neck lesions: assessment of vascularity by MR digital subtraction angiography. AJNR Am J Neuroradiol. 2004;25:1251–5.
53. Strecker R, Scheffler K, Klisch J, et al. Fast functional MRA using time-resolved projection MR angiography with correlation analysis. Magn Reson Med. 2000;43:303–9.
54. Castelijns JA, van den Brekel MW. Magnetic resonance imaging evaluation of extracranial head and neck tumors. Magn Reson Q. 1993;9:113–28.
55. Rabinov K, Weber AL. Radiology of the salivary glands. Boston, MA: G Hall & Co; 1985. p. 153–66.
56. Valvassori GE, Buckingham RA, Carter BL, et al. Head and neck imaging. Stuttgart: George Thieme Verlag; 1988.
57. Harnsberger HR, Mancuso AA, Muraki AS, et al. Branchial cleft anomalies and their mimic: computed tomographic evaluation. Radiology. 1984;152:739–48.
58. Bhaskar SN, Bernier JL. Histogenesis of branchial cyst: a report of 468 cases. Am J Pathol. 1959;35:407–23.
59. Siegel MJ, Glazer HS, St Amour TE, et al. Lymphangiomas in children: MR imaging. Radiology. 1989;170:467–70.
60. Tran L, Sadeghi A, Hanson DE, et al. Major salivary gland tumors: treatment results and prognostic factors. Laryngoscope. 1986;96:1139–44.
61. Kramer LA, Mafee MF. Salivary glands. In: Stark DD, Bradley WG, editors. Magnetic resonance imaging, vol. III. St. Louis, MO: Mosby-Year Book; 1999. p. 1771–83.
62. Mirich DR, McArdle CV, Kulkarni MY. Benign pleomorphic adenomas of the salivary glands: surface coil MR imaging versus CT. J Comput Assist Tomogr. 1987;11:620–3.
63. Thawley SE, Pange WR. Comprehensive management of head and neck tumors. Philadelphia, PA: WB Saunders; 1987.
64. Lawson W. Common tumors of the parapharyngeal space: refined imaging diagnosis. Radiology. 1988;169:81–5.
65. Som PM, Biller HF. High-grade malignancies of the parotid gland: identification with MR imaging. Radiology. 1989;173:823–6.
66. Swartz JD, Rothman MI, Marlowe FI, Berger AS. MR imaging of parotid mass lesions: attempts at histopathologic differentiation. J Comput Assist Tomogr. 1989;13:789–96.
67. Minami M, Tanioka H, Oyama K, Itai Y, Eguchi M, Yoshikawa K, Murakami T, Sasaki Y. Warthin tumor of the parotid gland: MR–pathologic correlation. Am J Neuroradiol. 1993;14:209–14.
68. Joe VQ, Westesson PL. Tumors of the parotid gland: MR imaging characteristics of various histologic types. Am J Roentgenol. 1994;163:433–8.
69. Sharafuddin MJ, Diemer DP, Levine RS, Thomasson JL, Williams AL. A comparison of MR sequences for lesions of the parotid gland. Am J Neuroradiol. 1995;16:1895–902.

70. Silver AR, Som PS. Salivary glands. Radiol Clin N Am. 1998;36:941–66.
71. Tabor EK, Curtin HD. MR of the salivary glands. Radiol Clin North Am. 1989;27:379–92.
72. Schellhas KP, Wilkes CH, Fritts HM, et al. Temporomandibular joint: MR imaging of internal derangements and postoperative changes. AJR Am J Roentgenol. 1988;150(2):381–9.
73. Katzberg RW. Temporomandibular joint imaging. Radiology. 1989;170(2):297–307.
74. Murphy W, Kaplan P. Temporomandibular joint. In: Resnick D, editor. Diagnosis of bone and joint disorders. Philadelphia, PA: Saunders; 1995. p. 1699–754.
75. Helms CA, Kaplan P. Diagnostic imaging of the temporomandibular joint: recommendations for use of the various techniques. AJR Am J Roentgenol. 1990;154(2):319–22.
76. Schwaighofer BW, Tanaka TT, Klein MV, et al. MR imaging of the temporomandibular joint: a cadaver study of the value of coronal images. AJR Am J Roentgenol. 1990;154(6):1245–9.
77. Larheim TA, Westesson P, Sano T. Temporomandibular joint disc displacement: comparison in asymptomatic volunteers and patients. Radiology. 2001;218(2):428–32.
78. Wilkes CH. Internal derangements of the temporomandibular joint. Pathological variations. Arch Otolaryngol Head Neck Surg. 1989;115(4):469–77.
79. Segami N, Nishimura M, Kaneyama K, et al. Does joint effusion on T2 magnetic resonance images reflect synovitis? Comparison of arthroscopic findings in internal derangements of the temporomandibular joint. Oral Surg Oral Med Oral Pathol Oral Radiol Endod. 2001;92(3):341–5.
80. Suenaga S, Abeyama K, Noikura T. Gadolinium enhanced MR imaging of temporomandibular disorders: improved lesion detection of the posterior disc attachment on T1-weighted images obtained with fat suppression. AJR Am J Roentgenol. 1998;171(2):511–7.
81. Kuseler A, Pedersen TK, Herlin T, et al. Contrast enhanced magnetic resonance imaging as a method to diagnose early inflammatory changes in the temporomandibular joint in children with juvenile chronic arthritis. J Rheumatol. 1998;25(7):1406–12.

4 Ultrasound Imaging and Its Craniofacial Applications

Madhanraj Selvaraj, Ramandeep Singh, Navdeep Kaur, and Sameer Peer

4.1 Introduction

To understand the craniofacial skeleton's complex anatomy and surrounding structures, radiographic imaging is critical for diagnosis and treatment planning. Two-dimensional radiographs like intraoral periapical radiographs (IOPA), occlusal radiographs, and cephalograms are most used in oral and maxillofacial imaging. The introduction of three-dimensional computed tomography (CT) in 1971 by Dr. Hounsfield in England was used for volumetric imaging that helped selective imaging of specific anatomic and pathologic structures and that craniofacial surgeons can use this technique for effective treatment planning. High radiation exposure to CT led to the development of cone beam CT(CBCT) in 1998, which created a revolution in dento-maxillofacial imaging. The resolution of CBCT images is measured in voxel size, which produces high-resolution and less distorted images. While the benefits of 2D and 3D have been reported widely, the repeated radiation dose to the patients has been a major concern [1–3].

M. Selvaraj
Division of Orthodontics and Dentofacial Orthopedics, Department of Dentistry, Jawaharlal Institute of Postgraduate Medical Education and Research, Puducherry, India

R. Singh · N. Kaur (✉) · S. Peer
Department of Radiodiagnosis, All India Institute of Medical Sciences, Bathinda, Punjab, India

Serial exposure to ionizing radiation causes biological damage, directly and indirectly disrupting the normal cell cycle. Magnetic resonance imaging (MRI) and Ultrasonography (USG) are evolving diagnostic methods in dento-maxillofacial imaging to overcome this limitation [4]. In the last few decades, technological developments allowed more enhancement in ultrasound signals and new ways of interpreting and displaying data, such as power Doppler, 3D, and 4D ultrasound.

The use of ultrasound in medical imaging was introduced by Dr. Karl Theodore Dussik in Austria in 1942 [5]. In 1951, Howry et al. demonstrated the first B mode 2D imaging using an 'immersion tank ultrasound system' [6]. With advancement, ultrasound's evolution improved from 2D to 3D and 4D, intracavitary probes, colour Doppler, spectral analyser, and many more. Ultrasound is a non-ionizing imaging technique that provides cost-effective, portable, real-time imaging with metal artefacts [7].

4.1.1 Ultrasound Imaging

It uses high-frequency sound waves beyond the human hearing range, i.e. 2–18 MHz and helps evaluate the patient's internal organs. Sound waves are transmitted through the body, vibrating back and forth, and are reflected back as echoes convert into images. The vibrations consist of

S. S. Rana et al. (eds.), *Applications of Three-dimensional Imaging for Craniofacial Region*,
https://doi.org/10.1007/978-981-97-4608-8_4

zones of high pressure (compression) and low pressure (rarefaction). Sound waves are described in terms of frequency, wavelength, and velocity. Frequency and wavelength are inversely proportional, whereas velocity is independent of frequency. High-frequency waves generate high-resolution images; however, the shorter wavelength cannot penetrate deeper structures and vice versa. Medical ultrasound imaging is broadly classified as diagnostic and therapeutic/interventional ultrasound. Diagnostic imaging produces images of internal body structures, whereas therapeutic types are used for physical therapy commonly [8].

4.2 Basics of Ultrasound Physics

4.2.1 Parts and Functioning of Ultrasound Machine

Transducer: The handheld component converts electrical energy into mechanical energy. Also, it acts as both a transmitter and receiver of sound waves. The structural components of a transducer are the following:

Piezoelectric material: *Lead zirconate titanate (PZT)* crystals are commonly used consisting of 128–512 crystals arranged in a linear or curvilinear pattern. Crystal thickness differs from 1.8 mm for a 1 MHz transducer to 0.18 mm for a 10 MHz transducer. Each crystal thickness is half the length of the wavelength to reduce impedance, and the length of the probe ranges from 5 to 15 cm. Also, other lead-free piezoelectric materials like potassium sodium niobate (KNN), lithium niobate, photoacoustic transducers involving polydimethylsiloxane (PDMS), carbon nanomaterials type, etc. are available [9, 10].

Acoustic insulator: Stops vibration of the transducer in the operator's hand.

Backing or damping material: Adhered to the back of crystals, dampens the transducer vibration creating a shorter and sharp spatial pulse determining the resolution of an image.

Matching layer: Improves energy transmission efficiency to the patient by reducing the impedance difference between the transducer material and the soft tissue. It is always one-quarter wavelength thick to reduce impedance difference. Ultrasound gel also improves energy transmission by eliminating the air between the transducer and the patient, which could otherwise attenuate and reflect the ultrasound beam.

A central processing unit (CPU): The computer processes all the information received from the transducer and the transducer pulse controls.

Display: Screening of image processed by the CPU.

Keyboard: Consists of various buttons for the machine control (Fig. 4.1).

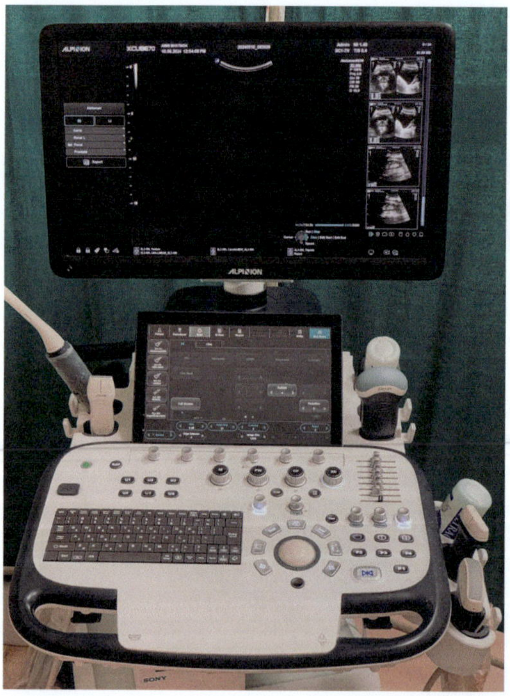

Fig. 4.1 A cart-based ultrasound system with display monitor (Alpinion e cube i 7, Mindray Medical International Limited, Shenzhen, China)

4.2.2 Production of the Ultrasound Beam and Image Formation

The principles behind ultrasound imaging are the piezoelectric effect and pulse echo principle. The ultrasound wave or beam is produced by the electrical current applied to PZT, causing them to deform and vibrate. This leads to the production of an ultrasound beam; generally, the wave frequency is determined by the PZT crystals present in the transducer. The sound wave is passed through the tissue surface, and the crystals wait for rebounding echoes to receive. The duration of the pulse is usually 1 μs repeated at intervals of 1 ms. The reflected waves excite the crystals and produce electrical signals converting them into images. The waves produced by crystals are 0.1% and receive 99.9% of the returning echoes. In addition, the intensity of sound waves depends upon the amount of voltage generated [8].

The acoustic impedance difference between tissues determines the amount of energy reflected from sound waves. The tissue's *acoustic impedance (Z)* is influenced by its velocity and the density at which waves pass through it. Bone has a higher density than soft tissue or water and is much higher than air. Therefore, the greater the impedance differential between two structures at the interface, the more energy will be reflected resulting in a brighter image. The tissue interface *depth(d)* must be calculated to obtain a two-dimensional image where ultrasound travels at an average *speed(c)* of 1540 ms^{-1}. The *time (t)* required for the ultrasound to traverse the *distance (d)* to interface and the reflected wave to return back to the transducer is computed

$$t = 2d / c$$

The energy of sound waves is progressively lost as they travel through the tissue surface, a process referred to as attenuation. It is caused by the *reflection, refraction, scattering,* and *absorption* of energy waves. Most attenuation happens through energy absorption, whereas reflection is important for the production of echoes. A combination of general attenuation leads to only a fraction of sound wave energy could reflect. Therefore, for restitution for this loss, the ultrasound machine employs a process known as *time gain compensation*, which amplifies the echoes and allows them to return faster and evenly [8, 11, 12].

4.3 Types of Transducers or Probes

Transducers are classified based on the arrangement of PZT crystals, frequency, and the aperture or footprint of the imaging field. The aperture or footprint is the probe portion that will contact the body surface. Throughout the year, various probes have been developed and marketed for medical use, among which point-of-care probes are mainly based on four designs (Table 4.1):

Table 4.1 Different types of ultrasound probes and its indications

Type of probe	Specifications	Indications
Linear	• Linear crystal arrangement • Rectangular shape of beam • Wide footprint with a central frequency of 6–15 MHz	• Best to view superficial structures like the thyroid, vascular, trachea, ocular, soft tissues, and musculoskeletal trauma • Also used guided procedures like needle aspiration and lumbar punctures
Curvilinear	• Also called a convex array probe provides a wide fan-shaped beam • Frequency ranging from 2 to 5 MHz	• Mostly used for deeper structures imaging like the abdomen, pelvis, and focused assessment with sonography in trauma (FAST)
Sector/phased	• Crystal arrangement at the Centre and pielike-shaped imaging • Smaller footprint • Frequency ranging from 1 to 5 MHz	• Echocardiography, abdomen, renal and paediatric patients

(continued)

Table 4.1 (continued)

Type of probe	Specifications	Indications
Intracavity	• Curvilinear crystal array with the wide view • Frequency ranging from 8 to 13 MHz • Resolution is higher	• Intra-oral pathology and transvaginal imaging

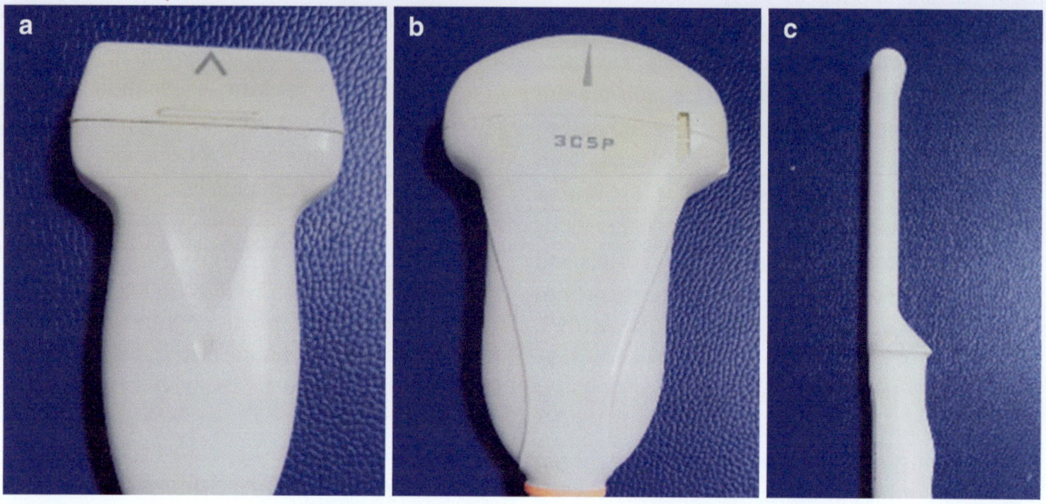

Fig. 4.2 Commonly used transducers: (**a**) linear probe; (**b**) curvilinear probe; (**c**) intracavity probe

- Linear (Fig. 4.2a).
- Curvilinear (Fig. 4.2b).
- Sector/phased.
- Intracavity (Fig. 4.2c).

4.4 Modes of Ultrasound

Depending on the context, real-time images of structures and motions can be produced using various *modes* of ultrasound scanning. There are mainly four basic modes of ultrasound imaging.

4.4.1 Amplitude or A-Mode

Its one-dimensional representation of reflected sound waves determines the depth and dimension of structures. It is graphically depicted as the amplitude (y-axis) and time (x-axis) needed for the echo to return back. Amplitude mode is a relatively simple method to differentiate solid and cystic masses [13]. Unfortunately, this method cannot picture the object's shape and the echo's direction. As a result, it has limited use other than echo-encephalography [14] to determine the orbital length and intraocular mass in the field of ophthalmology [15].

4.4.2 Brightness or B-Mode

It is the most extensively used greyscale ultrasound, displaying 2D images in a single plane. The sound waves reflected in the probe are depicted as a point on a greyscale. Therefore, the image's brightness is proportional to the reflected soundwave. With technological improvements, multiple B-mode images are created rapidly, conceiving real-time images and recording the same [16].

4.4.3 Motion or M-Mode

Commonly used in monitoring heart motion in both adult and foetal cardiac imaging. It displays a one-dimensional image of the amplitude of the echo. It is called a time-motion echo display along a preset ultrasound line. Movable echogenic structures stimulate line deflection, whereas static structures present flat lines, and interpretation depends on these variations. It is critical in the evaluation of heart valves, chambers, and vessel walls [16].

4.4.4 Doppler Ultrasound

Christian Andreas Doppler, an Austrian mathematician and physicist, found that the observed frequency of sound and light waves is affected by the relative motion of the source and the detector. This theory came to be known as the *Doppler effect,* and the change in frequency is called as *Doppler shift* in the year 1842. Conventional ultrasound images depend on the strength and time taken for an echo to remit back to the transducer. In addition, Doppler imaging measures the change or shift of the echoes received from moving objects like Red Blood Cells (RBCs). Surprisingly, any fluctuations in blood velocity Doppler frequency are audible, presenting the typical pulsating sound of blood flow.

Clinically, Doppler imaging can be in *pulsed* or *continuous* mode. Continuous modes are used for assessing peripheral vessels and foetal heart waves in cardiotocography (CTG). It is inexpensive, simple, and sensitive to flow; unfortunately, it cannot measure velocity and determine the depth of the signal. In comparison, the pulsed mode determines the direction, depth, and presence of flow from the Doppler signal. The pulsed mode is subclassified into three types: *colour, power, and spectral Doppler.* Colour Doppler is commonly used to visualise blood flow's speed, movement, and direction in different colours (Fig. 4.3). Power Doppler is a newer form providing more detailed blood flow without the direction of blood flow. Also, spectral Doppler provides graphical information on blood flow and determines the blood vessel blockage [16, 17].

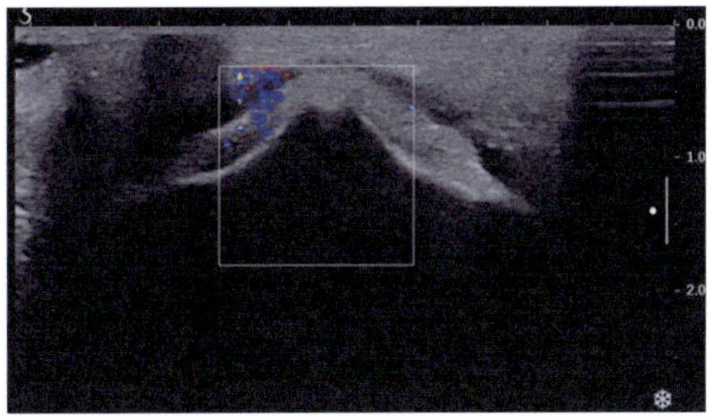

Fig. 4.3 Colour Doppler image of anterior palate region

4.5 3D and 4D Ultrasound

With advancements, high-quality 2D images are integrated or reconstructed to form volumetric images. A series of 2D data is acquired, followed by volumetric data analysis and displaying a 3D volumetric image. It helps to visualise morphology size and its relationship with related structures. Images can be displayed as volume-rendered or multiplanar images. In addition, they can also be displayed using the colour and power Doppler format. However, 4D ultrasound is live motion or streaming of video of 3D ultrasound. There are two commonly used methods to acquire 3D ultrasound, i.e. free-hand and automated techniques. The probe is moved manually in a free-hand technique, whereas the automated technique has a dedicated volumetric probe to acquire data [18–20].

Advantages

- Identification of congenital disabilities like cleft lip and palate and craniofacial syndromes.
- Periodic assessment of foetal growth, heartbeat, and well-being.
- Data storage for screening, expert review, or consult and teaching.
- Enhanced 3D and 4D (live streaming) volumetric or multiplanar view of a foetus.

Disadvantages

- Costly.
- Well-trained physician or expert to interpret.

- Low quality of image during foetal movements.
- Safety use of 3D and 4D ultrasound bioeffects.

4.6 Interpretation of Ultrasound Images

Thorough knowledge of applied anatomy in visualizing ultrasound images is fundamental for interpreting images. Ultrasound images differ from conventional radiographic methods, where images are radio-opaque or radio-lucent. At the same time, ultrasound is based on echogenicity, i.e. the ability of the tissue to reflect the sound waves. Some of the tissue absorbs the sound waves, while others reflect depending on the density of the tissue. Higher echogenicity tissues are *hyperechoic* and appear white on the screen. Less echogenic tissues are *hypoechoic* and look grey, while no echogenic tissues are *anechoic* and appear black [21]. Some of the basic anatomical structures appear on ultrasound (Table 4.2).

Table 4.2 Ultrasound image interpretation of different anatomical structures

Anatomical structure	Interpretation
Bone	Appears anechoic or black with hyperechoic(white) rim
Cartilage	Hypoechoic or grey
Blood vessels	Anechoic or black
Blood vessels on colour Doppler	Flow toward the probe is red and away is blue (BART-blue away, red toward)
Muscles	Hypoechoic with striate; fat is almost anechoic; fascia and connective tissue appear hyperechoic
Lymph nodes	Anechoic or hypoechoic
Nerves	Proximal nerves appear hypo-anechoic; distal nerves appear hyperechoic with stippling (honeycomb)
Ligaments and tendons	Hyperechoic

4.7 Ultrasound in Dentomaxillofacial Imaging

The major field of interest of imaging for a craniofacial surgeon is to assess maxillofacial injuries and pathology. The main applications of USG in dentistry in the past years have always been the diagnosis of intraoral soft tissue lesions, salivary gland pathologies, and cysts and tumours. Structural changes can be visualised as hypoechogenic, hyperechogenic, or anechogenic areas. Ultrasound has been used to assess fractures [22] and bone healing in distraction osteogenesis [23]. It has been proven reliable to determine the distraction gap and evaluate bone maturity, as ultrasound waves can pass through healing wounds devoid of cortical bone [23–25]. This is in addition to its growing popularity due to its power Doppler and colour Doppler features, which make it possible to evaluate the vascularisation of lesions, identify between cystic and solid lesions, and aid in identifying malignancy from benign lesions [26, 27].

The stability of the occlusion depends upon the surrounding orofacial soft tissue and tongue musculature. Therefore, it is imperative to understand the soft tissue changes during implant-prosthetic restoration and orthodontic treatment. Head and neck muscles have implied a major influence during treatment stages, such as the aetiology and active treatment of occlusal problems, jaw deformation, and treatment stability. USG has recently been a reliable imaging technique for precisely calculating changes in local cross-sectional parameters of the craniofacial muscle groups in real time and measuring the thickness and cross-sectional area of the masticatory muscles [28]. Tongue posture and volume have been related to the aetiology of malocclusion and facial anomalies. Swallowing patterns were investigated using B and M mode sonography [29, 30]. The majority of abnormal swallowing patterns and larger tongue were observed in class III or prognathic mandible [31].

Temporomandibular disorders affect the masticatory muscles, and it is essential to examine TMJ-related structures before and after orthodontic treatment. The prevalence of TMDs in the general population ranges from 10 to 70%, with various causes for the aetiology. Conventional radiographs, computed tomography (CT), and cone-beam CT (CBCT) are recommended for hard tissue visualisation. In contrast, magnetic resonance imaging (MRI) assesses soft tissue (TMJ disc) components [32]. Gateno et al. investigated the accuracy of USG to view the position of the mandibular condylar within the glenoid fossa. They concluded that USG could be used as an evaluation tool for reproducing the condylar position during orthognathic surgery [33]. However, according to Klatkiewicz et al., there are no standardised procedures for ultrasound scanning of the temporomandibular joint, and more research on both normal and abnormal TMJs is needed [34]. The use of ultrasound in different fields of dento-maxillofacial imaging has been summarised (Table 4.3).

Only a few studies have shown the use of ultrasonography in assessing the mid-palatal suture. For this, the patient is made to sit upright, and the ultrasound probe is positioned outside the mouth on the skin overlying the mid-palatal suture (a region between the nasal columella–labial junction and the upper lip), and the USG beam is oriented perpendicular to the bone surface [53, 54]. A real-time survey of the mid-palatal suture is then performed, producing axial slices (Fig. 4.4a and b).

It is necessary to conduct comparative studies of various imaging systems used in maxillofacial regions to obtain consensus or guidelines to provide clinicians with proper decision-making criteria. In addition, it is also essential to consider technological evolution to reduce the hazardous use of radiation imaging and consider non-ionizing imaging methods like USG and MRI. Innovation in USG intraoral and extraoral probes suitable for head and neck regions can reduce the usage of conventional imaging methods.

Table 4.3 Ultrasound diagnostic features of different pathological conditions in dento-maxillofacial region

Diagnosis in the dentomaxillofacial region	Ultrasound features
Maxillofacial fractures [22, 35]	Discontinuity in the hyperechoic cortical bone as small as 1 mm can be spotted using advanced high-resolution transducers
Distraction osteogenesis [23–25]	Ultrasound waves can pass through healing wounds, and bone maturation can be observed 3 weeks earlier than conventional radiographs Developing cysts in the distraction site is visualised better
Inflammatory lesion	A simple inflammatory lesion is seen as diffused hypoechoic areas and non-delineated margins
Facial abscess [36]	Observed as heterogeneous areas with unclear borders with posterior acoustic enhancement. Central liquefaction and debris may be seen as avascular areas, and abscess gases are seen as hyperechogenic areas Diagnostic accuracy of 90% can be observed
Paranasal and maxillary sinus [37, 38]	Anechoic to hypoechoic images with few isolated internal echoes and a homogeneous or heterogeneous, well-defined triangle shape (maxillary sinus) are seen when there is fluid accumulation in the paranasal sinus. In contrast, images with mucosal thickening show hypoechoic to echoic images with non-triangular shapes that have hazy borders
Oral submucous fibrosis [39, 40]	Early identification of feeble fibrotic bands A hyperechoic area is seen in fibrous bands with normal or reduced blood flow with peak systolic velocity
Ranula [41]	Appear as transparent, thin-walled hypoechoic lesions. Fine internal echoes may occasionally be seen in infected conditions

(continued)

Table 4.3 (continued)

Diagnosis in the dentomaxillofacial region	Ultrasound features
Salivary glands [42, 43]	Normal salivary glands are homogenous in echo structure, and the borders are clear Sialoliths appear hyperechoic with posterior shadowing Benign tumours appear well-defined lobulated hypoechoic lesions with microcystic or anechoic Sjogren's syndrome in chronic condition gives a 'tortoiseshell' appearance
Vascular lesions [44, 45]	Haemangiomas appear as hypoechoic sinusoidal compartments within lesions; high resistance waveform is seen in arterial flow Phleboliths were identified as hyperechoic with posterior shadowing
Lymphangiomas [46]	Appear as multilocular cystic masses with varying internal septa thickness Infected cysts consist of hyperechoic or anechoic
Periapical abscess [47–49]	A hypoechoic pattern with ill-defined or well-defined margins Increased vascularity is seen in the colour Doppler The periosteal reaction can also be seen in the USG sections
Soft tissue grafting [50, 51]	Used to measure connective tissue graft thickness, keratinised tissue around implants, masticatory mucosa, and gingival thickness during root coverage
Head and neck muscles [28]	Only superficial muscles are visualised by ultrasound Muscle thickness is measured between the outer and inner fascia Fascia appears echogenic compared to surrounding tissue, and deep fascia appears to be a thin hyperechoic band
Normal temporomandibular joint (TMJ) [33, 34]	Surface of the condyle appears hyperechoic Joint capsule, retrodiscal tissue and muscle are isoechogenic The articular disk in the sagittal plane is an inverted hypoechoic C-shaped structure
Mid-palatal suture (MPS) [52, 53]	Hyperechoic discontinuous line and the needle-like hyperechoic line, the non-homogenous zone seen in MPS, opened

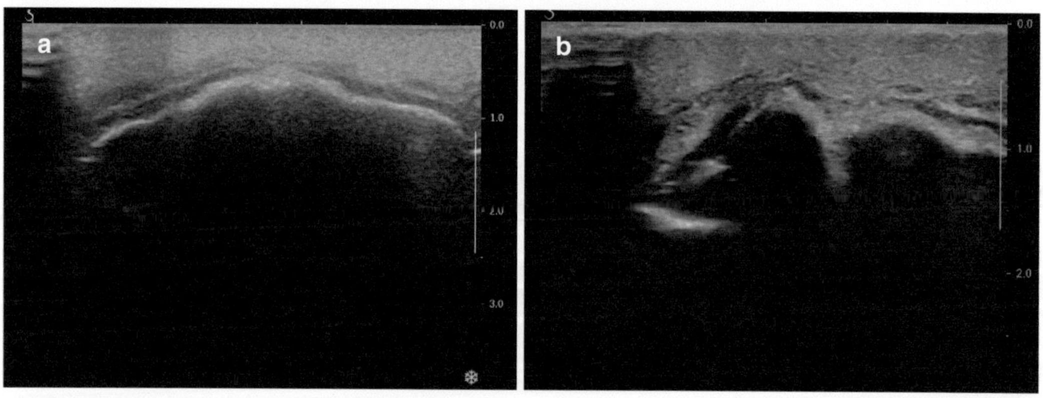

Fig. 4.4 Mid-palatal suture opening in a patient undergoing rapid maxillary expansion (RME): (**a**) before expansion; (**b**) after expansion

4.8 Summary

Ultrasonography is an excellent technique for assessing craniofacial morphology, but the views can be limited by shadowing from the ossified bone. 3D ultrasound may be helpful in the assessment of cleft palate and craniosynostosis. 3D printed models demonstrating foetal craniofacial abnormalities are obtained using data from prenatal surface-rendered sonographic data. In addition, the use of 3D/4D ultrasound for prenatal conditions may be useful in the assessment of cleft palate and craniosynostosis, but foetal magnetic resonance imaging can facilitate the diagnosis. Advanced imaging modalities, especially computer-aided, three-dimensional visualisation of the craniofacial complex, facilitate the diagnosis, planning, and treatment of craniofacial disorders.

References

1. Buzug TM. Computed tomography. In: Kramme R, Hoffmann KP, Pozos RS, editors. Springer handbook of medical technology [Internet]. Berlin, Heidelberg: Springer; 2011. p. 311–42. (Springer Handbooks).
2. Hans MG, Palomo JM, Valiathan M. History of imaging in orthodontics from Broadbent to cone-beam computed tomography. Am J Orthod Dentofacial Orthop. 2015;148(6):914–21.
3. Kapila SD, Nervina JM. CBCT in orthodontics: assessment of treatment outcomes and indications for its use. Dentomaxillofac Radiol. 2015;44(1):20140282.
4. Herfarth H, Palmer L. Risk of radiation and choice of imaging. Dig Dis. 2009;27(3):278–84.
5. Manbachi A, Cobbold RSC. Development and application of piezoelectric materials for ultrasound generation and detection. Ultrasound. 2011;19(4):187–96.
6. Howry DH, Bliss WR. Ultrasonic visualization of soft tissue structures of the body. J Lab Clin Med. 1952;40(4):579–92.
7. Marotti J, Heger S, Tinschert J, Tortamano P, Chuembou F, Radermacher K, et al. Recent advances of ultrasound imaging in dentistry—a review of the literature. Oral Surg Oral Med Oral Pathol Oral Radiol. 2013;115(6):819–32.
8. Aldrich JE. Basic physics of ultrasound imaging. Crit Care Med. 2007;35(5 Suppl):S131–7.
9. Wells PNT. Ultrasound imaging. Phys Med Biol. 2006;51(13):R83–98.
10. Chan J, Zheng Z, Bell K, Le M, Reza PH, Yeow JTW. Photoacoustic imaging with capacitive micromachined ultrasound transducers: principles and developments. Sensors (Basel). 2019;19(16):3617.
11. Martin DJ, Wells ITP, Goodwin CR. Physics of ultrasound. Anaesthes Intensive Care Med. 2015;16(3):132–5.
12. Powles AEJ, Martin DJ, Wells ITP, Goodwin CR. Physics of ultrasound. Anaesthes Intensive Care Med. 2018;19(4):202–5.
13. Ostrum BJ, Goldberg BB, Isard HJ. A-mode ultrasound differentiation of soft-tissue masses. Radiology. 1967;88(4):745–9.
14. Smith SW, Von Ramm OT, Kisslo JA, Thurstone FL. Real time ultrasound tomography of the adult brain. Stroke. 1978;9(2):117–22.
15. Silverman RH. Focused ultrasound in ophthalmology. Clin Ophthalmol. 2016;10:1865–75.
16. Moran CM, Thomson AJW. Preclinical ultrasound imaging—a review of techniques and imaging applications. Front Phys. 2020;8:124.
17. Katsi V, Felekos I, Kallikazaros I. Christian Andreas Doppler: a legendary man inspired by the dazzling light of the stars. Hippokratia. 2013;17(2):113–4.
18. Harvey CJ, Pilcher JM, Eckersley RJ, Blomley MJK, Cosgrove DO. Advances in ultrasound. Clin Radiol. 2002;57(3):157–77.
19. Yagel S, Cohen SM, Shapiro I, Valsky DV. 3D and 4D ultrasound in fetal cardiac scanning: a new look at the fetal heart. Ultrasound Obstet Gynecol. 2007;29(1):81–95.
20. Merz E, Abramowicz JS. 3D/4D ultrasound in prenatal diagnosis: is it time for routine use? Clin Obstet Gynecol. 2012;55(1):336.
21. Kehrer A, Sachanadani NS, Da Silva NPB, Lonic D, Heidekrueger P, Taeger CD, et al. Step-by-step guide to ultrasound-based design of alt flaps by the microsurgeon—basic and advanced applications and device settings. J Plast Reconstr Aesthet Surg. 2020;73(6):1081–90.
22. Adeyemo WL, Akadiri OA. A systematic review of the diagnostic role of ultrasonography in maxillofacial fractures. Int J Oral Maxillofac Surg. 2011;40(7):655–61.
23. Blane CE, Herzenberg JE, DiPietro MA. Radiographic imaging for Ilizarov limb lengthening in children. Pediatr Radiol. 1991;21(2):117–20.
24. Thurmüller P, Troulis M, O'Neill MJ, Kaban LB. Use of ultrasound to assess healing of a mandibular distraction wound. J Oral Maxillofac Surg. 2002;60(9):1038–44.
25. Andrade N, Aggrawal N, Jadhav G, Sahu V, Mathai PC. To determine the efficacy of ultrasonography in the evaluation of bone fill at the regenerate site for mandibular distraction osteogenesis over clinical and radiographic assessment - an in vivo prospective study. J Oral Biol Craniofac Res. 2018;8(2):89–93.
26. Ying M, Ahuja A, Brook F, Metreweli C. Vascularity and grey-scale sonographic features of normal cervical lymph nodes: variations with nodal size. Clin Radiol. 2001;56(5):416–9.
27. Ahuja AT, Ying M, Ho SY, Antonio G, Lee YP, King AD, et al. Ultrasound of malignant cervical lymph nodes. Cancer Imaging. 2008;8(1):48–56.
28. Benington PC, Gardener JE, Hunt NP. Masseter muscle volume measured using ultrasonography and its relationship with facial morphology. Eur J Orthod. 1999;21(6):659–70.
29. Peng CL, Jost-Brinkmann PG, Yoshida N, Miethke RR, Lin CT. Differential diagnosis between infantile and mature swallowing with ultrasonography. Eur J Orthod. 2003;25(5):451–6.

30. Peng CL, Miethke RR, Pong SJ, Lin CT. Investigation of tongue movements during swallowing with M-mode ultrasonography. J Orofac Orthop. 2007;68(1):17–25.
31. Ihan Hren N, Barbič U. Tongue volume in adults with skeletal class III dentofacial deformities. Head Face Med. 2016;12:12.
32. Murphy MK, MacBarb RF, Wong ME, Athanasiou KA. Temporomandibular disorders: a review of etiology, clinical management, and tissue engineering strategies. Int J Oral Maxillofac Implants. 2013;28(6):e393–414.
33. Gateno J, Miloro M, Hendler BH, Horrow M. The use of ultrasound to determine the position of the mandibular condyle. J Oral Maxillofac Surg. 1993;51(10):1081–6; discussion 1086–1087
34. Klatkiewicz T, Gawriołek K, Pobudek Radzikowska M, Czajka-Jakubowska A. Ultrasonography in the diagnosis of temporomandibular disorders: a meta-analysis. Med Sci Monit. 2018;24:812–7.
35. Sinha TP, Bhoi S, Kumar S, Ramchandani R, Goswami A, Kurrey L, et al. Diagnostic accuracy of bedside emergency ultrasound screening for fractures in pediatric trauma patients. J Emerg Trauma Shock. 2011;4(4):443–5.
36. Shah A, Ahmed I, Hassan S, Samoon A, Ali B. Evaluation of ultrasonography as a diagnostic tool in the management of head and neck facial space infections: a clinical study. Natl J Maxillofac Surg. 2015;6(1):55–61.
37. Reilly JS, Hotaling AJ, Chiponis D, Wald ER. Use of ultrasound in detection of sinus disease in children. Int J Pediatr Otorhinolaryngol. 1989;17(3):225–30.
38. Fufezan O, Asavoaie C, Chereches Panta P, Mihuţ G, Bursaşiu E, Anca I, et al. The role of ultrasonography in the evaluation of maxillary sinusitis in pediatrics. Med Ultrason. 2010;12(1):4–11.
39. Krithika C, Ramanathan S, Koteeswaran D, Sridhar C, Satheesh Krishna J, Shiva Shankar MP. Ultrasonographic evaluation of oral submucous fibrosis in habitual areca nut chewers. Dentomaxillofac Radiol. 2013;42(9):20120319.
40. Devathambi JR, Aswath N. Ultrasonographic evaluation of oral submucous fibrosis and masseteric hypertrophy. J Clin Imaging Sci. 2013;3(Suppl 1):12.
41. Jain P, Jain R. Types of sublingual gland herniation observed during sonography of plunging ranulas. J Ultrasound Med. 2014;33(8):1491–7.
42. Gritzmann N, Rettenbacher T, Hollerweger A, Macheiner P, Hübner E. Sonography of the salivary glands. Eur Radiol. 2003;13(5):964–75.
43. Zajkowski P, Ochal-Choińska A. Standards for the assessment of salivary glands—an update. J Ultrason. 2016;16(65):175–90.
44. Sugawara C, Takahashi A, Kawano F, Kudo Y, Ishimaru N, Miyamoto Y. Intraoral ultrasonography of tongue mass lesions. Dentomaxillofac Radiol. 2016;45(5):20150362.
45. Derindağ G, Sarıca İ, Çağlayan F. Examination of oral hemangiomas by intraoral ultrasonography. Oral Radiol. 2021;37(4):687–92.
46. Pui MH, Li ZP, Chen W, Chen JH. Lymphangioma: imaging diagnosis. Australas Radiol. 1997;41(4):324–8.
47. Rajendran N, Sundaresan B. Efficacy of ultrasound and color power Doppler as a monitoring tool in the healing of endodontic periapical lesions. J Endod. 2007;33(2):181–6.
48. Tikku AP, Kumar S, Loomba K, Chandra A, Verma P, Aggarwal R. Use of ultrasound, color Doppler imaging and radiography to monitor periapical healing after endodontic surgery. J Oral Sci. 2010;52(3):411–6.
49. Prince CN, Annapurna CS, Sivaraj S, Ali IM. Ultrasound imaging in the diagnosis of periapical lesions. J Pharm Bioallied Sci. 2012;4(Suppl 2):S369–72.
50. Tsiolis FI, Needleman IG, Griffiths GS. Periodontal ultrasonography. J Clin Periodontol. 2003;30(10):849–54.
51. Chifor R, Badea AF, Chifor I, Mitrea DA, Crisan M, Badea ME. Periodontal evaluation using a non-invasive imaging method (ultrasonography). Med Pharm Rep. 2019;92(Suppl 3):S20–32.
52. Sumer AP, Ozer M, Sumer M, Danaci M, Tokalak F, Telcioglu NT. Ultrasonography in the evaluation of midpalatal suture in surgically assisted rapid maxillary expansion. J Craniofac Surg. 2012;23(5):1375–7.
53. Gumussoy I, Miloglu O, Bayrakdar IS, Dagistan S, Caglayan F. Ultrasonography in the evaluation of the mid-palatal suture in rapid palatal expansion. Dentomaxillofac Radiol. 2014;43(8):20140167.
54. Selvaraj M, Duggal R, Manchanda S, Chaudhari PK, Bhalla AS. Comparison of Ultrasonography and Cone-beam Computed Tomography for Quantitative Assessment of Midpalatal Suture Opening after Rapid Palatal Expansion: A Pilot Study. J Med Ultrasound. 2024:10–4103.

5 Noninvasive 3D Facial Scanning

Edlira Zere, Raj Kumar Manas, Suraj Prasad Sinha, Shailendra Singh Rana, and Prabhat Kumar Chaudhari

5.1 Introduction of 3D Facial Scanning Technology

The craniofacial imaging clinical records include the hard tissues (upper and lower jaw with their teeth and TMJ complex) and soft tissues [1, 2]. Craniofacial imaging aims to provide a precise anatomic truth presentation of three-dimensional (3D) craniofacial structures with precise accuracy for diagnosis and treatment planning by giving insight and explaining the interconnection between craniofacial diagnosis, growth, effects of treatment, and stability [3]. Craniofacial imaging records help to clinically evaluate the form and size of human craniofacial structures in dental specialties including dentofacial orthopedics, orthodontics, maxillofacial surgery, facial clefts, and craniofacial anomalies [1–6].

The soft tissue paradigm of treatment emphasizes the importance of the soft tissues' function and esthetics in relation to the hard tissues during the clinical examination, which requires reliable record data of the external craniofacial soft tissues. 3D analysis of external craniofacial soft tissues, without being related to the skeletal and muscle components generates information about craniofacial surface morphology that the traditional direct craniofacial anthropometry, plaster models, and two-dimensional (2D) photography cannot truly represent due to their limitations and shortcomings [7, 8].

Three-dimensional surface imaging methods are divided in contact and noncontact methods [9]. The contact methods rely on mechanisms that interact with the surface such as the coordinate measuring machine (CMM), which performs the measurements using touch probes and arms with touching probes. The noncontact methods that avoid any pressure on surface or facial soft tissues without influencing the measurements' precision are preferred

E. Zere (✉)
Faculty of Medicine, Department of Orthodontics and Craniofacial Anomalies, Technion—Israel Institute of Technology, Rambam Health Care Campus, Haifa, Israel

Faculty of Medical Sciences, Department of Dentistry, Luarasi University, Tirana, Albania

R. K. Manas
Plastic Surgery, All India Institute of Medical Sciences, New Delhi, India

S. P. Sinha
Department of Craniofacial Orthodontics, Chang Gung Memorial Hospital, Taipei, Taiwan

Rutgers School of Dental Medicine, Newark, NJ, USA

S. S. Rana
Department of Dentistry, All India Institute of Medical Sciences, Bathinda, Punjab, India

P. K. Chaudhari
Division of Orthodontics and Dentofacial Deformities, Centre for Dental Education and Research (CDER), All India Institute of Medical Sciences, New Delhi, Delhi, India

S. S. Rana et al. (eds.), *Applications of Three-dimensional Imaging for Craniofacial Region*,
https://doi.org/10.1007/978-981-97-4608-8_5

for usage in facial soft tissue clinical and research practice [9].

The noncontact 3D facial surface imaging methods are based on transmission using the ionizing radiation (CT, MRI) and on reflection (optical and nonoptical) [9]. The optical methods can exploit the reflected energy, and the interaction is implemented through the light. The optical methods use light rays in some form to noninvasively capture and create a digital map of the facial surface information with a high speed of acquisition, improving the safety and enhancing patients' comfort.

Noninvasive 3D facial scanning represents a noncontact and nonionizing optical scanning method. It provides a digital photograph of the external facial soft tissues of craniofacial structures in three dimensions, which by using a 3D modeling software measures the surface points' Cartesian coordinates (x, y, z). This results in a 3D cloud of points called "virtual mesh" that represents the spatial model of the face overlaid by the color mapping and creating a virtual patient face with x-y-z coordinates being saved as a computer file in stereolithographic (STL) file format [10–13]. By using the 3D modeling software, STL files can be displayed on a 2D computer monitor as a 3D digital face or virtual facial surface that represents the original facial surface and can be used for further measurements. The resulting 3D file after being saved can be edited, measured, and 3D printed [9–13]. Optical 3D facial scanners are the most preferred devices to acquire the forms of the deformable human craniofacial, generate a 3D topography of craniofacial surface anatomy, and perform further analysis on a 3D model, i.e., measurement of the facial landmarks' distances, angles, ratios, and surface areas and facial portions' volumes and analysis of the soft tissues during movement.

Three-dimensional optical facial scanning methods are represented by the laser scanning, structured light projection, stereophotogrammetry, and 3D facial morphometry [14–19]. Each of them comes with its own specifics of accuracy and reliability, advantages, disadvantages, limitations, and costs [20–24].

5.2 Methods of 3D Facial Scanning

5.2.1 Laser Scanning System

"**L**ight **A**mplification by **S**timulated **E**mission of **R**adiation" known as **Laser** represents a light source of convergent, coherent, and monochromatic beam of electromagnetic radiation with wavelength ranging from ultraviolet to infrared.

The laser scanning system projects a laser beam at a known angle (i.e., alfa, α) onto a target facial surface to be measured. The 3D laser scanner device is combined with an electronic control unit, and a laser unit with one or more digital cameras to acquire the images can capture superficial data. A charge-coupled device (CCD) digital camera placed at a known offset from the laser captures the projected image. If the laser beam falls on a facial surface at point A or B, these will be seen in the image sensor of the laser scanner at the locations A′ or B′. Using the principle of laser triangulation, the system built in sensors calculates the 3D surface's coordinates of the light reflected by the facial surface (Fig. 5.1). From the resulting 3D point cloud, the available software package produces a meshed surface as a 3D triangle meshed geometry that accurately models the facial surface and calculates the distance to the object [15, 24–30].

During laser scanning, it is paramount to prevent the patient' movement and protect the clinicians and patients' eyes. If movements happen during acquisition with laser technology (related to the blinking reflex) [31], it will affect the accuracy of cloud of points gained with overlapping errors that will need a filtering operation to removing the extra information [32]. Laser facial scanning can obtain a complete facial image within a few seconds of approximately 10 seconds [32, 33] with high accuracy, validity and reliability as confirmed by several researches [18, 20, 27, 28, 34–36].

Three-dimensional laser scanners such as Minolta Vivid (900, 910) and 3D Scanner (Konica Minolta Sensing, Inc., Osaka, Japan) are used to digitize the facial morphology and facial landmarks marking on virtual model and have proven

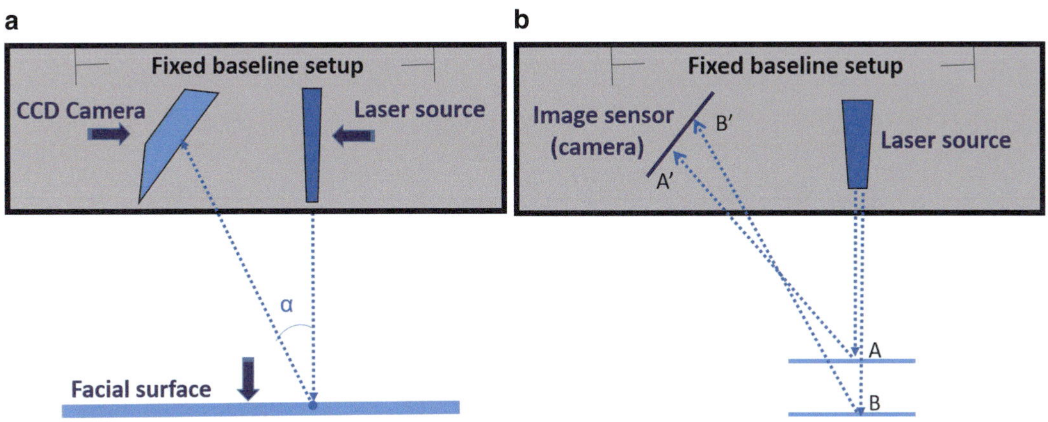

Fig. 5.1 (**a**) A typical laser triangulation setup. (**b**) Schematic presentation of principles of laser triangulation

to be precise and accurate to evaluate the facial morphology and symmetry and growth changes in plastic surgery and further clinical application [27–29, 33, 34].

5.2.2 Structured Light Projection

The structured light scanning technology uses an active illumination with designed 2D spatially varying intensity patterns of the white light expressed in grids, dots, or stripes, known as "structured light" projected on an object surface.

A single or two calibrated digital cameras being placed at a known distance from an object surface exploit the deformation of the light patterns projected from a video projector (Fig. 5.2). The system software captures and processes the distortion of the light pattern and using a standard triangulation method catches 3D data, calculates the depth, generates the geometric shape data, registers the 3D surface contour's color and texture information, and finally reconstructs the virtual 3D object image, i.e., a patient cranium and/or facial model [37–43].

The light patterns projected can be single pattern (short time with lower accuracy) used for dynamic objects or multi patterns (long capture time with higher accuracy) appropriate for static objects [34]. To acquire a patient's 3D virtual models with high accuracy, density, and quality, in clinical and research settings, the patient's craniofacial region or face needs to be illuminated several times with random patterns of light, which increases the capture time. Thus, patient collaboration is needed to avoid the risk of head movements. Also, to capture an ear to ear and complete craniofacial region captures, it may be needed to use several cameras to increase the accuracy and quality of 3D virtual patient [19, 41, 42].

Various structured light scanners have proven to provide facial scans with high resolution and accuracy and are available to evaluate facial soft tissues such as GIP 3D video camera (Geometric Image Processing Lab, Technion, Israel Institute of Technology) (Fig. 5.2) [15, 38], EinScan Pro 2X Plus (Shining 3D Tech. Co., Ltd. Hangzhou, China) [22], FaceScan3D (3D-Shape, Inc., Erlangen, Germany) [44], Morpheus 3D (Morpheus Inc., Seoul, Korea) [45], and Artec EVA (Artec EvaTM; Artec Group, Luxembourg) [46–48]. The last one is a handheld 3D scanner using Artec Studio 12 software to reconstruct 3D images with high-resolution textures, being useful and practical in medical 3D surface imaging.

5.2.3 Stereophotogrammetry

Stereophotogrammetry represents a facial scanning technique which captures two or more synchronous photographs of the face from different angles using as the light source simultaneous and coordinated stereoscopic pair of cameras that illuminate regular photographic flash to acquire rapid facial image without radiation [49,

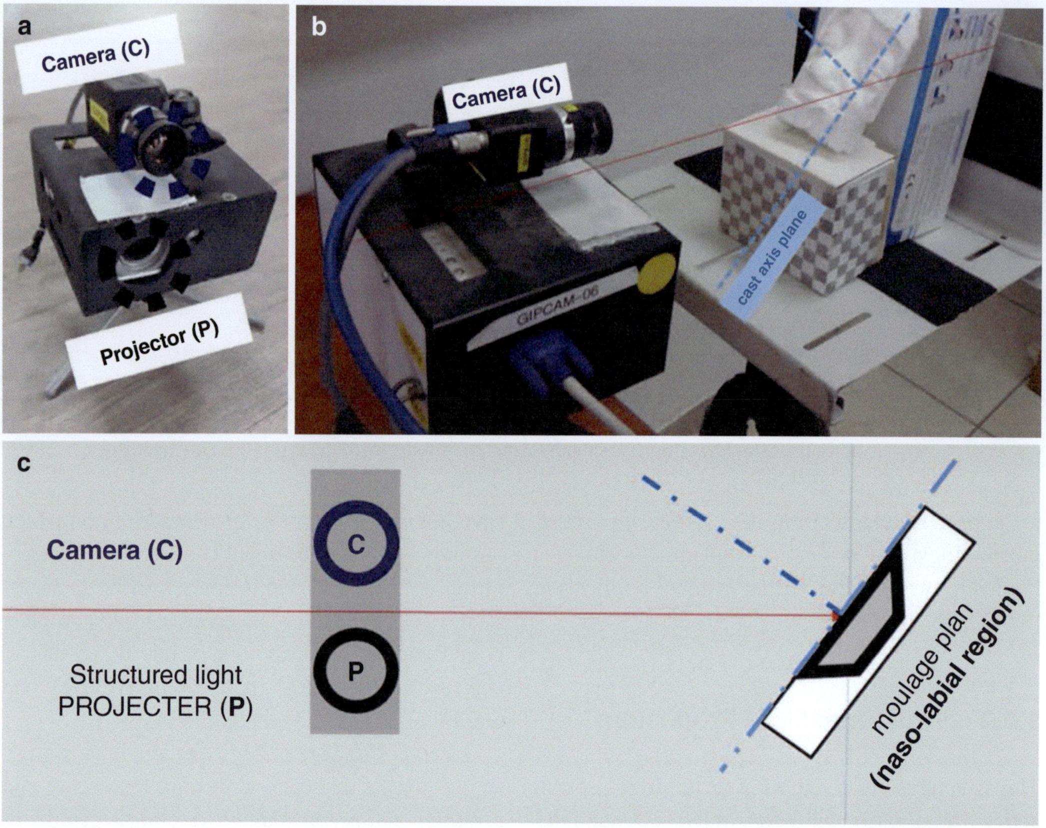

Fig. 5.2 (**a**) A noncontact structured light 3D surface scanning technology. (*Courtesy* of Geometric Image Processing (GIP) Laboratory, Faculty of Computer Science, Technion—Israel Institute of Technology, Haifa, Israel; with permission) [15]. (**b** and **c**) Structured light 3D surface imaging technique setup during plaster moulage scanning process. Redline represents a virtual line between the camera C (parallel to its optical axis) and projector P, for the most optimal view of the region of interest, the nasolabial region of plaster moulage

50]. The calibration of the system for the field of view to accurately set the relationship between cameras is performed using objects with known geometrical characteristics, which assists to compute the mathematical information and obtain a stereoscopic reconstruction of the face. The system software records the depths and using triangulation and fringe projection method merges it digitally generating a composite 3D geometric model that accurately represents a 3D face model with color and texture information that can be viewed and measured three dimensionally [15, 18]. Based on the type of triangulation algorithms, the stereophotogrammetry can be active or passive.

The active stereophotogrammetry projects on the facial surface a combination of a random unstructured light pattern with the visible natural facial light pattern. It depends less on external light to capture images but is recommended to darken the surroundings. The passive stereophotogrammetry is based only on the natural light patterns and is dependent on the external light for obtaining 3D geometry of the facial surface images. Thus, the passive stereophotogrammetry technology has more useful applications in doctors' offices and hospitals. The hybrid equipment uses both active and passive stereophotogrammetry [34].

Stereophotogrammetry is considered the most used and preferable among methods of 3D facial surface imaging for 3D facial analysis mainly in hospital and research settings [16, 51–54]. Several stereophotogrammetry systems (static or portable) are currently available, such as 3dMDface (3dMD, Atlanta, GA) [55], Scanify (Fuel 3D Technologies, Chinnor, UK) [56], Di3D (Dimensional Imaging, Hillington Park, Glasgow, UK) [57], and Vectra (Canfield Imaging Systems, Fairfield, NJ) [58–61].

3dMD technology (3dMD, Atlanta, USA) represents a stereophotogrammetry system that combines the stereophotometry and structured light being projected as a single constant light pattern on the facial surface. It is considered the gold standard, most accurate, and fastest system in 3D soft tissues evaluation that can be used in almost any clinical situations, even with uncooperative patients [62, 63]. 3dMDface system (3dMD Inc., Atlanta, GA, USA) uses six cameras positioned in different angles and connected to a computer (Fig. 5.3). The system's algorithm combines the taken images to create a 3D geometric facial data which is stored and used in 3dMD software for further linear, angular, and volumetric measurements [64]. As the development and improvements of 3dMD technology continue, the temporal 3dMDface and 3dMDtrio system represents the recent available commercial static 3D facial surface scanners [15]. Another stereophotogrammetric system named Canfield's Vectra imaging system merges 3D stereophotogrammetry and stereophotometry. The Canfield's Vectra scanners (Vectra H1, H2, XT, M3), static or portable, are considered valid and accurate clinical tools capable to capture accurate and reproducible images; even minor errors have been reported on the perioral region [60].

5.2.4 3D Facial Morphometry (3DFM)

Three-dimensional facial morphometry (3DFM) is a noninvasive system that can directly capture the soft tissues of a patient face having facial landmarks with reflective markers on it lightened up by an ultraviolet stroboscope. A two-side determination is applied to capture the whole face. Considered as a non-real "imaging system," 3DFM represents a system with two high-resolution infrared-sensitive video cameras, a hardware, and a software. The real-time hardware recognizes the markers, and the software reconstructs the landmarks' 3D coordinates relative to the reference system to calculate the 3D soft tissue measurements (linear, angular). Clinically, these data can add to the cephalometric measurements in analyzing the patient facial profile and facial skeleton [65, 66]. Ferrario et al. (1997) studied the growth and development of the nose using reflective landmarks on the soft tissue facial surface and using the 3DFM system [67]. This noninvasive system was used on young and non-patient subjects and provided real 3D

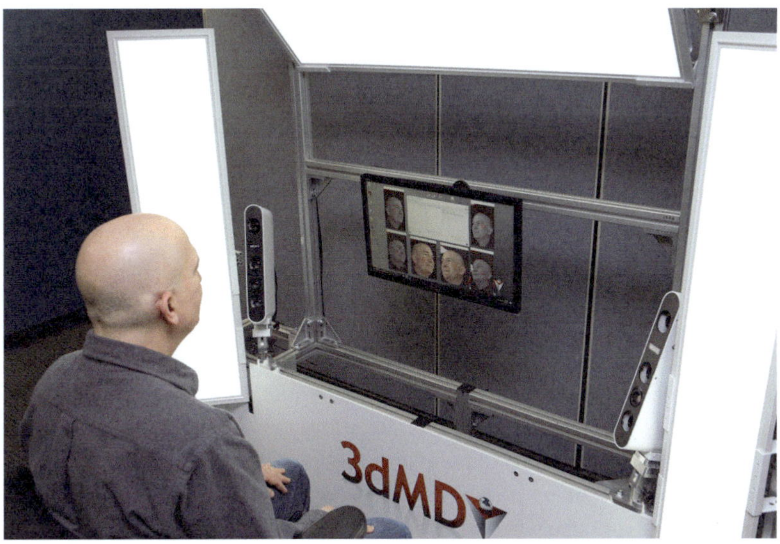

Fig. 5.3 Imaging acquisition with the 3dMDface system. (Courtesy of 3dMD LLC, Atlanta, GA, USA; with permission. ©2021 3dMD. All rights reserved)

data, independent of the head posture and projection error.

5.3 Advantages, Disadvantages, and Limitations of 3D Facial Scanning Methods

In general, all 3D optical facial scanning methods mentioned above (laser scanning, structured light projection, stereophotogrammetry, and 3D facial morphometry), when compare to the conventional techniques, have the advantages of being nonionizing, noninvasive, and noncontact (by eliminating compression, and any potential injuries during measurements); improve the safety without contamination, pain, or discomfort during acquisition; images can be frequently repeated as needed; being fast to collect 3D digital data of the facial morphology; being ease of the storage/archiving as a digital database; being ease of the visualization, simulation, communication clinicians-patients, and ease of the quantitative treatment assessment; of using advanced and reengineered computer-based software analysis to precisely and effectively collect, quantitatively assess and analyze 3D images and compare patients data for clinical and research purposes; and avoid the risk of data distortion, storage limitation and human mishandling. Furthermore, software programs are user-friendly due to the opportunities of zooming and rotation functions available. Each of the facial scanning methods (laser scanning, structured light projection, stereophotogrammetry, and 3D facial morphometry) has their advantages and disadvantages, which help clinicians to practically choose the most appropriate facial scanning system for their clinical research practice purposes (Table 5.1).

Laser scanning has the advantages of being high resolution and portable, but with disadvantage of not being able to clearly capture the difficult facial morphology around the nostrils, chin, and ears. Also, shadows may result in errors with a hampered 3D model scan if the subject may involuntarily move during acquisition such as in cases of noncompliant babies. Laser scanning requires long capture time and expensive equipment and is time-consuming. Especially in growing children, it must be kept in mind the risk of eye exposing to the laser beam [26, 30].

3D structured-light scanners can obtain the virtual patient with high speed and accuracy without radiation exposure using white light that is safe for the eyes [37]. Also, 3D structured-light scanners are cost-effective [40] and offer the advantage of easy operability and portability [38, 41] as used in long-term studies involving large population samples, especially children [39, 41]. However, when compared with the laser scanners, the resulting linear measurements of the structured light scanners have been shown to be relatively less accurate. Also, the inaccuracies of landmarks in the anteroposterior direction have shown to be greater; thus, the evaluation of the profile should be carefully to keep a proper head position to take an accurate image [43].

Stereophotogrammetry is a widely used method in plastic surgery and facial cosmetics for evaluation of volumes and distances for planning and follow-up [16] due to its high resolution, precision, and reproducibility for repeated measurements when compared to other imaging systems such as laser scanning [52]. Also, the digital stereophotogrammetry is easy to use and safe, can quickly capture (1.5 ms) the face's shape and texture being ideal to use in infants and children by decreasing the facial movement impact, and has a reported high accuracy (0.2–0.5 mm to identify landmarks and pre-labeled landmarks) in landmark recognition and wider facial soft tissue surface coverage (up to 360°) with high quality of facial surface data and information of texture. When compared with 3D laser scanning, the stereophotogrammetry has the ability to capture the color and texture of the face being not harmful for the patient's eyes avoiding motion artifacts in the orbital region caused by the blinking reflex. Ayaz et al. (2020) recommended 3D Vectra® H1 scanner as an accurate and reliable fixed 3D stereophotogrammetric system to evaluate the facial soft tissue morphology when compared to 2D imaging and laser scanning [31].

Main disadvantages of stereophotogrammetry that limit its popularity in clinical routine are the need to carefully control the condition of the

Table 5.1 Summary of the principles, advantages, and drawbacks of the different techniques available for 3D face scanning acquisition

Technology	Principle	Advantages	Disadvantages
Laser scanner	Laser beam steered across the face and reflected light detected	Nonionizing Noninvasive	Slow method/acquisition times (8–30 s)
	With a sensor (32)	High resolution	Distortion of the scanned image
			No texture/moderately photorealistic images
			Difficult landmark identification
			Costly
			Eye exposure issues,
			Especially in growing children Technicians and patients required to wear eye protection
Structured light scanner	Light pattern steered across the face whose distortion is recorded by	Nonionizing Noninvasive	Resolution varies between devices
	Cameras (21)	Textured image	
		Instantaneous acquisition	
		Relatively not costly	
Stereophotogrammetry	Multiple photographic images (49)	Nonionizing Noninvasive	Ears and submental region difficult to acquire
		Acquisition times (2 ms)	Stationary and complex system
		Ease of use	Continuous learning technical skills and update
		Photorealistic textured images	Costly
		High accuracy Avoid motion artifacts Coverage of the facial soft tissue of up to 360 degrees	
3D facial morphometry (3DFM)	Contour detection of reflective markers with infrared cameras (60)	Nonionizing Noninvasive	Time- and labor-consuming of face landmarks' placement
			Questionable reproducibility of landmark identification
			Change of facial expression between the two acquisitions
			Sessions increase the magnitude of error
			Two acquisition is usually needed to capture the whole face
			Produced no lifelike models
			Cannot be used as a 3D treatment-planning tool or media communication

lighting system during image acquisition, large footprint of the entire stereophotogrammetry equipment system which is static or relatively non-portable system with high-resolution multiple cameras, the large size of acquisition setting, increased cost, and requirements of a trained staff using the system software to analyze the images, together with frequent calibrations needed [53]. Also, to capture and analyze some special facial structures and regions such as the nostrils, ears, and chin known for their challenging 3D morphological features, it must be increased the number of cameras which may increase the investment cost. Another disadvantage is that the difficulty to prescribe the volume variations is due to the intervention or due to the growth in children and due to the edema in adults [54].

The disadvantages of static stereophotogrammetry equipment systems in any clinical settings such as the 3dMD system can be overcome by choosing portable stereophotogrammetry equipment system, which offers the ease of use, transfer, and storage with minimal training requirements [59]. However, research studies have concluded that if the scanning protocols are correctly followed, either stationary or portable 3D scanners offer the same range of accuracy without any significant clinical difference [68].

The computerized indirect anthropometry provided by 3DFM is less consuming than direct anthropometry, which is important in research with large number of subjects and in clinical settings with uncooperative patients. However, the 3DFM system has some disadvantages such as being time-consuming to place the facial landmarks, the marker dimension being a limiting factor of the number of landmarks collectable per unit of facial surface, the linear and angular measurements not being completely comparable to direct anthropometric measurements, a questionable repeatability of the facial landmark points, and finally being unable to produce models with displayed natural appearance and expression of the facial soft tissues. Therefore, the 3DFM system is not highly recommended for inter-clinicians or clinicians-patients communication and for orthodontic decision-making [67, 69, 70].

5.4 Craniofacial and Dental Uses of 3D Facial Scanning

Anthropometrical clinical assessment of craniofacial surface anatomy plays an important role for various dental specialists such as craniofacial and plastic surgeons, prosthodontists, and orthodontists to accurately diagnose the 3D soft tissue information, evaluate the growth, and plan craniofacial and plastic surgeries, dental rehabilitation, orthodontic treatment, and more sophisticated interdisciplinary treatments [29, 71, 72]. All the above can be achieved by using the 3D surface anthropometrical quantitative data combined with the hard tissue evaluation resulting in a 3D "virtual patient" to diagnose, evaluate preoperatively, plan the treatment, and further analyze the outcomes in long terms [73–75].

Nowadays, the ongoing advances in 3D surface imaging technology have improved the fast acquisition and ease of use of stereophotogrammetry, laser, and structured light methods. These noninvasive imaging modalities provide digital archives of the craniofacial surface data of patients and are becoming increasingly crucial, due to the improved accuracy and reliability. Noninvasive 3D facial scanning enables the collection of three-dimensional superficial data for indirect anthropometric assessments using computer graphics techniques to perform quantitative analysis and measurements of digital craniofacial face (angles, length, surface area, and volumes) and analyze morphological changes of the face [68]. Three-dimensional facial scanning continuously advancing allows a comprehensive analysis of the soft tissue with great importance in various field of medicine and dentistry such as in the following:

Anthropometry: Stereophotogrammetry has widely been used for clinical researches with healthy subjects to capture, define, quantify, and characterize the craniofacial human morphology of a certain population related to its development and normal growth [51, 76].

Craniofacial genetic research: Quantitative 3D facial imaging is an automated diagnostic tool for dysmorphic syndromes (syndrome-related facial shape variation) and facilitates the syndrome diagnosis related to dysmorphic craniofacial features to understand the aetiology of the craniofacial anomalies [77–79]. Also, it stimulates the use of facial phenotyping beyond clinical genetics and paediatrics craniofacial area to evaluate the growth of young children with and without craniofacial deformities, such as deformational plagiocephaly [80, 81].

Craniofacial syndromes and anomalies: Stereophotogrammetry and 3D soft tissue evaluation have been used to study and define the facial features of abnormal development and growth, identify the craniofacial features, plan the surgical repair, and evaluate the outcomes, for example, in patients with craniosynostosis [82] and cleft lip and/or palate (CL/P) [83, 84]. Stereophotogrammetry has also been helpful to study the facial movements and facial expression and further perform 3D surface and volumetric measurements for CLP infants [85, 86].

Facial reconstruction in forensic medicine: Forensic facial reconstruction is used to reconstruct the soft tissues onto the skull helping to obtain the image of an individual for his/her recognition and identification [87].

Orthodontics: Three-dimensional models of the face and facial soft tissue analysis are currently a reality with the recent ongoing development of 3D facial scanners, which are helpful tools for the orthodontic diagnosis, soft tissues comparisons before and after orthodontic treatment, and treatment outcomes evaluations in general [12, 19, 24, 36]. Optical laser scanning has been reported to accurately assess orthodontic treatment outcomes in extraction and non-extraction cases and to evaluate the functional treatment effects and changes on facial soft tissues [88, 89]. The facial soft tissue outcome of twin block treatment on Class II adolescents [90] and perioral facial movement characteristics of Class III patients with facial asymmetry had been accurately assessed using stereophotogrammetry [91]. Ferrario et al. (1999) applied the 3DFM technology in orthodontic and multidisciplinary dental researches [76]. Recently, the COVID-19 pandemic has widely influenced the use of 3D facial diagnosis in orthodontics with smartphones and 3D face-scanning apps promising a 3D face-scanning fast-expanding field [92].

Maxillofacial reconstructive and orthognathic surgery: Facial soft tissue changes and postoperative healing are crucial for evaluation of the success of orthognathic surgeries, where the resorption of postoperative edema remains a surgeons' concern. Three-dimensional facial imaging technologies help to objectively analyze the facial soft tissues in orthognathic patients and are a well-established protocol of virtual planning and follow-up [93]. Also, 3D imaging modalities are used to designate and construct individualized appliances, i.e., headgear, masks, respirators, custom-made cranial bands, and other medical devices [94, 95].

Plastic and facial cosmetic surgery: For the plastic surgeons, not only the 3D facial shape variations but also their visual elements dependent on the lighting or facial expressions do play a determinant role during planning the facial reconstructive surgery and succeeding the desired esthetic results [16, 72]. Also, plastic surgeons should pay attention not only to the physical but also to the visual variations of the shape that will change by the various projections of the light or facial expression [16, 72].

Facial recognition: Motion capture facial dynamics of human facial expression for facial behavior research, as represented by the 3dMD Face Dynamic Imaging System [96].

Human aging: Three-dimensional facial imaging technologies help to objectively analyze the facial soft tissues and evaluate the facial morphology and facial expression while aging [61, 97].

Human face sexual dimorphism: Stereophotogrammetry and 3D facial images have been used to categorize faces by sex [98, 99].

Dentistry in general: Extraoral 3D facial scans taken by non-static 3D facial scanners with mobile phone usage on the rise [100], and traditional static 3D facial scanners [101] assist general dentists, prosthodontists and implantologists in diagnosing, planning, designing and digitally visualising the patient's oral rehabilitation, especially of the aesthetic zone and his future smile. Also, 3D facial scanning serves as an important patient communication and education tool [100, 101].

5.5 Summary and Future Perspectives

The noninvasive facial scanning systems and the continuous development of their software programs enable precise and reliable analysis of the 3D craniofacial surface data. With current options for 3D noninvasive facial scanning, after careful balancing of strengths and weaknesses when compared by functionality, and being available at significantly different prices, the decision of choosing the right scanning technology depends on the requirements of the clinicians' specific applications. Three-dimensional noninvasive facial scanning systems should be a realistic and accurate solution to be used for craniofacial and dental purposes.

The emerging importance of telemedicine and tele-dentistry due to pandemic area is influencing the advancement in 3D technology and image analysis, with continuous speedy innovations in 3D that indirectly lowers their cost, all resulting toward a facilitated access of clinicians and patients to smartphones and 3D facial photogrammetry with improvements in their clinical decisions [68, 92]. Also, the recent integration of artificial intelligence (AI) based strategies in technological advancements offers future opportunities to improve and alleviate the 3D facial scanning systems toward a more individualized and anticipating diagnosis, treatment planning, and outcomes assessments [102, 103]. Further, the combined use of smartphones with AI is becoming the future practice of 3D facial scanning in medicine and dentistry [104], which has to be assessed by future studies and researches on this topic that may generate for sure interesting academic debates.

References

1. Sforza C, de Menezes M, Ferrario V. Soft- and hard-tissue facial anthropometry in three dimensions: what's new. J Anthropol Sci. 2013;91:159–84.
2. Lewyllie A, Cadenas De Llano-Pérula M, Verdonck A, Willems G. Three-dimensional imaging of soft and hard facial tissues in patients with craniofacial syndromes: a systematic review of methodological quality. Dentomaxillofac Radiol. 2018;47(3):20170154.
3. Jyothikiran H, Shanthara JR, Subbiah P, Thomas M. Craniofacial imaging in orthodontics—past present and future. Int J Orthod Milwaukee. 2014;25(1):21–6.
4. Ucar FI, Sekerci AE, Uysal T, Bengi AO. Standardization of records in orthodontics. Part 2: craniofacial imaging techniques. Turkish. J Orthod. 2012;25:167–87.
5. Da Silveira AC, Martinez O, Da Silveira D, Daw JL Jr, Cohen M. Three-dimensional technology for documentation and record keeping for patients with facial clefts. Clin Plast Surg. 2004;31(2):141–8.
6. Oberoi S, Nervina JM, Vargervik K. 3D imaging in diagnosis and treatment planning of craniofacial anomalies. Cone Beam Computed Tomography in Orthodontics: Indications, Insights, and Innovations. Wiley-Blackwell. 2014:485–508. https://doi.org/10.1002/9781118674888.ch23.
7. Holberg C, Schwenzer K, Mahaini L, Rudzki-Janson I. Accuracy of facial plaster casts. Angle Orthod. 2006;76(4):605–11.
8. Zogheib T, Jacobs R, Bornstein MM, et al. Comparison of 3D scanning versus 2D photography for the identification of facial soft-tissue landmarks. Open Dent J. 2018;12:61–71.
9. Bártolo PJ, et al. New challenges for reverse engineering in facial treatments: how can the new 3-D non-invasive surface measurements support diagnosis and treatment? London: Taylor & Francis Group; 2010.
10. Ireland AJ, McNamara C, Clover MJ, et al. 3D surface imaging in dentistry—what we are looking at. Br Dent J. 2008;205(7):387–92.
11. Karatas OH, Toy E. Three-dimensional imaging techniques: a literature review. Eur J Dent. 2014;8(1):132–40.
12. Hajeer MY, Millett DT, Ayoub AF, Siebert JP. Applications of 3D imaging in orthodontics: part I. J Orthod. 2004;31(1):62–70.
13. Hajeer MY, Millett DT, Ayoub AF, Siebert JP. Applications of 3D imaging in orthodontics: part II. J Orthod. 2004;31(2):154–62.
14. Quinzi V, Polizzi A, Ronsivalle V, Santonocito S, Conforte C, Manenti RJ, Isola G, Lo Giudice A. Facial scanning accuracy with stereophotogrammetry and smartphone technology in children: a systematic review. Children (Basel). 2022;9(9):1390.

15. Kim YJ, Jha N, Gupta S, Zvirin A, Qendro A, Zere E, Sokhi RK, KS N, Chaudhari PK. Principles and applications of various 3D scanning methods for image acquisition for 3D printing applications in oral health science. In: Chaudhari PK, Bhatia D, Sharan J, editors. 3D printing in oral health science. Cham: Springer; 2022. https://doi.org/10.1007/978-3-031-07369-4_2.
16. Lekakis G, Claes P, Hamilton G, Hellings P. Three-dimensional surface imaging and the continuous evolution of preoperative and postoperative assessment in rhinoplasty. Facial Plast Surg. 2016;32(1):088–94.
17. Sforza C, Dellavia C, De Menezes M, Rosati R, Ferrario VF. Three-dimensional facial morphometry: from anthropometry to digital morphology. In: Preedy V, editor. Handbook of anthropometry. New York, NY: Springer; 2012. https://doi.org/10.1007/978-1-4419-1788-1_32.
18. Gibelli D, Cappella A, Dolci C, Sforza C. 3D surface acquisition systems and their applications to facial anatomy: let's make a point. Ital J Anat Embryol. 2020;124(3):422–31.
19. Lane C, Harrell W Jr. Completing the 3-dimensional picture. Am J Orthod Dentofacial Orthop. 2008;133(4):612–20.
20. Gibelli D, Dolci C, Cappella A, Sforza C. Reliability of optical devices for three-dimensional facial anatomy description: a systematic review and meta-analysis. Int J Oral Maxillofac Surg. 2020;49(8):1092–106.
21. Ye H, Lv L, Liu Y, Liu Y, Zhou Y. Evaluation of the accuracy, reliability, and reproducibility of two different 3D face-scanning systems. Int J Prosthodont. 2016;29(3):213–8.
22. Amornvit P, Sanohkan S. The accuracy of digital face scans obtained from 3D scanners: an in vitro study. Int J Environ Res Public Health. 2019;16(24):5061.
23. Galantucci LM, Percoco G, Lavecchia F, Di Gioia E. Noninvasive computerized scanning method for the correlation between the facial soft and hard tissues for an integrated three-dimensional anthropometry and cephalometry. J Craniofac Surg. 2013;24(3):797–804.
24. Kusnoto B, Evans CA. Reliability of a 3D surface laser scanner for orthodontic applications. Am J Orthod Dentofacial Orthop. 2002;122:342–8.
25. Marmulla R, Hassfeld S, Luth T, Muhling J. Laser-scan-based navigation in cranio-maxillofacial surgery. J Craniomaxillofac Surg. 2003;31:267–77.
26. Majid Z, Chong AK, Ahmad AB, Setan H, Samsudin AR. Photogrammetry and 3D laser scanning as spatial data capture techniques for a national craniofacial database. Photogramm Rec. 2005;20(109):48–68.
27. Kau CH, Richmond S, Zhurov AI, Knox J, Chestnutt I, Hartles F, et al. Reliability of measuring facial morphology with a 3-dimensional laser scanning system. Am J Orthod Dentofacial Orthop. 2005;128:424–30.
28. Kovacs L, Zimmermann A, Brockmann G, Baurecht H, Schwenzer-Zimmerer K, Papadopulos NA, et al. Accuracy and precision of the three-dimensional assessment of the facial surface using a 3-Dlaser scanner. IEEE Trans Med Imaging. 2006;25:742–54.
29. Baik HS, Lee HJ, Lee KJ. A proposal for soft tissue landmarks for craniofacial analysis using 3-dimensional laser scan imaging. World J Orthod. 2006;7(1):7–14.
30. Schwenzer-Zimmerer K, Chaitidis D, Berg-Boerner I, Krol Z, Kovacs L, Schwenzer NF, Zimmerer S, Holberg C, Zeilhofer HF. Quantitative 3D soft tissue analysis of symmetry prior to and after unilateral cleft lip repair compared with non-cleft persons (performed in Cambodia). J Craniomaxillofac Surg. 2008;36(8):431–8.
31. Ayaz I, Shaheen E, Aly M, Shujaat S, Gallo G, Coucke W, Politis C, Jacobs R. Accuracy and reliability of 2-dimensional photography versus 3-dimensional soft tissue imaging. Imaging Sci Dent. 2020;50(1):15–22.
32. Galantucci LM. New challenges for reverse engineering in facial treatments: how can the new 3D non-invasive surface measures support diagnoses and cures? Virtual Phys Prototyp. 2010;5(1):3–12.
33. Germec-Cakan D, Canter HI, Nur B, Arun T. Comparison of facial soft tissue measurements on three-dimensional images and models obtained with different methods. J Craniofac Surg. 2010;21(5):1393–9.
34. Tzou CH, Artner NM, Pona I, Hold A, Placheta E, Kropatsch WG, Frey M. Comparison of three-dimensional surface-imaging systems. J Plast Reconstr Aesthet Surg. 2014;67(4):489–97.
35. Gibelli D, Pucciarelli V, Poppa P, Cummaudo M, Dolci C, Cattaneo C, Sforza C. Three-dimensional facial anatomy evaluation: reliability of laser scanner consecutive scans procedure in comparison with stereophotogrammetry. J Craniomaxillofac Surg. 2018;46(10):1807–13.
36. Erten O, Yılmaz BN. Three-dimensional imaging in orthodontics. Turk J Orthod. 2018;31(3):86–94.
37. Jason GJ. Structured-light 3D surface imaging: a tutorial. Adv Opt Photon. 2011;3:128–60.
38. Amirav I, Masumbuko CK, Hawkes MT, et al. 3D analysis of child facial dimensions for design of medical devices in low-middle income countries (LMIC). PLoS One. 2019;14(5):e0216548.
39. Yuan B, Jiang X, Liu Y, Dong J, Li D. Three-dimensional periorbital asymmetry assessment of congenital microphthalmia children with a structured light 3D scanning system. J Craniomaxillofac Surg. 2021;49(3):206–14.
40. Bakirman T, Gumusay MU, Reis HC, Selbesoglu MO, Yosmaoglu S, Yaras MC, Seker DZ, Bayram B. Comparison of low cost 3D structured light scanners for face modeling. Appl Opt. 2017;56(4):985–92.
41. Ma L, Xu T, Lin J. Validation of a three-dimensional facial scanning system based on structured light techniques. Comput Methods Prog Biomed. 2009;94(3):290–8.

42. Özsoy U, Sekerci R, Hizay A, Yildirim Y, Uysal H. Assessment of reproducibility and reliability of facial expressions using 3D handheld scanner. J Craniomaxillofac Surg. 2019;47(6):895–901.
43. Oh SH, Park JS, Ryu JJ, Song IS, Jung SK. Three-dimensional reproducibility of the soft tissue landmarks taken by structured-light facial scanner in accordance with the head position change. Healthcare (Basel). 2021;9(4):428.
44. Zhao YJ, Xiong YX, Wang Y. Three-dimensional accuracy of facial scan for facial deformities in clinics: a new evaluation method for facial scanner accuracy. PLoS One. 2017;12(1):e0169402.
45. Ahn HW, Chang YJ, Kim KA, Joo SH, Park YG, Park KH. Measurement of three-dimensional perioral soft tissue changes in dentoalveolar protrusion patients after orthodontic treatment using a structured light scanner. Angle Orthod. 2014;84(5):795–802.
46. Modabber A, Peters F, Kniha K, et al. Evaluation of the accuracy of a mobile and a stationary system for three-dimensional facial scanning. J Craniomaxillofac Surg. 2016;44(10):1719–24.
47. Alkhayer A, Becsei R, Hegedűs L, et al. Evaluation of the soft tissue changes after rapid maxillary expansion using a handheld three-dimensional scanner: a prospective study. Int J Environ Res Public Health. 2021;18(7):3379.
48. Koban KC, Perko P, Etzel L, Li Z, Schenck TL, Giunta RE. Validation of two handheld devices against a non-portable three-dimensional surface scanner and assessment of potential use for intraoperative facial imaging. J Plast Reconstr Aesthet Surg. 2020;73(1):141–8.
49. Ras F, Habets LL, van Ginkel FC, Prahl-Andersen B. Quantification of facial morphology using stereophotogrammetry—demonstration of a new concept. J Dent. 1996;24(5):369–74.
50. Miranda RE, Matayoshi S, JI B, Mijoshi LH. Use of stereophotogrammetry for measuring the volume of external facial anatomy: a systematic review. Rev Brasil Cirurgia. 2018;33(4):572–9.
51. Heike CL, Upson K, Stuhaug E, Weinberg SM. 3D digital stereophotogrammetry: a practical guide to facial image acquisition. Head Face Med. 2010;6:18.
52. Weinberg SM, Naidoo S, Govier DP, Martin RA, Kane AA, Marazita ML. Anthropometric precision and accuracy of digital three-dimensional photogrammetry: comparing the Genex and 3dMD imaging systems with one another and with direct anthropometry. J Craniofac Surg. 2006;17(3):477–83.
53. D'Ettorre G, Farronato M, Candida E, Quinzi V, Grippaudo C. A comparison between stereophotogrammetry and smartphone structured light technology for three-dimensional face scanning. Angle Orthod. 2022;92(3):358–63.
54. Miranda RE, Matayoshi S, Brabo JL, Miyoshi LH. Use of stereophotogrammetry or measuring the volume of external facial anatomy: a systematic review. Rev Bras Cir Plast. 2018;33(4):572–9.
55. Naini FB, Akram S, Kepinska J, Garagiola U, McDonald F, Wertheim D. Validation of a new three-dimensional imaging system using comparative craniofacial anthropometry. Maxillofac Plast Reconstr Surg. 2017;39(1):23.
56. Liu C, Artopoulos A. Validation of a low-cost portable 3-dimensional face scanner. Imaging Sci Dent. 2019;49(1):35–43.
57. Khambay B, Nairn N, Bell A, Miller J, Bowman A, Ayoub AF. Validation and reproducibility of a high-resolution three-dimensional facial imaging system. Br J Oral Maxillofac Surg. 2008;46(1):27–32.
58. Camison L, Bykowski M, Lee WW, Carlson JC, Roosenboom J, Goldstein JA, Losee JE, Weinberg SM. Validation of the Vectra H1 portable three-dimensional photogrammetry system for facial imaging. Int J Oral Maxillofac Surg. 2018;47(3):403–10.
59. Gibelli D, Pucciarelli V, Cappella A, Dolci C, Sforza C. Are portable stereophotogrammetric devices reliable in facial imaging? A validation study of VECTRA H1 device. J Oral Maxillofac Surg. 2018;76(8):1772–84.
60. De Stefani A, Barone M, Hatami Alamdari S, Barjami A, Baciliero U, Apolloni F, Gracco A, Bruno G. Validation of Vectra 3D imaging systems: a review. Int J Environ Res Public Health. 2022;19(14):8820.
61. Velemínská J, Jaklová LK, Kočandrlová K, Hoffmannová E, Koudelová J, Suchá B, Dupej J. Three-dimensional analysis of modeled facial aging and sexual dimorphism from juvenile to elderly age. Sci Rep. 2022;12(1):21821.
62. Petrides G, Clark JR, Low H, Lovell N, Eviston TJ. Three-dimensional scanners for soft-tissue facial assessment in clinical practice. J Plast Reconstr Aesthet Surg. 2021;74(3):605–14.
63. Quinzi V, Polizzi A, Ronsivalle V, Santonocito S, Conforte C, Manenti RJ, Isola G, Lo Giudice A. Facial scanning accuracy with stereophotogrammetry and smartphone technology in children: a systematic review. Children. 2022;9(9):1390.
64. Nord F, Ferjencik R, Seifert B, et al. The 3dMD photogrammetric photo system in cranio-maxillofacial surgery: validation of interexaminer variations and perceptions. J Craniomaxillofac Surg. 2015;43(9):1798–803.
65. Ferrario VF, Sforza C, Poggio CE, Tartaglia G. Distance from symmetry: a three-dimensional evaluation of facial asymmetry. J Oral Maxillofac Surg. 1994;52(11):1126–32.
66. Ferrario VF, Sforza C, Poggio CE, Serrao G. Facial three-dimensional morphometry. Am J Orthod Dentofacial Orthop. 1996;109(1):86–93.
67. Ferrario VF, Sforza C, Poggio CE, Schmitz JH. Three-dimensional study of growth and development of the nose. Cleft Palate Craniofac J. 1997;34(4):309–17.
68. Shujaat S, Bornstein MM, Price JB, Jacobs R. Integration of imaging modalities in digital dental workflows - possibilities, limitations, and poten-

tial future developments. Dentomaxillofac Radiol. 2021;50(7):20210268.
69. de Menezes M, Rosati R, Allievi C, Sforza C. A photographic system for the three-dimensional study of facial morphology. Angle Orthod. 2009;79(6):1070–7. https://doi.org/10.2319/111008-570.
70. Jayaratne YSN, Zwahlen RA, Lo J, Cheung LK. Three-dimensional color maps: a novel tool for assessing craniofacial changes. Surg Innov. 2010;17(3):198–205.
71. Maal TJ, Verhamme LM, van Loon B, Plooij JM, Rangel FA, Kho A, Bronkhorst EM, Bergé SJ. Variation of the face in rest using 3D stereophotogrammetry. Int J Oral Maxillofac Surg. 2011;40(11):1252–7.
72. Chang JB, Small KH, Choi M, Karp NS. Three-dimensional surface imaging in plastic surgery: foundation, practical applications, and beyond. Plast Reconstr Surg. 2015;135:1295–304.
73. Rasteau S, Sigaux N, Louvrier A, Bouletreau P. Three-dimensional acquisition technologies for facial soft tissues - applications and prospects in orthognathic surgery. J Stomatol Oral Maxillofac Surg. 2020;121(6):721–8.
74. Joda T, Brägger U, Gallucci G. Systematic literature review of digital three-dimensional superimposition techniques to create virtual dental patients. Int J Oral Maxillofac Implants. 2015;30:330–7.
75. Pérez-Giugovaz MG, Park SH, Revilla-León M. Three-dimensional virtual representation by superimposing facial and intraoral digital scans with an additively manufactured intraoral scan body. J Prosthet Dent. 2021;126(4):459–63.
76. Ferrario VF, Sforza C, Poggio CE, Schmitz JH. Soft-tissue facial morphometry from 6 years to adulthood: a three dimensional growth study using a new modeling. Plast Reconstr Surg. 1999;103:768–78.
77. Hammond P, Suttie M. Large-scale objective phenotyping of 3D facial morphology. Hum Mutat. 2012;33(5):817–25.
78. Richmond S, Howe LJ, Lewis S, Stergiakouli E, Zhurov A. Facial genetics: a brief overview. Front Genet. 2018;9:462.
79. Hallgrímsson B, Aponte JD, Katz DC, et al. Automated syndrome diagnosis by three-dimensional facial imaging. Genet Med. 2020;22(10):1682–93.
80. Kato R, Nagano N, Hashimoto S, Saito K, Miyabayashi H, Noto T, Morioka I. Three-dimensional versus two-dimensional evaluations of cranial asymmetry in deformational plagiocephaly using a three-dimensional scanner. Children (Basel). 2022;9(6):788.
81. Miyabayashi H, Nagano N, Kato R, Noto T, Hashimoto S, Saito K, Morioka I. Cranial shape in infants aged one month can predict the severity of deformational plagiocephaly at the age of six months. J Clin Med. 2022;11(7):1797.
82. Abdel-Alim T, Iping R, Wolvius EB, Mathijssen IMJ, Dirven CMF, Niessen WJ, van Veelen MC, Roshchupkin GV. Three-dimensional stereophotogrammetry in the evaluation of craniosynostosis: current and potential use cases. J Craniofac Surg. 2021;32(3):956–63.
83. McCance AM, Moss JP, Fright WR, Linney AD, James DR. Three-dimensional analysis techniques—part 1: three dimensional soft-tissue analysis of 24 adult cleft palate patients following Le Fort I maxillary advancement: a preliminary report. Cleft Palate Craniofac J. 1997;34:36–45.
84. Alpagan Ozdemir S, Esenlik E. Three-dimensional soft-tissue evaluation in patients with cleft lip and palate. Med Sci Monit. 2018;24:8608–20.
85. Brons S, Darroudi A, Nada R, Bronkhorst EM, Vreeken R, Berge SJ, Maal T, Kuijpers-Jagtman AM. Influence of involuntary facial expressions on reproducibility of 3D stereophotogrammetry in children with and without complete unilateral cleft lip and palate from 3 to 18 months of age. Clin Oral Investig. 2019;23(3):1041–50.
86. Hermann NV, Darvann TA, Larsen P, Lindholm P, Andersen M, Kreiborg S. A pilot study on the influence of facial expression on measurements in three-dimensional digital surfaces of the face in infants with cleft lip and palate. Cleft Palate Craniofac J. 2016;53(1):3–15.
87. Gupta S, Gupta V, Vij H, Vij R, Tyagi N. Forensic facial reconstruction: the final frontier. J Clin Diagn Res. 2015;9(9):ZE26–8.
88. Morris DO, Illing HM, Lee RT. A prospective evaluation of bass, bionator and twin block appliances. Part II—the soft tissues. Eur J Orthod. 1998;20(663–84):30.
89. Ismail SF, Moss JP, Hennessy R. Three-dimensional assessment of the effects of extraction and nonextraction orthodontic treatment on the face. Am J Orthod Dentofacial Orthop. 2002;121:244–56.
90. Bourne CO, Kerr WJ, Ayoub AF. Development of a three-dimensional imaging system for analysis of facial change. Clin Orthod Res. 2001;4(2):105–11.
91. Xue Z, Wu L, Qiu T, Li Z, Wang X, Liu X. Three-dimensional dynamic analysis of the facial movement symmetry of skeletal class III patients with facial asymmetry. J Oral Maxillofac Surg. 2020;78(2):267–74.
92. Thurzo A, Strunga M, Havlínová R, Reháková K, Urban R, Surovková J, Kurilová V. Smartphone-based facial scanning as a viable tool for facially driven orthodontics? Sensors (Basel). 2022;22(20):7752.
93. Reategui A, Phillips S, Dinis J, Junn A, Parsaei Y, Yang J, Lopez J, Steinbacher DM. Postoperative edema resolution post-orthognathic triple jaw surgery: a three-dimensional volumetric analysis. J Craniofac Surg. 2022;33(2):512–6.
94. Geoffroy M, Gardan J, Goodnough J, Mattie J. Cranial remodeling orthosis for infantile plagiocephaly created through a 3D scan, topological optimization, and 3D printing process. J Prosthet Orthot. 2018;30(4):247–58.

95. Franchi L, Vichi A, Marti P, Lampus F, Guercio S, Recupero A, Giuntini V, Goracci C. 3D printed customized facemask for maxillary protraction in the early treatment of a class III malocclusion: proof-of-concept clinical case. Materials (Basel). 2022;15(11):3747.
96. Yin L, Wei X, Sun Y, Wang J, Rosato MJ. A 3D facial expression database for facial behavior research. 7th International Conference on Automatic Face and Gesture Recognition (FGR06). 2006:211–216.
97. Lambros V, Amos G. Three-dimensional facial averaging: a tool for understanding facial aging. Plast Reconstr Surg. 2016;138(6):980e–2e.
98. Tanikawa C, Zere E, Takada K. Sexual dimorphism in the facial morphology of adult humans: a three-dimensional analysis. Homo. 2016;67(1):23–49.
99. Tanikawa C, Akcam MO, Gokalp H, Zere E, Takada K. Population affinity and variation of sexual dimorphism in three-dimensional facial forms: comparisons between Turkish and Japanese populations. Sci Rep. 2021;11(1):16634.
100. Daher R, Ardu S, Vjero O, Krejci I. 3D digital smile design with a Mobile phone and intraoral optical scanner. Compend Contin Educ Dent. 2018;39(6):e5–8.
101. Bynum JH, Mirelez JA. 3D facial scanning: dual-arch fixed prostheses from diagnosis to delivery. Compend Contin Educ Dent. 2021;42(5):230–5.
102. Jreige CS, Kimura RN, Segundo ÂRTC, Coachman C, Sesma N. Esthetic treatment planning with digital animation of the smile dynamics: a technique to create a 4-dimensional virtual patient. J Prosthet Dent. 2022;128(2):130–8.
103. Bouletreau P, Makaremi M, Ibrahim B, Louvrier A, Sigaux N. Artificial intelligence: applications in orthognathic surgery. J Stomatol Oral Maxillofac Surg. 2019;120(4):347–54.
104. Hung K, Yeung AWK, Tanaka R, Bornstein MM. Current applications, opportunities, and limitations of AI for 3D imaging in dental research and practice. Int J Environ Res Public Health. 2020;17(12):4424.

6 Nonionizing, Noninvasive Surface Imaging (Desktop and Intraoral Scanning) for Dentoalveolar Applications

Srirengalakshmi Muthuswamy Pandian, Q. Tabassum, and Prabhat Kumar Chaudhari

6.1 Introduction

Digital technology has transformed the oral health sector. The diagnosis and treatment planning have shifted from a conventional 2D planning to a 3D paradigm. Advancements in technology have reduced the dependence on paper, radiation, and dental casts in oral health practices. The implementation of digital scanners and additive manufacturing, along with the advancement of computer-aided design (CAD) and computer-aided manufacturing (CAM), has enhanced the precision, productivity, and predictability of treatment results [1]. Digitized models acquired via scanners serve for efficient recordkeeping, patient education, data exchange among experts to enhance communication, and the creation of personalized appliances such as aligners [2].

S. M. Pandian
Department of Orthodontics, Saveetha Dental College, Saveetha Institute of Medical and Technical Sciences, Saveetha University, Chennai, Tamil Nadu, India

Q. Tabassum
Department of Orthodontics, Faculty of Dentistry, Jamia Millia Islamia, Jamia Nagar, New Delhi, India

P. K. Chaudhari (✉)
Division of Orthodontics and Dentofacial Deformities, Centre for Dental Education and Research (CDER), All India Institute of Medical Sciences, New Delhi, Delhi, India

The utilization of CAD-CAM technology in oral health comprises three distinct phases: (1) data acquisition using scanners for both surface and bony data, (2) computer-aided design using various CAD software, and (3) manufacturing using 3D printing or milling. This chapter concentrates on obtaining surface data of dentoalveolar tissue with desktop and intraoral scanners.

6.2 Brief History

The concept of impression-taking was started in the eighteenth century. In 1856, Dr. Charles used impressions for constructing the oral prosthesis [3, 4]. The impression material used during that period had inherent problems of distortion and was difficult to use [5]. In 1937, elastic impression materials were introduced into dentistry. Agar was the first impression material used during crown preparation which was introduced by Sears [6]. The first elastomeric polyether material "Impregum" was introduced in 1965 [7]. Subsequently, condensation silicon was introduced, but the problem of dimensional stability and accuracy was seen in the impression. Later, the introduction of additional silicone vinyl polysiloxane impression material solved the problem of dimensional inaccuracy, odor, and poor taste. The impression material exhibited outstanding rip strength and a high modulus of elasticity [8].

S. S. Rana et al. (eds.), *Applications of Three-dimensional Imaging for Craniofacial Region*,
https://doi.org/10.1007/978-981-97-4608-8_6

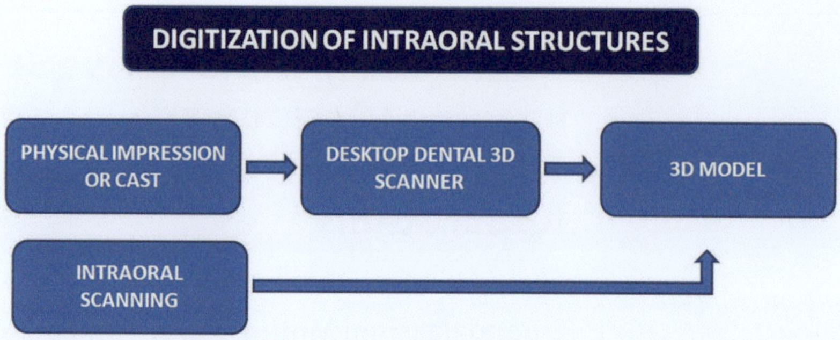

Fig. 6.1 Digitization of intraoral structures

The concept of CAD-CAM was first introduced in the year 1973 by Dr. Francois Duret in France for dental purposes [9, 10]. In 1987, the prototype device was introduced by the Sirona dental system in restorative dentistry for digital impressions which was known as CEREC (Chairside Economical Restoration for Esthetic Ceramics) [11]. The CEREC system was considered a pioneer of the CAD-CAM technique. The CEREC system was developed by Dr. Werner Moermann in Switzerland. Sirona Dental System 2 is another name for the CEREC system which is known today. After the introduction of CEREC 1, the CEREC 2, CEREC 3, and CEREC 3D were introduced in 1994, 2000, and 2003, respectively.

In 2006, the Lava chairside scanner system was introduced which was acquired by the 3M ESPE system. In the same year, Cadent launched the first iTero digital impression [12]. By 2008, it was announced that the iTero system was capable of full arch scanning [13]. Cadent launched the iTero system for users at the end of 2009. In 2011, Align Technology acquired Cadent and iTero for data transmission for aligner therapy. Simultaneously, it allowed the clinicians to submit the 3D scan for the Invisalign appliance therapy. At the end of 2012, a True definition scanner was introduced by 3M ESPE and enabled the orthodontist to submit 3D scans for custom lingual braces, Incognito system. Later Lythos digital impression system and clear guide system were introduced by Ormco in the same year [14]. In 2014, True definition scanners were permitted to be used for sending 3D impressions for Invisalign case submission and iTero scans for Incognito appliance systems. An international dental show was conducted in Cologne in the year 2017, where more than 14 scanners were demonstrated [15]. Despite the growing demand and popularity of intraoral scanners, there is always a question regarding applications and the differences among manufacturers.

Digitizing intraoral structures can be done in two ways: direct intraoral digitization and indirect digitization using desktop scanners (Fig. 6.1). Both the scanners are discussed below.

6.3 Desktop Scanners

Desktop scanners or dental lab scanners are commonly used for scanning dental impressions and models. This enables obtaining a digitized model that can be further processed. Desktop scanners commonly utilize structured light technology by displaying a series of patterns on the dental model's surface. The patterns are captured by one or more cameras to analyze the geometry of the part. Some scanners use lasers instead of structured light, but they operate on the same principle: the laser line appears distorted on surface details, and sensors analyze the lines to determine the geometry of the object. Most desktop dental 3D scanners can scan dental models, including whole arches and dies. The latest generation of scanners can capture negative dental impressions.

Desktop scanners can scan impressions, full arch models, dies, articulators, implants, and abutments.

Table 6.1 Commercially available desktop scanners

Scanner	Company	Technology	Accuracy	Cost
E40	3Shape	Blue light technology	4 µm	$26,000
Ceramill Map 200+	AmannGirrbach	White light technology	6 µm	$22,000
CS. Neo Pro	CADstar	White light technology	5 µm	19,000
7series	Dental Wings	Single laser line	15 µm	$20,000
inEos X5	Dentsply Sirona	Blue light technology	2.1 µm	$15,000
DScan 3	EG Solutions	Blue light technology	15 µm	$15,000
T500	Medit	Blue light technology	7 µm	$12,000
MDS500	Maestro	White light technology	8 µm	$12,000

6.3.1 Factors to Be Considered While Selecting a Desktop Scanner

(a) Technology used for the scanner: Several desktop scanners employ structured light technology, with blue light being the preferred option over white light. Laser line technology operates similarly but could have a slower pace.
(b) Scanner accuracy: 4–15 µm are recommended. Machines having ISO 12836 certification have undergone standardized testing to determine their level of accuracy.
(c) Resolution: Resolution up to 5 megapixels is acceptable.
(d) Speed: Many 3D scanners specify their speed based on the duration required to scan a complete arch model. Nevertheless, this could not be a dependable measure of productivity as software processing durations could exceed scanning durations. An ideal timeframe for full arch scanning is between 9 s and under 1 min.
(e) Software: Some scanners are compatible solely with included proprietary software, while others are compatible with third-party software such as Exocad.
(f) Output: STL, OBJ, and PLY are preferred. Scanners and software typically enable users to export files in standard formats suitable for 3D printing and milling.

A detailed comparison of the commercially available desktop scanners is given below (Table 6.1).

6.4 Intraoral Scanners

Intraoral scanners are used to directly digitize intraoral structures. Unlike desktop scanners, intraoral scanners can be used chairside. Intraoral scanners are a digital alternative to physical impressions. Details of the intraoral scanners are discussed below under the following headings:

- Physical Impression vs. Digital Impression
- The Technology Behind Intraoral Scanners
- In Vitro vs. In Vivo
- Factors to Be Considered While Procuring a Scanner
- Comparison of Commercially Available Scanners

6.4.1 Physical Impression vs. Digital Impression

Physical impressions in dentistry have been a mainstay in replicating the intraoral structures for a long time. They were used for a variety of purposes which include study models and fabrication of an appliance. In the last decade, intraoral scanning as a means to replicate oral structures is gaining popularity. One of the reasons for this transition is the greater efficiency and accuracy of the intraoral scans. It also helps in reducing the armamentarium required, the waste produced, and the overall cost incurred [15]. Considering the shift toward digital planning and appliance manufacture, intraoral scans are an ally in producing 3D stereolithographic models which are used in computerized designing and manufacturing.

Numerous literatures are available that compare physical and digital impressions in dental practice. Based on the studies, digital impressions produce less discomfort to the patients, whereas physical impression can cause gag reflex and discomfort in the patient due to the unpleasant taste and smell of the impression material [16]. However, digital impressions with intraoral scanners also can cause gag reflex if the wand size is large and is difficult in patients with limited mouth opening. Yilmaz et al. observed that youngsters found the digital impression approach more pleasant than the conventional method. Nevertheless, they observed no disparity in the time required to record the impression between the two approaches [17]. Anatomic details, particularly of the soft tissues, are more accurately captured in digital impressions compared to traditional impressions. It is also feasible to document the color for shade selection and for documenting clinical findings [18]. Recorded impressions can be quickly examined for flaws using rapid zoom features and corrected without having to redo the entire process, unlike actual impressions. Digital impressions are not affected by dimensional changes seen in physical impressions [15]. Physical impressions require storage space and have a risk of damage on long-term storage. Digital archiving saves space, but adequate storage backup is required to prevent loss of information. 3D-printed resin models are stronger and more resistant to damage and wear than stone models [19, 20]. Digital impression models have an advantage over physical models in terms of customization and simple reorder procedures for lost/damaged appliances and prostheses. Despite the advantages, digital impressions have some disadvantages. The high cost of the scanners and their maintenance and upgrade are important disadvantages. Due to the limited number of units that can be procured in a clinic, multiple patients cannot be scanned simultaneously. A systematic review and meta-analysis compared the accuracy of digital and physical impressions for implant prostheses. They found the digital impressions to have comparable 3D accuracy for partial and full mouth implant rehabilitation [21]. Digital impressions are also a powerful tool for patient communication, marketing, and communicating with the dental technician and the laboratory [22].

6.4.2 The Technology Behind Intraoral Scanners

Multiple brands of intraoral scanners are now on the market. Regardless of brand, the primary goal of an intraoral scanner is to precisely capture an object's 3D geometry by projecting light onto the object for scanning [23, 24]. The point clouds are created by processing the images that the imaging sensors take with scanning software. The software then triangulates these point clouds to create a virtual 3D surface model [25]. The primary factor affecting the scanner's performance is the image-acquiring technology and storage. The popular technologies include the following:

6.4.2.1 Optical Triangulation

Optical triangulation accurately calculates the distance to objects without physical contact, with precision ranging from a few millimeters to a few microns [26]. Optical triangulation involves three key points: the laser emitter, the sensor, and the object surface. The position of a point on a triangle can be determined by employing the locations and angles of two reference points. The scanner illuminates the object with a pattern of light stripes. The distance between the projected ray and the reflected ray is measured during the reflection of each light ray. The object's distance can be determined using the Pythagorean theorem, given that the fixed angle between the projector and sensor is known (Fig. 6.2). Thus, the term "triangulation" is derived from this concept [27]. For accurate scans, it is recommended to apply an opaque powder coating of titanium dioxide on surfaces with uneven light dispersion. The CEREC AC Bluecam,

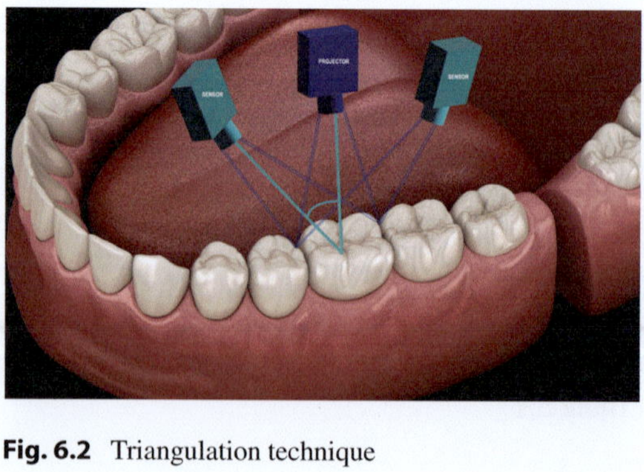

Fig. 6.2 Triangulation technique

a recent generation of CEREC scanners, uses LED blue diodes for illumination [23].

Scanners based on this technique: CEREC scanner.

6.4.2.2 Confocal Laser Scanning Microscopy

Confocal laser scanning microscopy (CLSM or LSCM) is an approach used to capture high-resolution pictures with precise depth selectivity. Images are recreated in three dimensions using a computer through a process known as "point and stitch reconstruction," where they are projected point-by-point, line-by-line, or multiple points simultaneously [23]. Confocal microscopy's main feature is its capability to generate high-resolution optical slices of objects at different depths in the x, y, and z coordinates with excellent contrast. The system exports digital picture files in STL format for sharing with other labs that have CAD/CAM systems [28] (Fig. 6.3).

Scanners based on this technique: iTero and TRIOS scanners.

6.4.2.3 Active Wavefront Sampling (3D-in-Motion Video Recording)

Active wavefront sampling (AWS) utilizes a 3D surface imaging method that involves a single optical route between an AWS module and only one camera to capture depth information [29]. Distance and depth data are determined and computed from the pattern created by each point generated by the revolving module along the optical axis (Fig. 6.4). AWS imaging enables any device equipped with a digital camera to operate in three dimensions. Therefore, it removes the necessity of using several

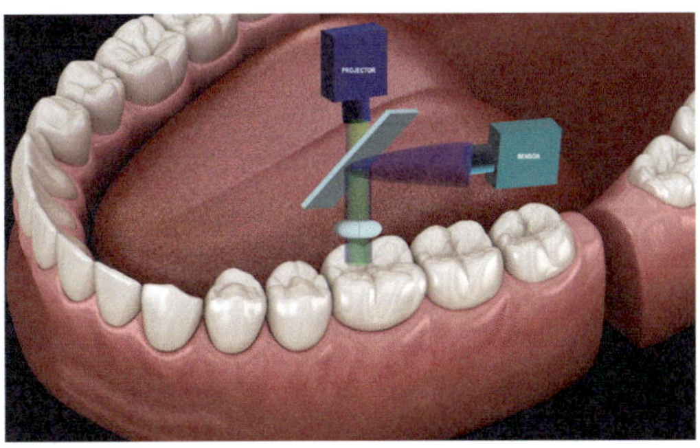

Fig. 6.3 Confocal laser scanning microscopy

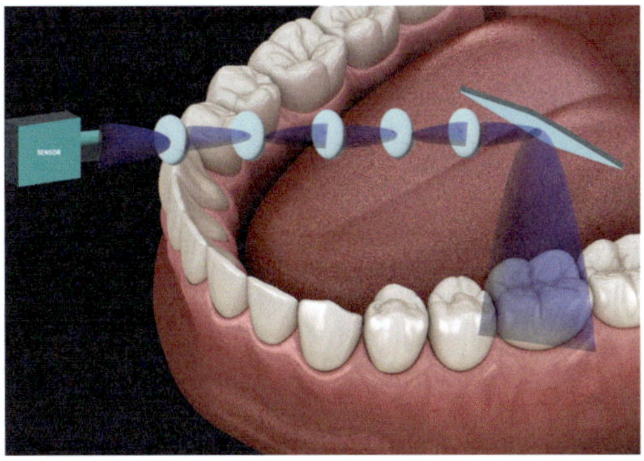

Fig. 6.4 Active wavefront sampling

cameras to capture 3D shapes. The primary feature of an AWS system is its ability to capture depth information using just one optical route [30].

Scanners based on this technique: LAVA Chairside Oral Scanner (COS).

6.4.2.4 Accordion Fringe Interferometry

AFI, or accordion fringe interferometry, is a three-dimensional extension of traditional linear laser interferometry. In AFI, an object is illuminated with two-point sources to create an interference fringe pattern. The curvature of the fringes is captured using a high-precision digital camera, albeit from an angle that is not perpendicular to the projector. By utilizing the apparent fringe curvature and the known geometry between the laser source and the camera, the AFI algorithms can digitize the surface of the object being scanned (Fig. 6.5). The X, Y, and Z coordinates of every pixel in the camera are recorded by AFI-based imagers [30, 31].

Scanners using the DPI-3D scanning method.

6.4.2.5 Optical Coherence Tomography

Optical coherence tomography is an interferometric imaging approach that offers cross-sectional images of the subsurface microstructure of certain objects, such as biological tissues [32]. It is similar to ultrasound imaging but uses light instead of sound. Micron-scale distance and microstructure measurements are acquired in real time and in vivo using backscattered or back-reflected light waves [33].

Scanners based on this technique: E4D by DAD Technologies

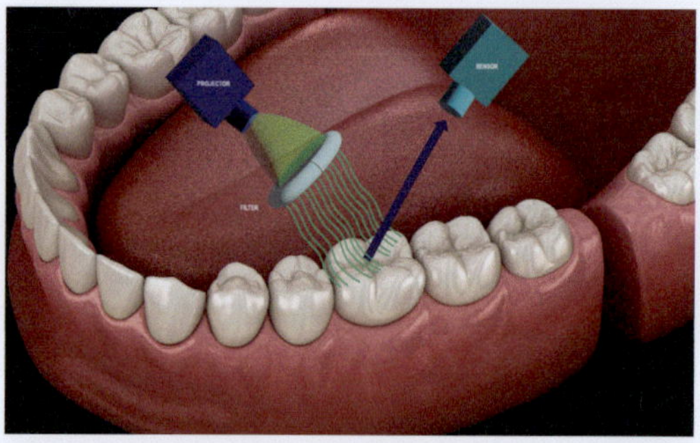

Fig. 6.5 Accordion fringe interferometry

6.4.3 In Vitro vs. In Vivo

Various studies are available that compare the accuracy and reproducibility of the scans both in vitro and in vivo. Tooth-width measurements on digital models and intraoral scans did not differ significantly from caliper measurements acquired from the corresponding plaster models, as demonstrated by Wiranto et al. [34] and Naidu and Freer [35]. In a study conducted by Akyalcin et al. [36], it was discovered that intraoral scan measurements of tooth width were more accurate than cone-beam computed tomographic measurements and closely matched caliper measurements on dry skulls.

Key factors in evaluating an intraoral scanner are its precision and accuracy. Accuracy/trueness refers to how closely a test or measurement result aligns with the true value. To determine the accuracy of a scan, an experimental model is scanned using both the intraoral scanner and a reference scanner. The virtual casts produced by each scanner are then compared. This method has been utilized to evaluate accuracy in laboratory conditions; however, the accuracy of intraoral scanners has been noted to diminish while capturing an entire dental arch in comparison with a smaller section [37]. The reduced accuracy of intraoral scans in comparison with extraoral scans is due to factors such as moisture, salivary flow, and limited space within the mouth, which can make it challenging to capture precise intraoral images [38]. Pellitteri et al. [39] conducted a study comparing the accuracy of full-arch digital imprints from several intraoral scanning systems in vivo. They also compared this with a traditional polyvinyl siloxane (PVS) impression. The most accurate single-tooth scanner was found to be the Trios 3Shape; however, when compared to PVS impressions, the Carestream CS 3600 performed better in terms of inter-arch diameter.

6.4.4 Factors to Be Considered While Procuring a Scanner

Many intraoral scanners are available commercially. Selection of the intraoral scanner should be based on the scanner's features and application. The various factors to be considered are as follows:

(a) Accuracy
(b) Reproducibility
(c) Scanning speed and flow
(d) Overall ease of use
(e) Scanner size and tips
(f) Patient comfort
(g) Software and additional features
(h) Cost
(i) Applicability

6.4.4.1 Accuracy

The quality of a scan involves various factors, with precision being the foremost concern [40]. ISO 5725-1 defines accuracy as the combination of trueness and precision. Most scanners exhibit great precision in vivo, with no significant variations among them [41]. Kierl et al's investigation indicates that both the iTero Element and the 3Shape TRIOS intraoral scanners were found to have clinically acceptable accuracy [42]. Another study found that TRI-OS had greater accuracy compared to CEREC [43]. Diverse scanning technologies impact accuracy in varying manners.

The accuracy of an impression might be influenced by the surface type being scanned. This comprises metal crowns, prostheses, and orthodontic brackets. Park et al. conducted a study on bracket accuracy in vitro, finding that lingual brackets are less precise than buccal brackets. Both TRIOS and iTero outperformed in these situations [44]. Edentulous regions are another clinical condition that can affect accuracy. It is challenging to obtain correct digital impressions due to the absence of teeth as clear anatomical cues for registration [45].

6.4.4.2 Reproducibility

Several investigations have demonstrated the good reproducibility and reliability of intraoral scanners [35, 46, 47].

6.4.4.3 Scanning Speed and Flow

Goracci et al. [48] in their systematic review revealed that the scanning duration can change among research for the same models due to variations in how it is measured, either from machine activation or when scanning begins. Typically, the time taken for scanning decreases as the operator gains more experience. Operators need to acquaint themselves with the specific functions of each machine [49]. According to a study, iTero might scan more slowly than the traditional imprint method because of its lengthier scanning period. Clinical expertise, however, strengthens this restriction. However, TRIOS takes less time to scan than conventional technologies and is easier to use even for untrained operators [45]. Currently, a reliable scanner can capture a whole arch scan in less than 60 s, and newer scanners with even shorter scan periods are being developed. Table 6.1 displays the scanning times for different commercially available scanners.

6.4.4.4 Overall Ease of Use

Common challenges affecting the user experience of scanners are scan duration, expenses, and the format of the files produced by the scanner [47]. The operator's experience and convenience of use are crucial factors to consider when selecting a scanner.

According to Kim et al.'s research, iTero had a faster learning rate and a longer average scanning duration than TRIOS. While the mean scanning time was shorter and unaffected by clinical experience, TRIOS had a slow learning rate [45]. It can be difficult to achieve impartiality because, according to studies, practitioners more used to older procedures and less familiar with digital scanners may find it difficult to use the devices and associated software. On the other hand, intraoral scanning allows dental practitioners and students who are more accustomed to digital techniques to become clinically competent and faster [50]. The learning curve for each clinician differs depending on age, previous digital equipment experience, capacity to adjust to new technology, and patient involvement [51].

Operators typically favored the TRIOS intraoral scanner over iTero due to its ease of use and clinical utility [52]. In a questionnaire survey conducted by Park et al. [53] among practicing orthodontists, it was discovered that 56% of digital users reported utilizing digital scanners in their offices, with zero being the most preferred choice at 86%.

6.4.4.5 Scanner Size and Tips

When choosing a new scanner for the dental office, it is important to evaluate its size to ensure it suits the office area and can be readily relocated. All intraoral scanners, regardless of their size, come in a standard form with wheel stands. The TRIOS Pod and Mobile True definition are lightweight and portable choices designed for offices with limited space that cannot accommodate a huge trolley. Older scanners had tips that were too large for people with restricted mouth openings. A scanner with a smaller tip is typically favored for increased patient comfort and easier scanning in the posterior regions [15, 22].

About the infection control of the scanner tips, operator guidelines need to be followed. Carestream recommends chemical sterilization of the scanner tips. However, they do not recommend solutions containing iodophors or phenol as it may damage the surface coating of the scanner. iTero and TRIOS scanners have an autoclavable tip.

6.4.4.6 Patient Comfort

The digital impressions were more comfortable compared to conventional procedures, as previously discussed [22, 54–57]. The intraoral scanners received higher ratings for comfort, gag reflex, and breathing problems [22]. Using powder during intraoral scanning significantly influences the comfort level of patients. The powder was seen by 64% of patients scanned with LAVA and 74% of patients scanned with CEREC; 14% and 18% of patients, respectively, reported discomfort as a result of the powder [16]. In terms of patient comfort and convenience, iTero received higher ratings than TRI-OS [52]. Forty-four precent of patients preferred CEREC over LAVA when comparing the two scanners, while 39% had no preference at all [16].

6.4.4.7 Software and Additional Features

During the selection of a scanner and the brand, it is essential to look for additional software and features that may not be available in others. These include proprietary CAD software, caries detection software, ortho simulation, model builder, and smile design. It is essential to check if the scanner comes with the software package or software subscription cost is separate. Many scanners have yearly subscriptions for upgrades, maintenance, and support.

Additionally, some scanners have a wireless option, which improves ergonomics and seamfreeness. Of the intraoral scanners that have been studied, 3Shape has gained the most reputation in the literature for producing software that is easy to use. 3Shape's Ortho Analyzer can do analysis, generate a standardized digital model, and provide virtual model settings. By using a 3D printer, clinicians can design customized clear aligners and accessories. Other businesses also have unique advantages. Invisalign provides strong technological support for iTero. With a wealth of experience in CAD/CAM and restorative dentistry, CEREC offers technician, assistant, and physician educational training programs.

The requirement for powder and opacization is common in first-generation intraoral scanners. However, the latest devices are powderless. It is preferred to procure a scanner that does not require opacization as it may be an inconvenience for the patient. Using an incorrect opacization approach might lead to uneven layer thicknesses on different parts of the teeth, increasing the likelihood of mistakes that lower the scan's quality [24, 58, 59].

6.4.4.8 Cost

The price of obtaining an IOS can range from 7500 USD to 45,000 USD, depending on the model. In recent years, new models have been introduced to the market, potentially leading to a decrease in prices. The expense of an intraoral scanner might be offset over time by incorporating the technology into the clinical workflow in different dental specialties [22]. The scanners need frequent maintenance for hardware calibration and software upgrades [60]. The associated costs should be considered before purchasing a scanner.

Finally, a scanner should be compatible with an open workflow. An intraoral scanner often requires two outputs: a proprietary file with legal validity and an open-format file such as STL, OBJ, or PLY. Open-format files can be promptly accessed and utilized by all CAD prosthetic systems [23–25, 58, 61]. Open systems offer versatility and the opportunity to reduce expenses by eliminating the requirement to purchase individual CAD licenses or pay to unlock files. Some level of experience may be necessary at first to interact with the various software and milling equipment. This issue does not occur in a closed system. The scanners produce output files that are proprietary and can only be accessed and manipulated by a specific CAD software from the same manufacturer. The main limitations of closed systems are the inability to freely access and use STL files, as well as the requirement to pay fees to unlock them [23–25, 58, 61].

6.4.4.9 Applicability

Assessment of the applicability of the scanner is an important criterion before selecting it for dental practice. The clinician should assess the type of practice and patient flow. For example, a practice that uses digital scans for orthodontic treatment should prefer scanners with good full arch scan accuracy. The TRIOS scanner is more precise when scanning a single dental element compared to the entire arch, making it a preferred choice for prosthodontists working on partial fixed prosthesis reconstructions.

6.4.5 Comparison of Commercially Available Scanners

Based on the features, the commercially available scanners and their features are tabulated (Table 6.2).

Table 6.2 Comparison of commercially available intraoral scanners

Intraoral scanners	TRIOS (TRIOS 4)	CEREC primescan	Emarald S	i700	iTero element 5D plus	CS 3700	Virtuo vivo	Heron IOS	WOW scanner	Runyes-3DS
Company	3Shape	Dentsply sirona	Planmeca	Medit	Align Technology	Carestream Dental	Dental wings/ straumann	**3DISC**	**Biotech dental**	**Ningbo Runyes Medical**
Technology used	Confocal laser scanning microscopy	High-resolution Sensors and Shortwave Light with Optical High Frequency Contrast Analysis for Dynamic Deep Scan	Optical Triangulation	Active Wavefront sampling (3D-in-motion video technology)	Confocal laser scanning microscopy	Active Triangulation with Smart-shade Matchingvia Bidirectional Reflectance Distribution Function	Blue laser-Multiscan Imaging Technology	**Continuously scanning and accumulating (stitching) depth and color data**		**Synchronous 3D Video Quick Technology**
Weight	345 g (wired) or 375g (wireless with a battery)	Primescan weighs 457 g/524 g depending on what scanner sleeve is used, (disposable plastic or metal).	Scanner with Tip-229 g	245 g	500 g	316 g	130 g	**150 g**	**110 g**	**210 g**
Scanning time	Full arch scan under 45 s	Full arch scan under 45 s	65 frames/s	Full-arch scans under 40 s	Full arch scan under 45 s	Full arch scan in 60 s	Full arch scan in 1 min	**Full arch scans in 60 s**	**2–3 min for full arch scan**	**40 s per quadrant**
Output	Open STL, DCM	Open STL	Open STL and PLY	Open STL, OBJ and PLY	Open STL and PLY	Open STL, PLY, OBJ	Open STL and PLY	**Open STL, PLY and OBJ**	**Open STL and PLY**	**Open STL, PLY and OBJ**
Software	Smile designing Patient monitoring Ortho planning Treatment simulation	CAD CAM software Smile design	Caries detection CAD CAM software	Smile Design Ortho Simulation Model builder	Can be integrated with EXOCAD only Patient simulation Ortho simulation Caries detection	No CAD software	Basic CAD software CoDiagnostix implant software	**Relies on third party software foe CAD**	**Scan only**	**Scan only**

(continued)

Table 6.2 (continued)

Intraoral scanners	TRIOS (TRIOS 4)	CEREC primescan	Emarald S	i700	iTero element 5D plus	CS 3700	Virtuo vivo	Heron IOS	WOW scanner	Runyes-3DS
Cost										
Wireless scanner	Yes	No	No	No	No	Yes (CS 3800)	No	**No**	**No**	**No**
Method of sterilization	Autoclavable—one tip lasts upto 150 cycles of sterilization	Three sleeves-steel sleeve—cold disinfection and dry heat sterilization Disposable single use sleeve Autoclavable sleeve with a disposable scanning window	Two autoclavable scanning tip options: Standard and SlimLine	Autoclavable tips—100 cycles per tip	Single use non—autoclavable tips only	Autoclavable tips—60 cycles per tip	Autoclavable tips—250 cycles per tip	**Autoclavable tips—250 cycles per tip**	**Cold sterilization**	**Autoclavable tips—50 cycles per tip**
Advantages	Very fast Wireless and ergonomic Software apps Powerful CAD software	Very fast Unbeaten CAD CAM workflow Best foe chairside CAD/CAM	Fast scanner Subscription free Affordable Decent CAD CAM workflow	Very fast Low cost Subscription free	Fast Scanner Best Orthodontic simulator Best caries detection technology	Decent speed Excellent shade matching Smaller tip sizes available for pediatric patients and patients with TMJ issues	Lightweight Ergonomic pen design	**Good scan speed** **Ergonomic and light weight** **Low cost and no yearly fee**	**Smallest scanner in market and ergonomic** **Low cost and comes with a high performance laptop**	**Low cost** **No subscriptions** **Lightweight**
Disadvantages	Expensive Multiple costly subscriptions	No software apps Big size of scanner and tip	Software apps are limited and basic	Requires an internet connection to work No CAD/CAM software	Expensive cost and yearly subscription Large size and cumbersome Single use scanner heads No CAD software	No CAD design software Basic scan analysis/manipulation tools No patient motivation applications Relatively expensive for a scanner-only with no CAD	Technique sensitive scanning strategy Lack of scanner apps Software UI needs improvement Mandatory subscription fee	**Basic software** **No apps foe smile design and ortho simulation** **No CAD software**	**No available CAD software** **Hard to use** **Scan modification and cleanup tools are lacking**	**No software applications** **Cannot be used in edentulous patients** **Lacking AI**

6.5 Summary

Intraoral scanning may be the best way to take impressions now because of the widespread availability of digital devices. Manufacturers are continuously improving the precision of these gadgets, which opens up a wide range of potential uses. They also help speed up and make the clinical process more pleasant for both patients and dentists. A wide variety of individualized orthodontic appliances can be created using digital imprints. Although no scanner is without flaws, there are several that stand out from the pack. Factors including available funds, the primary emphasis of your business, and existing third-party equipment should all be considered when settling on an intraoral scanner.

Acknowledgments The authors would like to acknowledge Dr. Shwetha and Dr. Shruthi for their contribution toward the literature search and illustrations.

References

1. Chaudhari PK, Bhatia D, Sharan J, editors. 3D printing in oral health science. Cham: Springer; 2022. https://doi.org/10.1007/978-3-031-07369-4_2.
2. Koch GK, Gallucci GO, Lee SJ. Accuracy in the digital workflow: from data acquisition to the digitally milled cast. J Prosthet Dent. 2016;115:749–54.
3. Guerini V. Historia tes odontiatrikes [History of dentists]. Odontostomatol Proodos. 1981;35(6):198–204.
4. Bremner MDK. The story of dentistry. New York & London: Dental Items of Interest Pub Co., Inc.; 1954.
5. Ring ME. How a dentist's name became a synonym for a life-saving device: the story of Dr. Charles stent. J Hist Dent. 2001;49(2):77–80.
6. Jacobson B. Taking the headache out of impressions. Dent Today. 2007;26:74–6.
7. Donovan TE, Chee WW. A review of contemporary impression materials and techniques. Dent Clin N Am. 2004;48(2):vi–vii, 445–70.
8. Al-Zarea BK, Sughaireen MG. Comparative analysis of dimensional precision of different silicone impression materials. J Contemp Dent Pract. 2011;12(3):208–15.
9. Duret F. The optical impression. Universite Claude Bernard; 1973.
10. Logozzo S, Franceschini G, Kilpelä A, Caponi M, Governi L, Blois L. A comparative analysis of intraoral 3d digital scanners for restorative dentistry. Internet J Med Technol. 2008;5:1–18.
11. Rekow ED. Dental CAD/CAM systems: a 20-year success story. J Am Dent Assoc. 2006;137:5S–6S.
12. Cadent debuts. "Next generation" iTero digital impression system. Implant Tribune. 2007;1:14.
13. Kravitz ND, Groth C, Jones PE, Graham JW, Redmond WR. Intraoral digital scanners. J Clin Orthod. 2014;48(6):337–47.
14. Kim YJ, et al. Principles and applications of various 3D scanning methods for image acquisition for 3D printing applications in oral health science. In: Chaudhari PK, Bhatia D, Sharan J, editors. 3D printing in oral health science. Cham: Springer; 2022. https://doi.org/10.1007/978-3-031-07369-4_2.
15. Hann-Min HH, Chi-Wei C, Yi-Jane C, Jane YC-C. An overview of digital intraoral scanners: past, present and future—from an orthodontic perspective. Taiwanese J Orthod. 2018;30(3):148–61.
16. Burhardt L, Livas C, Kerdijk W, van der Meer WJ, Ren Y. Treatment comfort, time perception, and preference for conventional and digital impression techniques: a comparative study in young patients. Am J Orthod Dentofacial Orthop. 2016;150:261–7.
17. Yilmaz H, Aydin MN. Digital versus conventional impression method in children: comfort, preference and time. Int J Paediatr Dent. 2019;29:728–35.
18. Deferm JT, Schreurs R, Baan F, Bruggink R, Merkx MAW, Xi T, et al. Validation of 3D documentation of palatal soft tissue shape, color, and irregularity with intraoral scanning. Clin Oral Investig. 2018;22:1303–9.
19. Martin CB, Chalmers EV, McIntyre GT, Cochrane H, Mossey PA. Orthodontic scanners: what's available? J Orthod. 2015;42:136–43.
20. De Luca CG, Pacheco-Pereira C, Lagravere MO, Flores-Mir C, Major PW. Intra-arch dimensional measurement validity of laser-scanned digital dental models compared with the original plaster models: a systematic review. Orthod Craniofac Res. 2015;18:65–76.
21. Papaspyridakos P, Vazouras K, Chen YW, Kotina E, Natto Z, Kang K, Chochlidakis K. Digital vs conventional implant impressions: a systematic review and meta-analysis. J Prosthodont. 2020;29(8):660–78.
22. Mangano F, Gandolfi A, Luongo G, Logozzo S. Intraoral scanners in dentistry: a review of the current literature. BMC Oral Health. 2017;17(1):149.
23. Ting-Shu S, Jian S. Intraoral digital impression technique: a review. J Prosthodont. 2015;24:313–21.
24. Zimmermann M, Mehl A, Mörmann WH, Reich S. Intraoral scanning systems: a current overview. Int J Comput Dent. 2015;18:101–29.
25. Imburgia M, Logozzo S, Hauschild U, Veronesi G, Mangano C, Mangano FG. Accuracy of four intraoral scanners in oral implantology: a comparative in vitro study. BMC Oral Health. 2017;17(1):92.
26. van der Meer WJ, Andriessen FS, Wismeijer D, Ren Y. Application of intra-oral dental scanners in the digital workflow of implantology. PLoS One. 2012;7:e43312.
27. Ji Z, Leu MC. Design of optical triangulation devices. Opt Laser Technol. 1989;21(5):339–41.
28. Carlsson K, Danielsson PE, Lenz R, Liljeborg A, Majlöf L, Aslund N. Three-dimensional microscopy

using a confocal laser scanning microscope. Opt Lett. 1985;10(2):53–5.
29. Frigerio F. Methods and apparatus for 3D surface imaging using active wave-front sampling. U.S. Patent No. 8,369,579. 5; 2013.
30. Logozzo S, Zanetti EM, Franceschini G, Kilpelä A, Mäkynen A. Recent advances in dental optics—part I: 3D intraoral scanners for restorative dentistry. Opt Lasers Eng. 2014;54:203–21.
31. FARO. FARO—brochures—accordion fringe interferometry. http://www.faro.com/site/resources/details/912.
32. Schmitt JM. Optical coherence tomography (OCT): a review. IEEE J Selected Topics Quantum Electron. 1999;5:1205–15.
33. Taneva E, Kusnoto B, Evans CA. 3D scanning, imaging, and printing in orthodontics. Issues Contemp Orthod. 2015;3:148–9.
34. Wiranto MG, Engelbrecht WP, Tutein Nolthenius HE, van der Meer WJ, Ren Y. Validity, reliability, and reproducibility of linear measurements on digital models obtained from intraoral and cone-beam computed tomography scans of alginate impressions. Am J Orthod Dentofacial Orthop. 2013;143:140–7.
35. Naidu D, Freer TJ. Validity, reliability, and reproducibility of the iOC intraoral scanner: a comparison of tooth widths and Bolton ratios. Am J Orthod Dentofacial Orthop. 2013;144:304–10.
36. Akyalcin S, Cozad BE, English JD, Colville CD, Laman S. Diagnostic accuracy of impression-free digital models. Am J Orthod Dentofacial Orthop. 2013;144:916–22.
37. Kernen F, Schlager S, Seidel Alvarez V, Mehrhof J, Vach K, Kohal R, Nelson K, Flügge T. Accuracy of intraoral scans: an in vivo study of different scanning devices. J Prosthet Dent. 2022;128(6):1303–9.
38. Flugge TV, Att W, Metzger MC, Nelson K. Precision of dental implant digitization using intraoral scanners. J Prosthodont. 2016;29(3):277–83.
39. Pellitteri F, Albertini P, Vogrig A, Spedicato GA, Siciliani G, Lombardo L. Comparative analysis of intraoral scanners accuracy using 3D software: an in vivo study. Prog Orthod. 2022;23(1):21.
40. Atieh MA, Ritter AV, Ko CC, Duqum I. Accuracy evaluation of intraoral optical impressions: a clinical study using a reference appliance. J Prosthet Dent. 2017;118:400–5.
41. Ender A, Attin T, Mehl A. In vivo precision of conventional and digital methods of obtaining complete-arch dental impressions. J Prosthet Dent. 2016;115:313–20.
42. Kierl JM Accuracy of digital models acquired from two different intraoral scanners: an in vivo study. Master's Thesis, University of Oklahoma Health Sciences Center, Oklahoma, OK; 2018.
43. Nedelcu R, Olsson P, Nystrom I, Ryden J, Thor A. Accuracy and precision of 3 intraoral scanners and accuracy of conventional impressions: a novel in vivo analysis method. J Dent. 2018;69:110–8.
44. Park JM, Choi SA, Myung JY, Chun YS, Kim M. Impact of orthodontic brackets on the intraoral scan data accuracy. Biomed Res Int. 2016;2016:5075182.
45. Kim JE, Amelya A, Shin Y, Shim JS. Accuracy of intraoral digital impressions using an artificial landmark. J Prosthet Dent. 2017;117:755–61.
46. Duvert R, Gebeille-Chauty S. La précision des empreintes numériques intra-orales en orthodontie est-elle suffisante? Int Orthod. 2017;88:347–54.
47. Sun LJ, Lee JS, Choo HH, Hwang HS, Lee KM. Reproducibility of an intraoral scanner: a comparison between in-vivo and ex-vivo scans. Am J Orthod Dentofacial Orthop. 2018;154:305–10.
48. Goracci C, Franchi L, Vichi A, Ferrari M. Accuracy, reliability, and efficiency of intraoral scanners for full-arch impressions: a systematic review of the clinical evidence. Eur J Orthod. 2016;38:422–8.
49. Yi-lun X, Gang S. Accuracy and reproducibility of intraoral scanning in vivo. Shanghai J Stomatol. 2016;25:593–9.
50. Marti AM, Harris BT, Metz MJ, Morton D, Scarfe WC, Metz CJ, Lin WS. Comparison of digital scanning and polyvinyl siloxane impression techniques by dental students: instructional efficiency and attitudes towards technology. Eur J Dent Educ. 2017;21:200–5.
51. Christopoulou I, Kaklamanos EG, Makrygiannakis MA, Bitsanis I, Perlea P, Tsolakis AI. Intraoral scanners in orthodontics: a critical review. Int J Environ Res Public Health. 2022;19(3):1407.
52. Park HR, Park JM, Chun YS, Lee KN, Kim M. Changes in views on digital intraoral scanners among dental hygienistsafter training in digital impression taking. BMC Oral Health. 2015;15:151.
53. Park JH, Laslovich J. Trends in the use of digital study models and other technologies among practicing orthodontists. J Clin Orthod. 2016;50:413–9.
54. Grunheid T, Mc Carthy SD, Larson BE. Clinical use of a direct chairside oral scanner: an assessment of accuracy, time, and patient acceptance. Am J Orthod Dentofacial Orthop. 2014;146:673–82.
55. Sfondrini MF, Gandini P, Malfatto M, Di Corato F, Trovati F, Scribante A. Computerized casts for orthodontic purpose using powder-free intraoral scanners: accuracy, execution time, and patient feedback. Biomed Res Int. 2018;2018:4103232.
56. Glisic O, Hoejbjerre L, Sonnesen L. A comparison of patient experience, chair-side time, accuracy of dental arch measurements and costs of acquisition of dental models. Angle Orthod. 2019;89:868–75.
57. Christensen L. Digital work flows digital orthodontic forum 2017. Singapore; 2017.
58. Zaruba M, Mehl A. Chairside systems: a current review. Int J Comput Dent. 2017;20(2):123–49.
59. Prudente MS, Davi LR, Nabbout KO, Prado CJ, Pereira LM, Zancopé K, Neves FD. Influence of scanner, powder application, and adjustments on CAD-CAM crown misfit. J Prosthet Dent. 2018;119(3):377–83.
60. Rehmann P, Sichwardt V, Wostmann B. Intraoral scanning systems: need for maintenance. Int J Prosthodont. 2017;30:27–9.
61. Mangano FG, Veronesi G, Hauschild U, Mijiritsky E, Mangano C. Trueness and precision of four intraoral scanners in oral implantology: a comparative in vitro study. PLoS One. 2016;11(9):e0163107.

7 CAD/CAM Technology and Their Applications in Craniofacial Surgery

Babu Lal, Ragavi Alagarsamy, and Shailendra Singh Rana

7.1 Introduction

Congenital and acquired deformities of the cranio-maxillofacial skeleton are usually complex and require meticulous planning and execution to achieve optimal outcomes. Before the advent of advanced imaging techniques, surgeons arbitrarily performed the procedures. With advanced technology, diagnostic imaging has become an integral part of cranio-maxillofacial surgery. These imaging techniques provide valuable insights regarding the intricate anatomy of the region. Sometimes, in patients with complex issues, suboptimal results following surgical management were observed due to planning with a two-dimensional image for a three-dimensional problem.

The requisite for precision in surgical procedures in cranio-maxillofacial surgery led to novel technological evolution, to provide improved outcomes and quality of life [1]. The introduction of three-dimensional (3D) imaging technologies like computed tomography (CT), cone-beam computed tomography (CBCT), ultrasound sonography (USG), and magnetic resonance imaging (MRI) paved the way for emergent computer-aided designing (CAD) and computer-aided manufacturing (CAM) technology in medicine and dentistry [2, 3]. These invariant data sets can be virtually manipulated by segmentation to assist in the accurate positioning of bony and soft tissue constructs. Then, the data can be utilized to create a 3D model or patient-specific implants. The 3D tangible models of real-anatomic sizes are known as biomodels [4]. In addition, the surgical guide and/or positioning jig or mold can be constructed based on virtual surgical planning using CAM technology. These 3D artifacts act as presurgical and surgical tools and have a significant impact on the accuracy and precision of surgery, ultimately leading to profound increase in the postoperative predictability. Specifically, these solutions increase the surgeons' confidence and reduce overall time in the operating room.

The realm of medical imaging has undergone revolution by the advent of 3D imaging technology which has superseded the conventional imaging. This paradigm shift to 3D imaging and further its conversion to a tangible form in medicine changed the entire gamut of diagnosis, treatment planning, and management. In this chapter, we will discuss the workflow for fabricating the

B. Lal (✉)
Department of Trauma and Emergency Medicine, All India Institute of Medical Sciences, Bhopal, Madhya Pradesh, India
e-mail: blsoni.tem@aiimsbhopal.edu.in

R. Alagarsamy
Department of Burns, Plastic and Maxillofacial Surgery, VMMC and Safdarjung Hospital, New Delhi, India

S. S. Rana
Department of Dentistry, All India Institute of Medical Sciences, Bathinda, Punjab, India

S. S. Rana et al. (eds.), *Applications of Three-dimensional Imaging for Craniofacial Region*,
https://doi.org/10.1007/978-981-97-4608-8_7

physical artifact from the virtual 3D image while briefing about cutting-edge CAD and CAM technologies that have led to significant impact in the medicine and dentistry; furthermore, we will overview the common applications of these technologies in cranio-maxillofacial surgery.

7.2 CAD/CAM Technology

CAD/CAM technology has opened the doors for the healthcare professionals aiding in manufacture of physical artifacts. They have become a revolutionary approach with the advent of sophisticated software and automation tool. The conversion of raw data to tangible form involves three steps including conversion of the medical scan to 3D image, CAD which consists of digital manipulation of 3D image and bespoke designing, and CAM which is by additive or subtractive method.

7.2.1 Technical Needs

The fundamental technical requirements include a computer system with a minimum of 8GB RAM and a 2GB graphics card. Various software are used, each serving a distinct function including image processing software for the conversion of medical raw data to 3D image, software for the repair of a digital file, CAD software for virtual surgery, and custom designing and slicing software for G-code generation. CAM technology encompasses hardware such as a 3D printer, computer numeric control (CNC) machine, and a post-processing unit.

7.2.2 Raw Data Maturation

The entire workflow begins with data acquisition. This entails gathering the raw data in Digital Imaging and Communications in Medicine (DICOM) format, which includes various medical imaging such as CT, MRI, CBCT, and USG. It is then imported into the image processing software, where it undergoes a series of processing steps and the virtual 3D image of the region of interest can be obtained. This virtual image is further subjected to additional processing in CAD software. The data from other sources like 3D scanners or specific CAD files in the form of .stl or .obj can directly be imported into CAD software.

7.2.3 Computer-Aided Design (CAD)

Three-dimensional images obtained from imaging software or 3D scanner file have to be imported into CAD software for virtual surgical planning (VSP) and bespoke designing. VSP aids to inspect the intricate anatomic details, digital manipulation of data, surgical simulation, and envisioning surgical outcomes, thus minimizing the surgeons' uncertainty [5]. CAD includes creation, inspection, alteration, and optimization of models. Bespoke designing includes the virtual construction and design of surgical guides, jigs, molds, and custom implants. These CAD files can be exported as .stl, .obj, etc. format for subsequent CAM process.

7.2.4 Pre-CAM Processing

Three-dimensional printers and CNC machine do not understand CAD files in .stl, .obj, etc. format directly. The CAD file needs to be converted into G-code for recognition. G-code is digital instruction in the form of codes to produce a physical object of interest. In other words, G-code tells the position of the heated nozzle in XYZ coordinates in the 3D printer and directs the path of the cutting tool in CNC machine.

Sometimes, the CAD file generated from medical data is suboptimal and contains various errors making it unfit for an accurate CAM process. These errors could encompass deficiencies such as holes (e.g., spaces/interstices between triangular facets), inverted normal (which distinguishes the internal and external aspect of the print), and application of local and/or global smoothing technique to the model. These errors have to be removed by using specified software. It is crucial to assess the precision/validity of the processed file prior to CAM. Subjective evaluation can be done by superimposition of 3D model onto the DICOM image slices for visual inspection to determine the accuracy in pertinent regions. However, the accuracy of printing or milling depends on many factors including expertise in segmentation, the ability to comprehend human anatomy and pathology, and the number of triangles in the particular CAD file [6].

7.2.5 Computer-Aided Manufacturing (CAM)

VSP stand-alone does not suffice in the execution of complex cases. Three-dimensional models aid in haptic feedback, and tangible surgical guides assist in the transfer of a virtual desktop plan to the operation theater [5]. The 3D artifacts including models, guides, jigs, molds, and custom implants can be produced by using CAM technology either 3D printing or CNC machining. The entire technical process for converting raw medical imaging data into physical objects is summarized in Fig. 7.1.

7.2.5.1 3D Printing

Three-dimensional printing is the layer-by-layer manufacture of a physical construct from a CAD

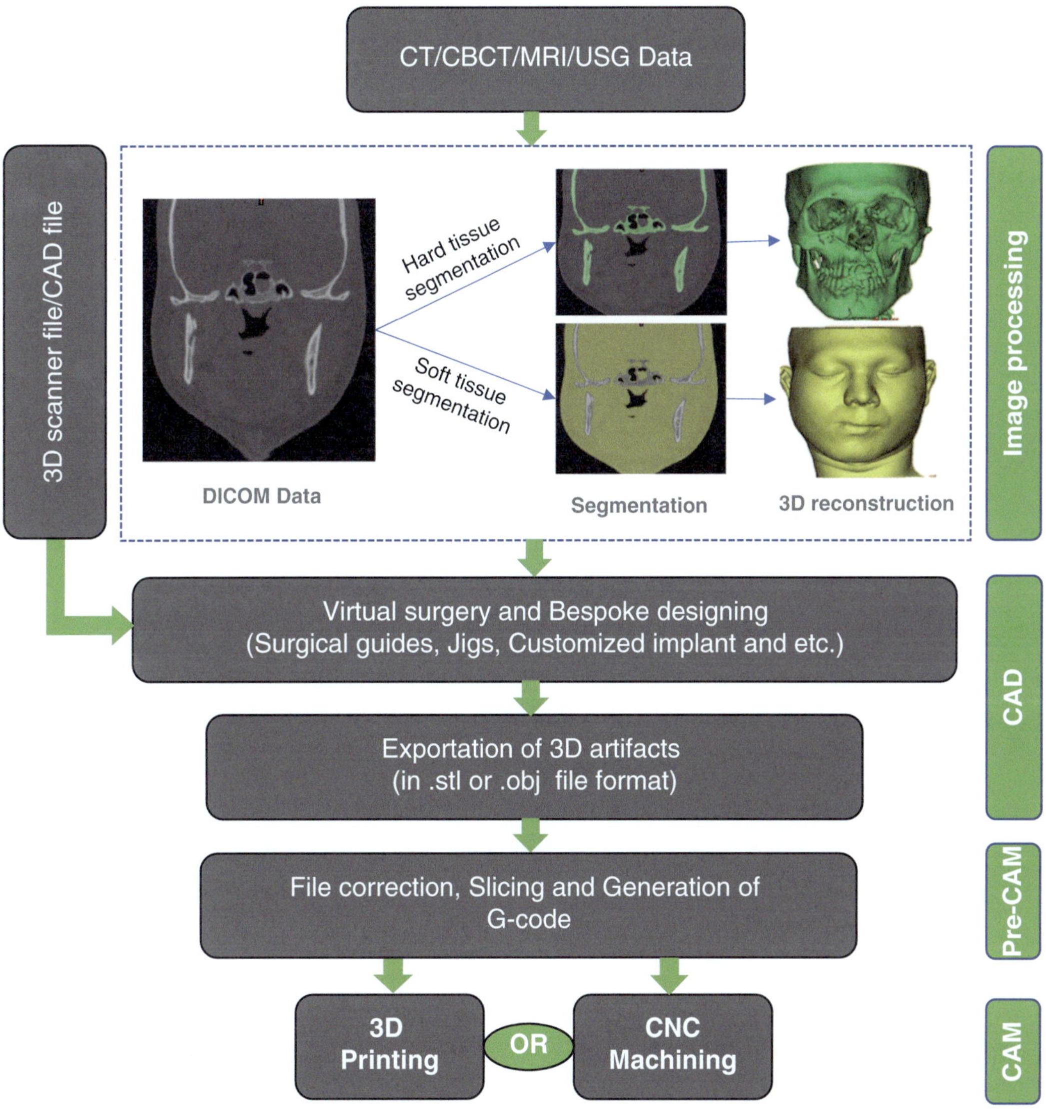

Fig. 7.1 Flow diagram showing CAD/CAM process

model [7] (Fig. 7.2). It is also referred to as additive manufacturing (AM), a terminology widely used in industry. Many times, it is used interchangeably with rapid prototyping (RP) as it is commonly used to create a prototype for new product development. However, the advent of technologies permits acceptance as an efficient way for rapid manufacturing.

Even since its introduction, 3D printing found potential applications in craniofacial surgery aiding in the manufacture of physical artifacts from a plethora of materials like polymers, metals, composites, ceramics, and biological substances. They have spectacular potential to produce precise objects of complex and irregular morphology marking the fourth revolution of personalization. A 3D printer can be used for the fabrication of patient-specific models (region of interest), guides or templates for osteotomy and repositioning of osteotomized parts, a guide for drill or position of screw and mold for fabrication customized implant, etc. Currently, there are various 3D printing technologies. The selection of particular technology for medical use depends on the individual case requirement.

According to the American Society of Testing and Materials, the seven major types of 3D printing technology are as follows:

- Vat polymerization-stereolithography (SLA)
- Material extrusion
- Powder bed fusion
- Material jetting
- Binder jetting
- Sheet lamination
- Directed energy deposition

The first three types are most commonly used in the medical field, and comparative analysis is enumerated in Table 7.1. The details of other types of 3D technologies are beyond the scope of the current chapter. It is important to note that Table 7.1 is a general comparison and that specific results may vary depending on the specific application and the use of the printed object.

7.2.5.2 CNC Machining

CNC machining is an example of subtractive manufacturing (SM). SM is the traditional manufacturing process that involves the removal of material from a solid block to create the desired artifact (Fig. 7.3). Like a 3D printer, a CNC machine is also operated by commands in G-code form [8].

CNC machine work complexity depends on the number of axes. Usually, three axes machine is used for simple industrial applications. In three axes the cutter can allow movement along the three directions, i.e., X, Y, and Z (side to side, back and forth, up and down).

Lately, the use of multi-axis machines, those that possess more than three axes, has been adopted in the medical industry to fabricate both artifacts and bespoke implants. These additional axes enable rotation around one or two of the X, Y, and Z axes, thereby taking into consideration not only the position but also the orientation. This can be accomplished either by rotating the cutting tool or by tilting the table that supports the work piece. The utilization of a multi-axis CNC machine (>3) presents several benefits including a decrease in the overall manufacturing time, the

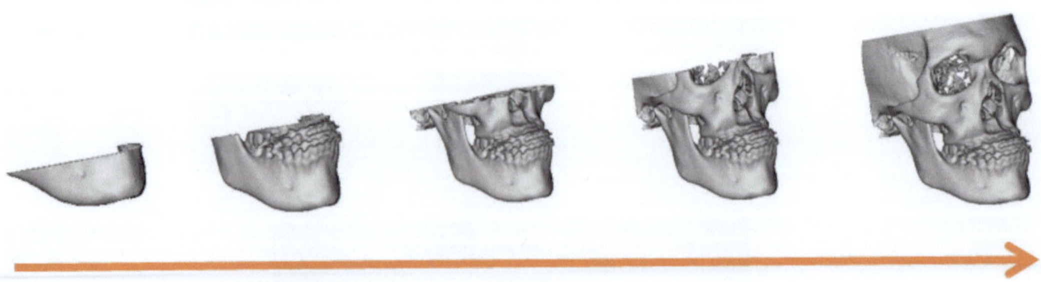

Fig. 7.2 Representation of 3D printing concept

Table 7.1 Comparative analysis of commonly used 3D printing technologies

	FDM printing	Vat polymerization printing	Powder bed fusion printing
Synonyms/ subtypes	Fused deposition modeling (FDM) or fused filament fabrication (FFF)	SLA/DLP type	Selective laser sintering (SLS), direct metal laser sintering (DMLS), selective laser melting (SLM), and electron beam melting (EBM)
Raw material	Mainly thermoplastics like acrylonitrile butadiene styrene (ABS) and polylactic acid (PLA)	Photo-curable resin	Nylon (polyamide) and metal powder
Material strength	Better	Relatively weaker	Best
Accuracy (approx. in mm)	Moderate (±0.5 mm)	Highest (±0.1 mm)	High (±0.3 mm)
Ease of use	Minimal training required	Moderate training required	Highly skilled personnel required
Cost and maintenance	Lower	Moderate	Higher
Limitation	Lower resolution and accuracy and a high risk of printing failure	Low strength and prone to distortion	Limited material option and large space requirement
Applications	3D model for clinical and training purposes	Surgical guides, dental model, temporary restoration, aligners, retainers, castable crown, and bridge	3D model and guides

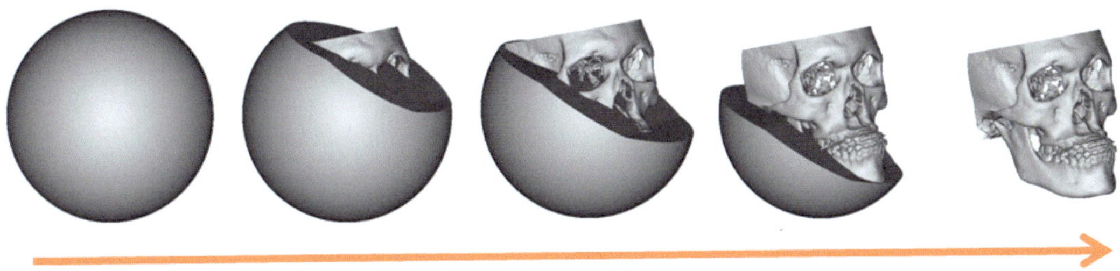

Fig. 7.3 Representation of CNC machining concept

elimination of misalignment errors, and a reduction in the need for intricate fixtures.

While CNC machines have many potential applications in the medical field [9], there are still limitations with their precision in certain areas, such as reproducing thin walls and undercuts. Milled models cannot replicate the displaced thin bony fragments or closed cavities, like paranasal sinuses. In contrast, 3D printing is often preferred for creating detailed models of the face. However, when it comes to custom implant fabrication, CNC machines are often considered to be more suitable. The advantages and disadvantages of each method can be seen in a comparison (Table 7.2).

Table 7.2 Comparative advantages and disadvantages of 3D printing and CNC machining

	3D printing	CNC machining
Advantages	Cost-effective prototyping Complex customization Mass production Fewer space requirements	Repeatable and high accuracy Ability to run 24/7 without stopping Wide range of material options Does not change the material properties Required less post-processing
Disadvantages	Limited material options Inaccuracy due to geometric error Questionable final strength Problem of warping Requires post-processing	Raw material wastage Impossible to construct hollow cavities High initial setup cost

7.2.6 Post-CAM Processing and Sterilization

The physical artifacts manufactured by 3D printing and CNC machining technology require post-processing and standard sterilization before final clinical use. The process of final finishing after manufacturing by various methods is known as post-processing.

The common post-processing procedures include the removal of the support structure, cleaning, gap filling, curing, heating (annealing), polishing, and protective coating to achieve desired material properties [10]. The procedure required for each object depends on the material and CAM technique. The artifacts fabricated by CNC machining have better surface finish and accuracy, hence requiring fewer post-processing treatments in comparison with objects fabricated by 3D printing.

The most commonly used 3D printing technologies for medical model and guide fabrication include FDM, SLA/DLP, and SLS/SLM. ABS and PLA are two materials used in FDM. The parts manufactured by FDM technology have limited mechanical properties and low surface finish. They require the removal of support structures by cutting or dissolving them in warm water depending on the support material used. The anisotropy and defective adhesion between the various additive layers results in voids in FDM-printed artifacts. Gap filling is performed to mask such defects. FDM-printed objects have striations that remain recognizable leading to the rough texture of the model. This is known as staircase effect or Z-stepping and it entails surface polishing. Treatments in acetone and epoxy solutions are done to decrease the surface roughness and reinforce material strength, respectively. Painting and electroplating coating are done to improve the mechanical and electrical properties of the printed parts [11]. PLA-made object might require annealing (heating treatment) for increasing their strength [12].

For SLA or DLP printed parts, the first post-processing typically involves washing with an organic solvent like isopropyl alcohol or isopropanol to remove the uncured resin that remains on the surface of the object. After washing, the object is cured with UV light to ensure a complete polymerization process. The additional post-processing steps may include the removal of support material with hand and cutting tools, protecting coating with paint, ancillary UV curing, and polishing with mineral oil to enhance appearance [13].

The common post-processing techniques for objects manufactured by SLS technology include cleaning the powder, vapor smoothing, heat treatments (annealing), finishing, coating or painting, and polishing. Annealing is the exposure of printed objects to controlled temperatures to improve their strength and durability [10].

Special heat treatments like isostatic pressure sintering, homogenization, and aging are done for metallic objects printed by SLM technology. Isostatic pressure sintering is performed to decrease the porosity and increase the overall mechanical strength [14]. Procedures like homogenization and aging further increase the strength of the objects. Special processes like shot peening and ultrasonic impact treatment can also be used to improve the surface texture and surface stresses reducing the likeliness of fatigue failure. Overall, the benefits of post-processing in 3D-printed objects are enhancement of thermo-mechanical properties, durability, and esthetic appearance. One should take extra care not to alter any dimension of the object during the post-processing procedure.

CNC machining is known for its high precision and accuracy. The CNC-made products are relatively finished. Hence, they require minimal post-processing involving minor finishing or polishing procedures.

Following post-processing, standard sterilization techniques must be adopted before the final use of physical artifacts in a clinical setup. The use of sterilization method depends on the material and available facility. Low-temperature sterilization methods such as gas plasma or ethylene oxide (EtO) are routinely used for plastic (ABS or PLA) artifacts to prevent deformation. Gas plasma is suitable for solid models and prints that are created in sterile environments, such as under a laminar flow hood. EtO sterilization is appropriate for all nonsolid items fabricated from low-temperature thermoplastic material, including biomodels and surgical guides [15]. Metal and high thermoplastic materials can be sterilized using the standard autoclave method. For low-temperature thermoplastic materials such as PLA-based surgical guides, cold sterilization with a 2.4% glutaraldehyde solution can be used [16]. Gamma irradiation sterilization is also an option for implantable devices.

7.3 Applications in Craniofacial Surgery

The CAD/CAM process aids in the fabrication of various tangible forms, ranging from 3D models to bespoke implants, depending upon individualized requirements in cranio-maxillofacial surgeries. These forms have multiple uses, including clinical care, research, education, and training, and can be deployed in forensic medicine as well. With the advancement in technological integrity, they have become relatively affordable and accessible due to expeditious industrialization and commercialization. The following section discusses the various applications of CAD/CAM in the cranio-maxillofacial region.

7.3.1 Dentistry

The use of CAD/CAM technology in dentistry is well-known to any dental surgeon. Applications are varied from education, training, research, and clinical solutions. From simple periodontal defects to complex prosthetic rehabilitation [17] and esthetic procedures in endodontics or orthodontics, CAM/CAM technology has found profound applications in dentistry. Three-dimensional printed tooth models assist in preclinical education in dental residency for the preparation of cavity, crown, and root canals [18]. A surgical template or guide can be used for orthodontic mini-screws and miniplate placement, root canal treatment in the calcified canal, and apicoectomy [19, 20]. In the current era of personalized medicine, even dentistry is not untouched. Inlays, onlays, veneer, temporary or permanent crowns, bridge, partial or complete denture frameworks, and splints can be fabricated by 3D printing or CNC milling [21]. Fabrication of dental restorations with complex hierarchical structure can be done by additive manufacturing with maximum accuracy and minimum wastage of material. 3D-printed space maintainer and stainless-steel crown can be fabricated using digital impression with better compliance in the pediatric group.

The clear aligners have revolutionized the field of orthodontics. These aligners are fabricated from a series of virtually modified 3D-printed dental models which are hassle-free and reduce the follow-up visits of the patient in comparison with conventional orthodontic treatment.

Dental implant is a complex array in dentistry demanding high practical skills and achieving parallel alignment, while placement of multiple adjacent implants is challenging. In the dental implant surgical process, 3D-printed guide helps in placing the implant in a planned position, depth, and angulation [22]. Three-dimensional templates can help in the harvesting of bone grafts for local sites and also assist in sinus lift procedures. A 3D jaw model can be utilized for implant placement practice and training.

7.3.2 Trauma

In the case of craniofacial trauma, 3D models aid in the identification and direct visualization of the displaced bone fragments and inter-fragment relations. The 3D-printed models can be used for resident training reducing errors in patients. The patient-specific models can be used in residual deformity cases to assess the exact status of the malunited segments and rehearsal of planned surgery [23]. Customized models can be used for pre-bending, adaptation, or contouring of the hardware [24, 25]. Custom-made implants for the reconstruction of the mandible, zygoma, orbit, or frontal region can be fabricated by either 3D printing or CNC machining [26].

7.3.3 Pathology

The reconstruction of craniofacial region is challenging due to the presence of various types of tissue and their complexity within a confined region. In the case of pathological lesions, VSP aids in 3D visualization of the pathology and helps in deciding the resection margins and forecasting the defect to result after resection. Customized 3D model for pre-bending of metal plates to be placed after removal of pathological bone and 3D-printed bespoke guides for resection and reconstruction can be fabricated [27]. In free fibular reconstruction cases, free fibula graft harvesting guides for accurate length and sectioning of fibula part for precise reconstruction [28].

7.3.4 Temporomandibular Joint

In the temporomandibular joint (TMJ), 3D models aid in understanding the normal anatomy and direct visualization or evaluation of dimension of the bony chunk in TMJ ankylosis cases [29]. Cutting guides can be used for the precise cutting of the ankylotic chunk. Surgical simulation, fabrication, and verification of customized TMJ prostheses can be done on tangible 3D models [30, 31]. 3D-printed templates specific to patient anatomy can be used for arthrocentesis or prolotherapy [32]. Custom-made alloplastic total TMJ prostheses can be fabricated using both 3D printing and CNC machining for end-stage TMJ disorders.

7.3.5 Orthognathic Surgery

In jaw corrective surgeries, 3D evaluation of existing jaw discrepancy, measurement of important surgical landmarks, rehearsal of planned surgery, and visualization of predicted results can be done on 3D tangible patient-specific models [33]. These models can also be utilized for the pre-bending of the plates. 3D-printed surgical cutting guides of planning osteotomy levels, repositioning jigs of required advancements or setbacks, and occlusal splints of optimal occlusal relations are used for the replication of the virtual plan to the operating room [34]. Currently, titanium-based customized 3D-printed or CNC milled hardware is being used for cutting as well as fixation purposes.

7.3.6 Distraction Osteogenesis

Distraction osteogenesis is an effective method of achieving bone lengthening. The 3D model of the particular patient aids in the preoperative analysis of bone anatomy and bone stock and osteotomy planning with greater accuracy. The model can help in distractor adaptation and determine the pin location ensuring their exact placement during surgery. Mock surgery can be executed on 3D models to evaluate the vector of the distraction and distraction simulation prior to planned surgery [35]. 3D-printed guides for planned osteotomy sites help in the exact transfer of the vector for distraction [36]. Additionally, these models can be used to fabricate custom-made distractors. In syndromic cases requiring distraction, patient-specific surgical guides help in the transfer of planned osteotomy and pin location in case of rigid external distractor placement [37].

7.3.7 Facial Esthetics

Custom guides have been increasingly used for soft tissue correction, rhinoplasty, and gender correction surgeries [38–40]. High fidelity custom facial implants can be fabricated for any area of the facial skeleton like the chin, malar, mandibular angle, and infraorbital regions, which can be tailored to the patient's specific anatomic features [41]. A bone contouring guide can be manufactured to aid in the accurate transfer of virtual plans and achieve harmonious results.

7.3.8 Cleft Lip and Palate

Patients with cleft lip and palate require a multidisciplinary approach, and each procedure demands precision to achieve an optimal outcome. Presurgical orthopedic plates can be fabricated for patients with cleft lip and palate [42]. The preoperative evaluation of the three-dimensional bony defect, relative teeth position with respect to the defect, and quantification of bone graft can be done virtually as well as in a 3D model [43, 44]. Custom-made appliances such as jaw expanders and special splints can also be created using metal 3D printing technology.

7.3.9 Cranio-Maxillofacial Prosthesis

The cranio-maxillofacial prosthesis fabrication demands highly artistic and skilled workers. VSP along with the 3D printing has notably changed the prosthetic rehabilitation enabling manufacture of replica with improved form and minimal turnaround time. 3D-printed custom molds enable the creation of highly precise and customized prosthetic solutions for individuals with deformities in the ears, nose, eyes, and other facial regions. These act as templates for the final prosthesis which can be fabricated by either printing techniques or CNC milling [45].

7.4 Potential Benefits

- Benefits before surgery
  - Adjunct in diagnosis, treatment planning, and interdisciplinary discussion
  - Direct 3D visualization of anatomic structures
  - Preoperative adaptation or pre-bending of reconstruction plates
  - Rehearsal of planned surgery
  - Verification of custom-made implant fit and device testing
- Benefits during surgery
  - Decrease the surgical, anesthesia, and wound exposure time.
  - Reference 3D model for anatomical relations between risk areas and the final target of the operation
  - Improved overall outcome
- Auxiliary benefits
  - Develops confidence in operating surgeon due to familiarity with anatomy from the tangible artifact
  - Patient and relative education for disease understanding and operative strategy
  - Helps in taking informed consent
  - Useful for instrumentation trial and resident training
  - Rare disease models which can be used for the academic library
  - Three-dimensional models and other bespoke which can be utilized for research purposes

7.5 Challenges

The integration of CAD/CAM technology in the cranio-maxillofacial region has been a versatile and encumbered process. However, every advancing technology is bound to have limitations. The challenges include high initial costs and turnover times which are overcome by cost-effective 3D printers and industrialization. A clinicians' lack of technical knowledge regarding the CAD/CAM, limited awareness about the clinical benefits, and miscommunication between the surgeon and engineer can result in inaccuracy due to human errors. Surgeons should be well informed about recent software and be aware of their potential uses. There is a lack of established standards of procedures (SOPs) for the bespoke designing of models and guides which creates nuance in planned execution. With continued technological improvements and refinement of techniques, outcomes can be improved substantially in the future. In addition, the system needs proper legislation and guidelines for the usage of the personalized medicine approach.

7.6 Future Perspective

In the last three decades, the application of CAD/CAM technology in the medical or dental field grew exponentially with continued research and innovations in software, hardware, and raw materials. CAD software is being developed that utilizes artificial intelligence (AI) algorithms to automatically segment and generate 3D images. The future is not far when virtual surgical planning, automated guides, and prosthesis can be fabricated with a click of a button based on inputs and constraints given by the surgeon.

The future of CAD software is envisaged to be characterized by enhanced automation, integration of AI, and the use of augmented reality. Cloud-based software is predicted to gain popularity as it will allow access from anywhere and collaborate in real time. Software with parametric functionality can aid in faster design processes and revisions [46].

In CAM, newer generation 3D printers and CNC machines are more efficient and require less maintenance. Recently, low-budget desktop printers have been proven for clinical use. The use of 3D printing and CNC machining in combination with bioprinting could aid in the fabrication of living tissue replacements. 3D-printed scaffolds can be generated for cell seeding, culturing, and allowing them to grow and mature to form tissue constructs [47]. Currently, bioprinting is in the nascent stage; however, technological advancements will revolutionize its use in cranio-maxillofacial surgery.

7.7 Summary

The conversion of medical images (CT/CBCT/MRI/USG/3D scan) into 3D virtual images and then further into a tangible form requires a series of complex CAD/CAM procedures. These tangible models help in the 3D visualization and analysis of normal or altered anatomy. In addition, 3D artifacts like guides or templates further help the transferring of the whole virtual surgical plan to the operating room. Literature evidence proved that 3D-printed assisted surgeries have a better outcome and also show significant decreases in the surgical, anesthesia, and wound exposure time intraoperatively. Tangible artifacts help the treating surgeon not only with the accurate diagnosis but also in the execution of complex surgeries with a minimally invasive approach. Additionally, the patient can understand their disease or defect in a simple and better way. It further improves the patient's overall outcome and quality of life. Patients also prefer advanced technology-based digitally assisted surgical procedures that are less invasive. Hence, it is beneficial to both doctors and patients. Except for clinical applications, CAD/CAM solutions are also valuable in research and academic applications.

For the precise outcome, the quality of the 3D-printed artifact is an important factor to be considered. These medical 3D artifacts are considered medical devices; hence, it is strongly recommended to follow standard manufacturing protocol followed by appropriate sterilization methods before use.

However, CAD-/CAM-based artifacts have a few challenges like initial high cost, long turnaround time, the learning curve for virtual planning, etc. This can be overcome by doing regular awareness and training programs, establishing an in-house lab, and working as a team in an interdisciplinary field. In conclusion, recent advances in CAD/CAM technology with reduced costs, widespread uses, and increasing awareness among medical specialists have changed the entire gamut of surgical management of complex cases with a minimally invasive approach.

References

1. Ahmed KS, Ibad H, Suchal ZA, Gosain AK. Implementation of 3D printing and computer-aided design and manufacturing (CAD/CAM) in craniofacial reconstruction. J Craniofac Surg. 2022;33(6):1714–9.
2. Malik HH, Darwood ARJ, Shaunak S, Kulatilake P, El-Hilly AA, Mulki O, et al. Three-dimensional printing in surgery: a review of current surgical applications. J Surg Res. 2015;199(2):512–22.
3. Dawood A, Marti Marti B, Sauret-Jackson V, Darwood A. 3D printing in dentistry. Br Dent J. 2015;219(11):521–9.
4. Mazzoli A. Selective laser sintering in biomedical engineering. Med Biol Eng Comput. 2013;51(3):245–56.
5. Ostaş D, Almăşan O, Ileşan RR, Andrei V, Thieringer FM, Hedeşiu M, et al. Point-of-care virtual surgical planning and 3D printing in oral and cranio-maxillofacial surgery: a narrative review. J Clin Med. 2022;11.
6. Huotilainen E, Jaanimets R, Valášek J, Marcián P, Salmi M, Tuomi J, et al. Inaccuracies in additive manufactured medical skull models caused by the DICOM to STL conversion process. J Cranio-Maxillofacial Surg. 2014;42(5):e259–65.
7. Marro A, Bandukwala T, Mak W. Three-dimensional printing and medical imaging: a review of the methods and applications. Curr Probl Diagn Radiol. 2016;45(1):2–9.
8. Xu XW, Newman ST. Making CNC machine tools more open, interoperable and intelligent—a review of the technologies. Comput Ind. 2006;57(2):141–52.
9. Asiltürk İ, Neşeli S, İnce MA. Optimization of parameters affecting surface roughness of Co28Cr6Mo medical material during CNC lathe machining by using the Taguchi and RSM methods. Measurement. 2016;78:120–8.
10. Dizon JRC, Gache CCL, Cascolan HMS, Cancino LT, Advincula RC. Post-processing of 3D-printed polymers, vol. 9. Technologies; 2021.
11. Nguyen TK, Lee B-K. Post-processing of FDM parts to improve surface and thermal properties. Rapid Prototyp J. 2018;24(7):1091–100.
12. Takayama T, Todo M, Tsuji H. Effect of annealing on the mechanical properties of PLA/PCL and PLA/PCL/LTI polymer blends. J Mech Behav Biomed Mater. 2011;4(3):255–60.
13. Phillips BT, Allder J, Bolan G, Nagle RS, Redington A, Hellebrekers T, et al. Additive manufacturing aboard a moving vessel at sea using passively stabilized stereolithography (SLA) 3D printing. Addit Manuf. 2020;31:100969.
14. Peng X, Kong L, Fuh JYH, Wang H. A review of post-processing technologies in additive manufacturing. J Manuf Mater Process. 2021;5(2).
15. Aguado-Maestro I, De Frutos-Serna M, González-Nava A, Merino-De Santos AB, García-Alonso M. Are the common sterilization methods completely effective for our in-house 3D printed biomodels and surgical guides? Injury. 2021;52(6):1341–5.
16. Rankin TM, Giovinco NA, Cucher DJ, Watts G, Hurwitz B, Armstrong DG. Three-dimensional printing surgical instruments: are we there yet? J Surg Res. 2014;189(2):193–7.
17. Torabi K, Farjood E, Hamedani S. Rapid prototyping technologies and their applications in prosthodontics, a review of literature. J Dent (Shiraz, Iran). 2015;16(1):1–9.
18. Marty M, Broutin A, Vergnes J-N, Vaysse F. Comparison of student's perceptions between 3D printed models versus series models in pediatric dentistry hands-on session. Eur J Dent Educ. 2019;23(1):68–72.
19. Anderson J, Wealleans J, Ray J. Endodontic applications of 3D printing. Int Endod J. 2018;51(9):1005–18.
20. Liu H, Liu D, Wang G, Wang C, Zhao Z. Accuracy of surgical positioning of orthodontic miniscrews with a computer-aided design and manufacturing template. Am J Orthod Dentofacial Orthop. 2010;137(6):728.e1–728.e10.
21. Lin L, Fang Y, Liao Y, Chen G, Gao C, Zhu P. 3D printing and digital processing techniques in dentistry: a review of literature. Adv Eng Mater. 2019;21(6):1801013.
22. Flügge TV, Nelson K, Schmelzeisen R, Metzger MC. Three-dimensional plotting and printing of an implant drilling guide: simplifying guided implant surgery. J Oral Maxillofac Surg. 2013;71(8):1340–6.
23. Herlin C, Koppe M, Béziat J-L, Gleizal A. Rapid prototyping in craniofacial surgery: using a positioning guide after zygomatic osteotomy—a case report. J Cranio-Maxillofacial Surg. 2011;39(5):376–9.
24. Elegbede A, Diaconu SC, McNichols CHL, Seu M, Rasko YM, Grant MP, et al. Office-based three-dimensional printing workflow for craniomaxillofacial fracture repair. J Craniofac Surg. 2018;29(5):e440.
25. Alagarsamy R, Lal B, Sagar S, Roychoudhury A, Yadav R. Digital workflow for treating comminuted anterior mandibular fracture—a technical note. J Stomatol Oral Maxillofac Surg. 2021;122(4):453–5.
26. Hartmann A, Kämmerer P, Ortolano LC, Sagheb K, Seiler M. Customised products for orbital wall reconstruction: a systematic review. Br J Oral Maxillofac Surg. 2022;60(5):e702–11.

27. Tarsitano A, Battaglia S, Ricotta F, Bortolani B, Cercenelli L, Marcelli E, et al. Accuracy of CAD/CAM mandibular reconstruction: a three-dimensional, fully virtual outcome evaluation method. J Cranio-Maxillo-Facial Surg. 2018;46(7):1121–5.
28. Yang W-F, Choi WS, Leung YY, Curtin JP, Du R, Zhang C-Y, et al. Three-dimensional printing of patient-specific surgical plates in head and neck reconstruction: a prospective pilot study. Oral Oncol. 2018;78:31–6.
29. Alagarsamy R, Roychoudhury A, Bhutia O, Lal B, Yadav R, Bhalla AS. Evaluation of fit feasibility of stock total joint replacement in temporomandibular joint ankylosis patients. Br J Oral Maxillofac Surg. 2021;59(7):792–7.
30. Movahed R, Wolford LM. Protocol for concomitant temporomandibular joint custom-fitted total joint reconstruction and orthognathic surgery using computer-assisted surgical simulation. Oral Maxillofac Surg Clin North Am. 2015;27(1):37–45.
31. Mercuri LG. Alloplastic temporomandibular joint replacement: rationale for the use of custom devices. Int J Oral Maxillofac Surg. 2012;41(9):1033–40.
32. Mahmoud K, Galal N, Ali S, Gibaly A, Elbehairy MS, Mounir M. Computer-guided arthrocentesis using patient-specific guides: a novel protocol for treatment of internal derangement of the temporomandibular joint. J Oral Maxillofac Surg. 2020;78(3):372.e1–7.
33. Zhang N, Liu S, Hu Z, Hu J, Zhu S, Li Y. Accuracy of virtual surgical planning in two-jaw orthognathic surgery: comparison of planned and actual results. Oral Surg Oral Med Oral Pathol Oral Radiol. 2016;122(2):143–51.
34. Metzger MC, Hohlweg-Majert B, Schwarz U, Teschner M, Hammer B, Schmelzeisen R. Manufacturing splints for orthognathic surgery using a three-dimensional printer. Oral Surg Oral Med Oral Pathol Oral Radiol Endodontol. 2008;105(2):e1–7.
35. Hany HE-D, El Hadidi YN, Sleem H, Taha M, El Kassaby M. Novel technique and step-by-step construction of a computer-guided stent for mandibular distraction osteogenesis. J Craniofac Surg. 2019;30(7):2271–4.
36. Seeberger R, Davids R, Kater W, Thiele OC. Use of stereolithographic drilling and cutting guides in bilateral mandibular distraction. J Craniofac Surg. 2011;22(6):2031–5.
37. Lal B, Alagarsamy R, Agarwal B, Bhutia O, Roychoudhury A. Patient-specific three-dimensional printed template for halo frame pin placement for multiple skull bone defects after cranioplasty. Br J Oral Maxillofac Surg. 2021;59(7):847–9.
38. Arias E, Huang Y-H, Zhao L, Seelaus R, Patel P, Cohen M. Virtual surgical planning and three-dimensional printed guide for soft tissue correction in facial asymmetry. J Craniofac Surg. 2019;30(3):846.
39. Bekisz JM, Liss HA, Maliha SG, Witek L, Coelho PG, Flores RL. In-house manufacture of Sterilizable, scaled, patient-specific 3D-printed models for rhinoplasty. Aesthetic Surg J. 2019;39(3):254–63.
40. La Padula S, Hersant B, Chatel H, Aguilar P, Bosc R, Roccaro G, et al. One-step facial feminization surgery: the importance of a custom-made preoperative planning and patient satisfaction assessment. J Plast Reconstr Aesthet Surg. 2019;72(10):1694–9.
41. Chang P-C. Computer-assisted planning and 3D printing-assisted modeling for Chin augmentation. Aesthetic Surg J. 2017;38(1):1–10.
42. Zarean P, Zarean P, Thieringer FM, Mueller AA, Kressmann S, Erismann M, et al. A point-of-care digital workflow for 3D printed passive presurgical orthopedic plates in cleft care. Child (Basel, Switzerland). 2022;9(8).
43. Shirota T, Kurabayashi H, Ogura H, Seki K, Maki K, Shintani S. Analysis of bone volume using computer simulation system for secondary bone graft in alveolar cleft. Int J Oral Maxillofac Surg. 2010;39(9):904–8.
44. Van der Meij AJW, Baart JA, Prahl-Andersen B, Valk J, Kostense PJ, Tuinzing DB. Bone volume after secondary bone grafting in unilateral and bilateral clefts determined by computed tomography scans. Oral Surg Oral Med Oral Pathol Oral Radiol Endodontol. 2001;92(2):136–41.
45. Lal B, Ghosh M, Agarwal B, Gupta D, Roychoudhury A. A novel economically viable solution for 3D printing-assisted cranioplast fabrication. Br J Neurosurg. 2020;34(3):280–3.
46. Hirz M, Rossbacher P, Gulanová J. Future trends in CAD—from the perspective of automotive industry. Comput Aided Des Appl. 2017;14(6):734–41.
47. Bishop ES, Mostafa S, Pakvasa M, Luu HH, Lee MJ, Wolf JM, et al. 3-D bioprinting technologies in tissue engineering and regenerative medicine: current and future trends. Genes Dis. 2017;4(4):185–95.

Computational Analysis of 3D Craniofacial Imaging

8

Kausalya Neelavara Makkithaya, Sindhoora Kaniyala Melanthota, Rajib Biswas, Shailendra Singh Rana, Manikanth Karnati, and Nirmal Mazumder

8.1 Introduction

Three-dimensional imaging produces the perception of depth inside an image by converting 2D data into a 3D format. In craniofacial research, 3D imaging is focused on the diagnosis and treatment of traumatic injuries, congenital defects, and malformations. Thus, the field has evolved to be multidisciplinary, contributed by oral and maxillofacial surgeons, orthodontists, geneticists, epidemiologists, developmental biologists, and, more recently, computer scientists. Accurate representation of the human skull is important to facilitate appropriate diagnosis and treatment plans to be provided by the clinician. However, reading and assimilation of the data is quite challenging on a day-to-day basis.

Three-dimensional imaging uses cutting-edge technology to gather anatomical data, handle it by a computer, and show the illusion of depth on a 2D monitor [1]. Hence, the field of medical imaging is codependent on the technology and undergoing constant changes. There is a recent surge in the application of artificial intelligence (AI) due to the development of deep learning (DL) based tools and the advantages offered by the technology [2].

Advances made in the field of computer science and 3D imaging technology have enabled the application of computational methods for the analysis of the craniofacial region. Computational analysis strategies enable the researcher to analyze the images and predict treatment outcomes more effectively through simulations. The application of computational analysis methods also enables researchers to use the digitally available data to innovate new approaches for craniofacial image analysis. This chapter discusses the computational techniques employed for image processing and analysis of images from the craniofacial region, their applications in craniofacial research, and their drawbacks.

8.2 Analysis Techniques

Data modeling and analysis play a crucial role in many applied sciences, including finance, engineering, and many others. With the expanding amount of clinical data, the demand for support in data analysis has also increased. Thereby, combining emerging data science technologies and AI, gathered data can produce new results

K. N. Makkithaya · S. K. Melanthota · M. Karnati · N. Mazumder (✉)
Department of Biophysics, Manipal School of Life Sciences, Manipal Academy of Higher Education, Manipal, Karnataka, India
e-mail: nirmal.mazumder@manipal.edu

R. Biswas
Department of Physics, Tezpur University, Tezpur, Assam, India

S. S. Rana
Department of Dentistry, All India Institute of Medical Sciences, Bathinda, Punjab, India

S. S. Rana et al. (eds.), *Applications of Three-dimensional Imaging for Craniofacial Region*, https://doi.org/10.1007/978-981-97-4608-8_8

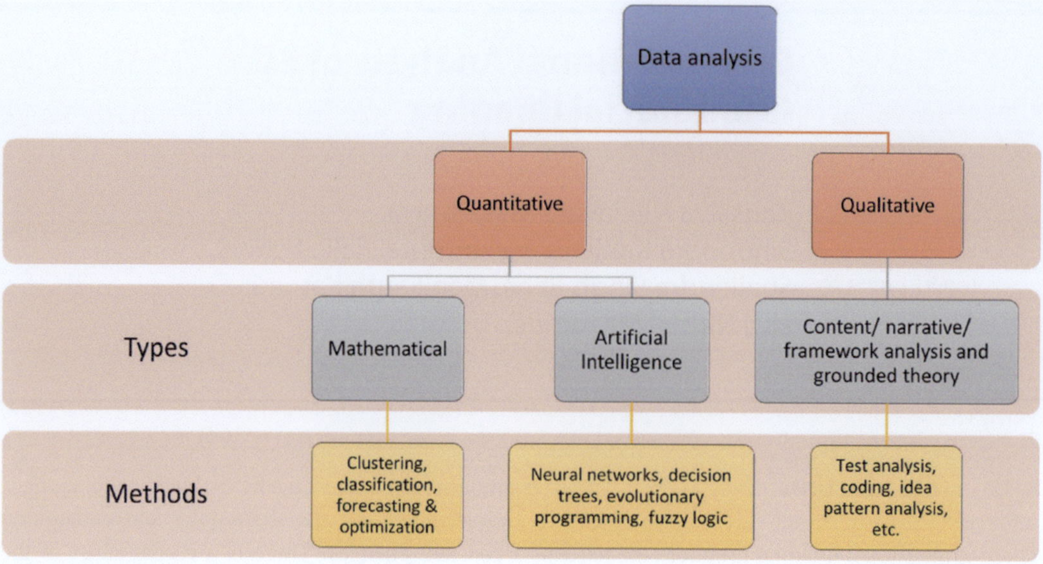

Fig. 8.1 Flowchart of data analysis: types, methods, and techniques

[3]. Numerous algorithms find applications in statistics, machine learning, and related disciplines. However, the decision regarding which algorithm to employ hinges on the specific distribution utilized for modeling the data [4]. Because of its complicated morphology, delineating the craniofacial structure is difficult, and manual elucidation has low repeatability and might take a long period. Of all available techniques of data analysis (Fig. 8.1), few computational analytical algorithms have paved the way in aiding clinicians and researchers, particularly in the field of craniofacial radiology, surgery, and orthodontics, which are discussed below.

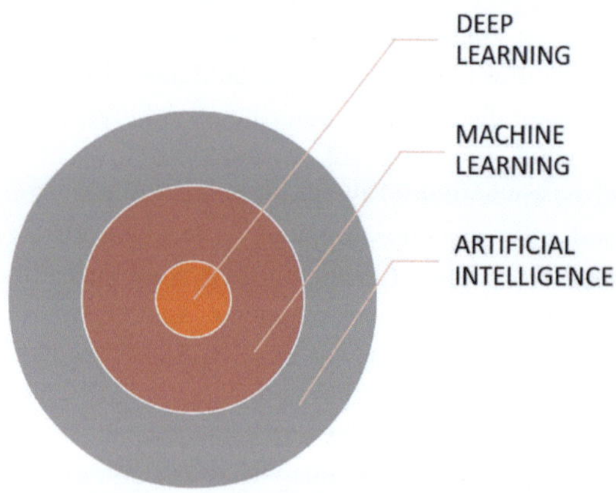

Fig. 8.2 Conceptual relationship between artificial intelligence, machine learning, and deep learning

8.2.1 Machine Learning

Automatic picture segmentation from machine learning and artificial intelligence (AI) techniques relieves the stress of manual processing while increasing reliability [5]. Understanding the conceptual connections between AI, machine learning, and deep learning is crucial for comprehending the definition and application of AI (Fig. 8.2). Machine learning is the use of AI in an engineering environment, but the phrase "AI" has a very broad meaning.

Machine learning constitutes a data analysis technique that significantly automates the analytical process. Falling within the domain of artificial intelligence, it operates on the premise that machines can acquire knowledge from provided datasets, discern patterns, and render decisions with minimal human intervention. It involves the writing of algorithms that are trained to analyze or "learn" a set of existing data and use it to analyze a new dataset similar to the trained data. Machine learning algorithms are mostly based on statistical problem-solving techniques and mathematical probability. However, the additional computational techniques allow machine learning algorithms to outperform the established statistical approaches [6]. Machine learning algorithms can predict patterns or classify data points in unseen data based on a set of parameters. The algorithm is trained on the features of a dataset. The accuracy of the prediction or classification performed by the algorithm depends on the quality of the features the algorithm is trained on. The development and deployment of a machine learning algorithm have the following steps: a) training, b) testing, and c) validation. The training stage of the process is of utmost importance because the performance of the algorithm in the further stages depends on it. The accuracy of the algorithm could be improved by increasing the size of the dataset used for training. The algorithm's performance is evaluated in the testing phase, using the testing dataset. Here, the accuracy and bias of the algorithm are determined, and steps are taken to reduce the bias and increase the variance, to achieve a nearly accurate algorithm. The performance of the algorithm is assessed using a validation dataset [7]. Machine learning is categorized into three distinct groups—supervised learning, unsupervised learning, and reinforcement learning—which are determined by the nature of the dataset employed to train the algorithms [8] (Fig. 8.3).

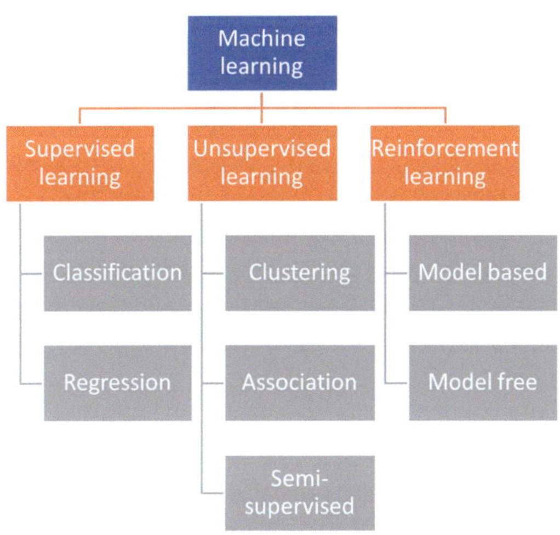

Fig. 8.3 Flowchart showing types of machine learning algorithms

8.2.1.1 Supervised Learning

In supervised machine learning, an algorithm undergoes training using a meticulously labeled dataset, allowing the system to acquire the capacity to predict and classify instances based on the information contained within the training dataset. The labeled data here shows the inputs that have already been mapped to their specific outputs. After being trained with the input and matching output, machines are told to predict the output using the test dataset. Correlating the input variable (x) with the outcome (y) is the main goal of the supervised learning approach. (a) Classification techniques are used to solve problems where the output variable is categorical, i.e., "yes" or "no," red or blue, etc. The classification algorithms forecast the categories that are present in the dataset. There are now systems in place for classifying emails, like spam detection and filtering. (b) The regression techniques are used to tackle regression problems where there is a linear relationship between the input and output variables. They are used to predict continuous output variables, such as market movements, weather prediction, etc.

8.2.1.2 Unsupervised Learning

The unsupervised learning algorithm is trained using a non-labeled dataset, and the algorithm clusters data points based on the patterns identified. The primary objective of the unsupervised learning approach is to classify or combine the unsorted dataset based on patterns, similarities, and differences. The input dataset's hidden patterns are to be discovered by the algorithm. (a) Clustering: The natural groups in the data are located using the clustering technique. It's a method of organizing things so that those closest to each other stay in that group and don't resemble anything in other groupings at all. (b) Association: Intriguing connections between variables in a huge dataset are found using the unsupervised learning technique association rule learning. To map the variables in a way that maximizes profit, this learning algorithm's main objective is to find the dependencies between data items. In continuous production, market basket analysis, web usage mining, etc., this technique is frequently employed. (c) Semi-supervised learning: This machine learning approach that is in between supervised and unsupervised learning is called semi-supervised learning. It bridges the gap between supervised learning algorithms, which use labeled training data, and unsupervised learning algorithms, which do not, by utilizing both labeled and unlabeled datasets during the training phase. Although semi-supervised learning is a middle ground between supervised and unsupervised learning, it typically uses unlabeled data. It operates on data that contains a few labels. It is completely different from supervised and unsupervised learning, which depend on the presence or absence of labels. The idea of semi-supervised learning is presented to address the shortcomings of supervised learning and unsupervised learning algorithms. Instead of using solely labeled data, the primary goal of semi-supervised learning is to make optimal use of all accessible data. An unsupervised learning technique is first used to cluster comparable data, and it also aids in labeling the unlabeled data into labeled data. This happens since the labeled data is a comparatively more expensive acquisition than unlabeled data.

8.2.1.3 Reinforcement Learning

Reinforcement learning algorithms improve the output based on reward-dependent learning. Here the algorithm is involved in learning from the environment, and this process is continuous [9].

8.2.2 Finite Element Analysis

To fully comprehend and quantify physical phenomena, such as the behavior of structures or fluids, thermal transfer, wave propagation, or the development of biological cells, mathematics has been required. These phenomena are described through partial differential equations (PDEs). The advancement of computers and computational technologies have allowed the PDEs to be solved computationally through many numerical strategies. One of the methodologies employed is the finite element method (FEM), a prevalent computational approach utilized in addressing problems within applied mathematics and engineering, notably through finite element analysis (FEA). It deals with physical systems that are exposed to certain external forces under a specific set of conditions.

The foundation of FEM is the minimization principle, which asserts that when a boundary condition (such as displacement or force) is applied, only that configuration of the body's many possible configurations—where the total energy is lowest—is selected. The simulation will produce the same results no matter how many times it is run (R). Courant invented this technique in 1943 to explore the torsion on a cylinder. The method has experienced significant advancement owing to its applicability in various domains such as thermal, electromagnetic, fluid, and structural analysis under working conditions. The core principle underlying finite element analysis posits that intricate geometries can be decomposed into a finite set of simpler components, each representing the complex geometry. This partitioning encompasses diverse material properties and local features [10]. To understand the concept of FEM, consider a body through which the distribution of a field variable, e.g., displacement or stress, is required (Fig. 8.4). The body can be either a one-, two-, or three-dimensional solid that can be split into an assembly of smaller "finite" elements. The model's degrees of freedom must be limited to a finite quantity. Interconnected joints called "nodes" link the finite elements together. There are no spaces or surfaces between elements because they are conceptually small regions rather than distinct objects. A mesh is the collective term for the entire set or assemblage of elements. The process of representing a component as a group of finite elements is known as discretization. When the model has been discretized, or broken down into discrete pieces, the governing equations for each element are calculated and then combined to generate system equations (the mesh). After the general structure of the equations for that element type (such as a linear distribution element) has been established, calculating the equations for each instance of a specific element in the body is straightforward. Nodal coordinates,

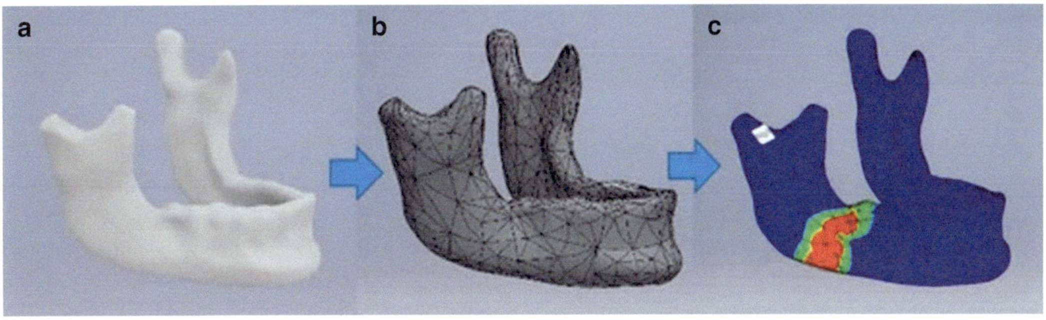

Fig. 8.4 Finite element analysis (FEA): (**a**) numerical model of the lower jaw, (**b**) division into finite elements, (**c**) FEA of simulated forces at different regions of the numerical model. (This figure was reproduced with permission (Lisiak-Myszke M et al. 2020) [13])

material properties, and element loading conditions can all be simply substituted in the general format. Equations of each element given are used to derive the equations to describe the entire system as an entity. However, some kind of boundary condition must be used before the equation may be "inverted" and solved. The body must be stopped from rigid body action when experiencing stress. Once the matrix equations have been created, the system of equations is solved by passing the equations to a solver. Direct or iterative problem-solvers are usually applied, depending on the type of problem.

Since experimental investigations necessitate the use of living animals in laboratories, ethical committees frequently object to them. FEM makes it possible to foresee how the tissue will react to the use of orthodontic mechanics. In orthodontics and craniofacial imaging, a geometrical model is created based on digital equivalents such as CBCT images, CAD software images, microtomography, etc. Material properties such as Young's modulus or Poisson's ratio are assigned to each dissected element. These mechanical properties are a result of a set of experimental studies. Finally, the model is simulated such that it receives forces at different regions. The specific stresses and strains of the model in response to the simulated forces are then studied [11]. Knowledge of the biomechanics of craniofacial structures is important to ensure optimal treatment. FEA models allow the surgeon to analyze and determine the impact of various stresses and strains that occur on the craniofacial structures and the adjacent soft tissues, due to several biomechanical changes. The simulations performed on the FEA models also aid in determining an appropriate fixation system, thus reducing the cases of failed fixation caused due to improper selection or positioning [12, 13].

8.2.3 Computational Fluid Dynamics

Being the field of aerodynamic engineering, computational fluid dynamics (CFD) uses computer-based simulation to analyze fluid flow, energy transfer, and related processes in their whole [14]. CFD is a widely used approach for resolving difficult issues in engineering fields, and its application is also being acknowledged in several sectors of medical sciences involving airway and circulatory studies. Computational fluid dynamics (CFD) is widely used in many engineering and biomedical domains, including vehicle aerodynamics and hydrodynamics, power plants (including turbines), electronic and chemical engineering, exterior and interior architectural design, marine and environmental engineering, hydrology, and meteorology [15].

The CFD technique has been frequently used to examine airflow in both healthy and problematic human airways. It performs the function of computer-based software that simulates fluid movement. The ability to use experimental simulation to evaluate extremely complicated systems or circumstances is one advantage of the

CFD methodology over other fluid mechanics analysis methodologies (e.g., airways). Fluid motion and how processes are impacted by fluid flow behavior can be assessed using CFD software. The physical characteristics of fluid mobility are described by basic mathematical equations. These equations, which typically take the form of partial differential equations, control the process of interest. As a result, the equations are frequently referred to as the governing equations. Supercomputer programming languages are used to decipher the Navier-Stroke equation. Numerical simulations used in the study of fluid flow are produced as a result of high-speed supercomputer algorithms that seek out numerical solutions [16, 17].

Medical researchers can evaluate and standardize the basic principles of respiration, circulation, and body fluid flow, as well as the expected performance of system components, for research studies. The models can be modified in any way, making it possible to produce biomedical interventions with more definitive oversight.

8.3 Applications

8.3.1 Machine Learning

AI and ML are seeing an increased application for the analysis of data. Machine learning tools developed are applied for image analysis increasingly in the medical sector. Numerous investigations have been conducted on the utilization of machine learning for the identification, diagnosis, and prediction of cancer and allied ailments in the craniofacial region.

8.3.1.1 Cephalometric Landmark Identification

The application of computer-aided analysis of skeletal landmarks for cephalometric analysis was first used in 1984 [18]. This paved the way for the use of computers for the analysis of cephalometric data. Cephalometric landmark detection and annotation is an important procedure in orthodontics. The quantitative evaluation of these landmarks provides information on the skull and the surrounding soft tissues. Cephalometric landmark annotation is performed on the two-dimensional cephalogram. The procedure is tedious and subject to random errors when performed manually, thus giving rise to the need for computational techniques for the automation of the process [19, 20]. Several models were introduced to assist in analyzing the cephalometric landmarks accurately. Yue et al. put forth an active shape model (ASM) for the identification of lateral landmarks in the cephalometric radiograph. The model applied principal component analysis and gray pattern matching for landmark identification in cephalograms. The model was however limited due to the limited resolution of the cephalogram. It was also found that the accuracy of the model was dependent on the quality of the images, thus limiting the application of the proposed model for cephalometric analysis [21]. This limitation was overcome in another model proposed by Kunz et al. [22] The authors applied convoluted neural networks (CNNs) for image analysis of the cephalograms. The CNN model was trained using manually positioned lateral cephalometric graphs. The model was also based on only look once algorithm, which has proven to be computationally efficient in previous studies [23, 24]. The accuracy of the model was also optimized based on the opinions of the experts, thus leading to an effective and robust model.

Two-dimensional imaging was popular in the earlier stages of craniofacial imaging. However, with the advent of three-dimensional imaging techniques like CBCT imaging, it is possible to obtain a more accurate spatial representation of the oral and craniofacial structures with precise cephalometric measurements. The landmark marking of these three-dimensional images is challenging, due to its time-consuming nature and the requirement of significant experience to do so manually. The advances in the field of computer science have led to the integration of computational tools for the automation of such analyses [25]. In this regard, Gupta et al. have proposed an algorithm based on MATLAB programming for cephalometric landmark identification from CBCT images. The algorithm was successful in detecting 20 landmarks with an overall mean error of 2.01 mm. When compared to manual detection and other existing algorithms, the proposed algorithm showed a detection range of 90.33% within a 4 mm error range of manually marked landmarks [26]. Ma et al. mechanized the landmarking process using a variety of machine learning approaches, including principal component analysis (PCA) and convolutional neural networks (CNNs). PCA was used to consider the correlation and anatomical relationships between the different cephalometric landmarks and create a shape model which was used as a part of the training model for the CNN network. The results showed that the accuracy of the automated model was within 5.785 mm, thereby indicating that the model had a distinctive advantage over the traditional landmarking methods [27]. Despite the progress from using manual cephalometric landmarking to the application of machine learning to do the same, there are some issues with the handling of the dimensionality of the 3D cephalometric images such as 3D CT scans that are yet to be tackled by the scientific world. In their work, Lee et al. have attempted to solve this issue by using multiple shadowed 2D images in a layer-by-layer manner to generate a two-dimensional image with three-dimensional cues. These cues were then used to train a deep learning network to obtain the cephalometric landmarks [28]. Li et al. have demonstrated the application of artificial neural networks (ANNs) to assess all possibilities of orthodontic treatment plans. This included scenarios of determination of extraction, non-extraction, the patterns of extraction, and the existing anchorage patterns. The developed model was able to aid the doctor in making decisions regarding the orthodontic treatment plan with an accuracy of 94%, sensitivity of 94.6%, and 93.8% (Fig. 8.5) [29].

8.3.1.2 Orthognathic Surgery

Correct diagnosis and treatment planning are some of the key factors for successful orthognathic surgery. A correct and timely diagnosis and an effective treatment plan by a clinician would

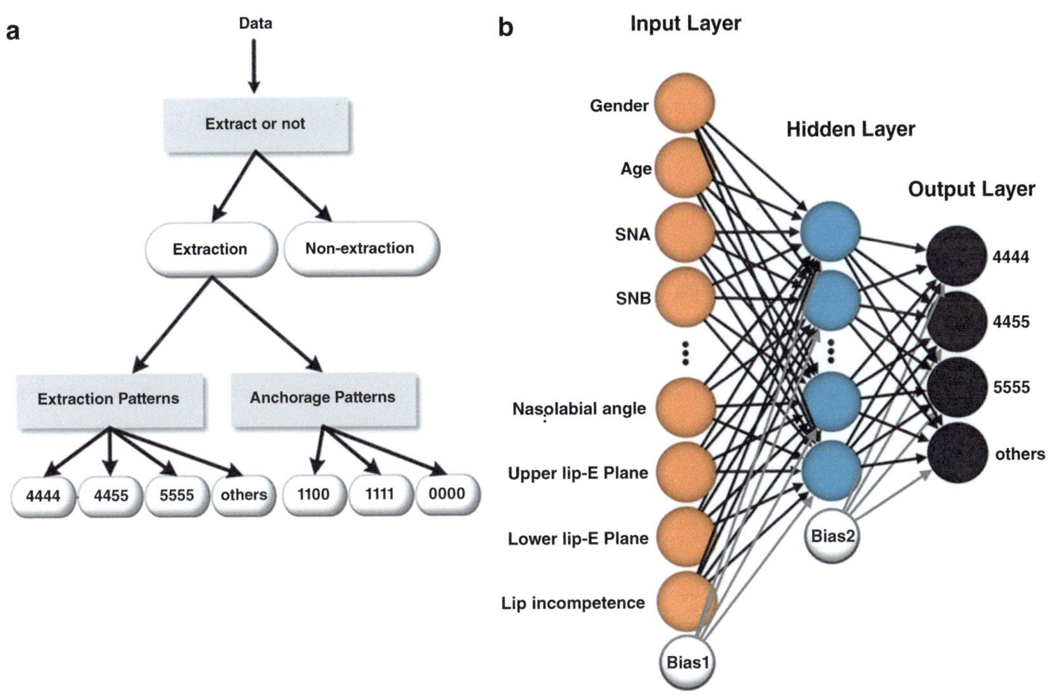

Fig. 8.5 (**a**) Methodology followed for data processing and (**b**) structure of neural network developed to predict extraction patterns in orthodontic treatment plans. (This figure was reproduced with permission from (Li P et al. 2019) [29])

go a long way in ensuring the well-being of the patient. The advances made in the computational field enable the incorporation of computational techniques for effective and speedy decision-making in the medical field as well. Choi et al. have proposed the application of artificial neural networks to aid in the effective planning of orthognathic surgery. The model developed was trained with cephalometric landmarks of individuals requiring the surgery and those not requiring the surgery. The diagnosis of the developed model was compared to that of a trained expert in the field. It was found that the model was able to diagnose surgeries/non-surgeries for the patients with an accuracy of 96%. The model was also able to give a detailed diagnosis of the type of surgery to be employed with an accuracy of 91% [30]. Deep learning was applied by Jeong et al., to study the soft tissue profiles of the craniofacial area before orthognathic surgery. The CNN model developed was able to classify the patients who needed an orthognathic surgery and those who did not need the surgery with an accuracy of 89.3% by judging them based on the soft tissue profiles of the patients [31]. In another study, Lin et al. applied CNN and transfer learning methods to evaluate the facial symmetry of the patients before and after the orthognathic surgery, thereby allowing the doctors to enhance the medical treatments offered to their patients. CBCT scans were used to train the deep learning model, and transfer learning was applied to amplify the dataset without compromising the integrity of the images and to optimize and adjust various parameters of the model [32]. Detection of periapical lesions is an important step for the diagnosis of apical periodontitis. Apical periodontitis is currently detected by the interpretation of CBCT images which is performed by a clinician, making this a tedious task and also resulting in a low rate of agreement between clinical observers. This issue was addressed by Setzer et al. in their work wherein a deep learning model developed by the authors was trained for the identification of lesions in the CBCT images. The model was also used to segment and classify the lesions like the periapical lesions, tooth structure, bone, and restorative materials. In the segmentation phase, the model attained 93% accuracy and 88% specificity [33].

8.3.1.3 Applications of Supervised Learning

A few of the common applications of supervised learning are given below [8]:

- Image segmentation

  Picture or image segmentation employs supervised learning algorithms. This approach does picture classification on a variety of image data using preestablished labels.
- Medical diagnosis

  In the medical field, supervised algorithms are frequently employed for diagnostic purposes. Using historical data, which includes labeling for medical images and disease scenarios, it is finished. The computer might be able to diagnose a disease in new patients using this technique.
- Fraud detection

  To detect fraudulent clients, transactions, etc., algorithms for supervised learning are used. Historical data is utilized to identify patterns that could indicate probable fraud.
- Spam detection

  Classification algorithms are used for spam identification and filtering. These algorithms determine whether or not an email is spam. The spam folder receives the emails.
- Speech recognition

  Speech recognition also makes use of supervised learning techniques. Voice data was used to train the system, which can now recognize a variety of objects, including passwords and voice-activated commands.

8.3.1.4 Applications of Unsupervised Learning

Network analysis: While analyzing text data for scholarly papers using document network analysis, unsupervised learning is utilized to detect plagiarism and copyright.

Recommendation systems: Recommendation systems commonly use unsupervised learning approaches to generate suggestion applications for different online applications and e-commerce websites.

Anomaly detection: Anomaly detection, which may identify out-of-the-ordinary data points in the dataset, such as to uncover fraudulent transactions, is another use of unsupervised learning.

Singular value decomposition: Singular value decomposition, or SVD for short, is a technique for retrieving specific information from databases. Compiling information about every user in a specific area is an example of SVD.

8.3.2 Finite Element Analysis

8.3.2.1 Trauma Surgery

Investigating the impact of facial trauma in vivo is a daunting task due to ethical considerations. A trustworthy physical test model that accurately represents the complexity of the mechanical parameters of the facial soft tissue and bones is difficult to develop. This endeavor is also costly mainly due to its single-use nature, thus making the application of virtual models like FEA for stress analysis practical and cost-effective.

A virtual platform of the human cranium was developed by Perestrelo et al., to analyze cranial injuries and head trauma. The virtual platform was implemented with a BioCAD protocol, including CT (computed tomography) software, CAD (computer-aided design) software, and FEA. The results of the virtual platform were found to be by the literature describing the simulated injuries [34]. FEA has also been used for the analysis of the strength or weakness of the mandibular bone, which is extremely susceptible to damage due to trauma. The influence of the presence of a third molar on the mandibular weakness was also examined through finite element analysis (FEA) [35]. The possibility of occurrence of an iatrogenic fracture on the excess removal of the bone around the impacted third molar was also investigated using FEA. It was concluded that during surgical procedures that involve removing the external oblique ridge, mandibular stress is extremely high during normal clenching, thus suggesting that the surgeons could modify their approach to such surgeries [36]. Mandibular fractures are some of the most common facial injuries that occur due to falls in elderly patients making it a major healthcare concern requiring immediate assistance. An earlier response in situations of trauma is of importance. FEA has enabled Santos et al. to map the exact distribution of stress in the geriatric edentulous mandible, due to trauma in the symphyseal region, parasymphyseal region, and the mandible itself. This is potentially useful to emergency responders facing a similar situation of mandibular fractures among the elderly [37].

8.3.2.2 Orthognathic Surgery

FEA is also helpful in performing orthognathic surgeries to assess the stress and strains in the region of surgery, thereby aiding the surgeon in treating the patients more effectively (Fig. 8.6). Bridging elements are a key component in orthognathic surgeries that treat splits and other maxillary trauma. The use of an appropriate bridging material for such surgeries is a crucial factor that decides the success of the surgery and the overall well-being of the patient. FEA has been applied in numerous scenarios to test the effectiveness and stability of various materials available to perform a bilateral split osteotomy. Larson et al. analyzed the stability and stress distribution of the techniques used to fix a sliding plate and a conventional miniplate through FEA [38]. In another study, Ghorashi et al. applied FEA to construct a model to deduce an effective fixation method used in bilateral sagittal split osteotomy surgery [39]. The studies demonstrated the application of FEA to gain an understanding and analyze the effect of various surgical techniques on the bones of the craniofacial region and the stress distribution overall [40, 41].

FEA was also found to be useful in analyzing and simulating the risk of fractures that may occur during an osteotomy. In a study by Fujii et al., the authors constructed a 3D FEA model using the imaging data and were able to simulate the pterygomaxillary disjunctions. The model was successfully used for the simulation of fracture lines and prediction of pterygomaxillary disjunction patterns that occur during various

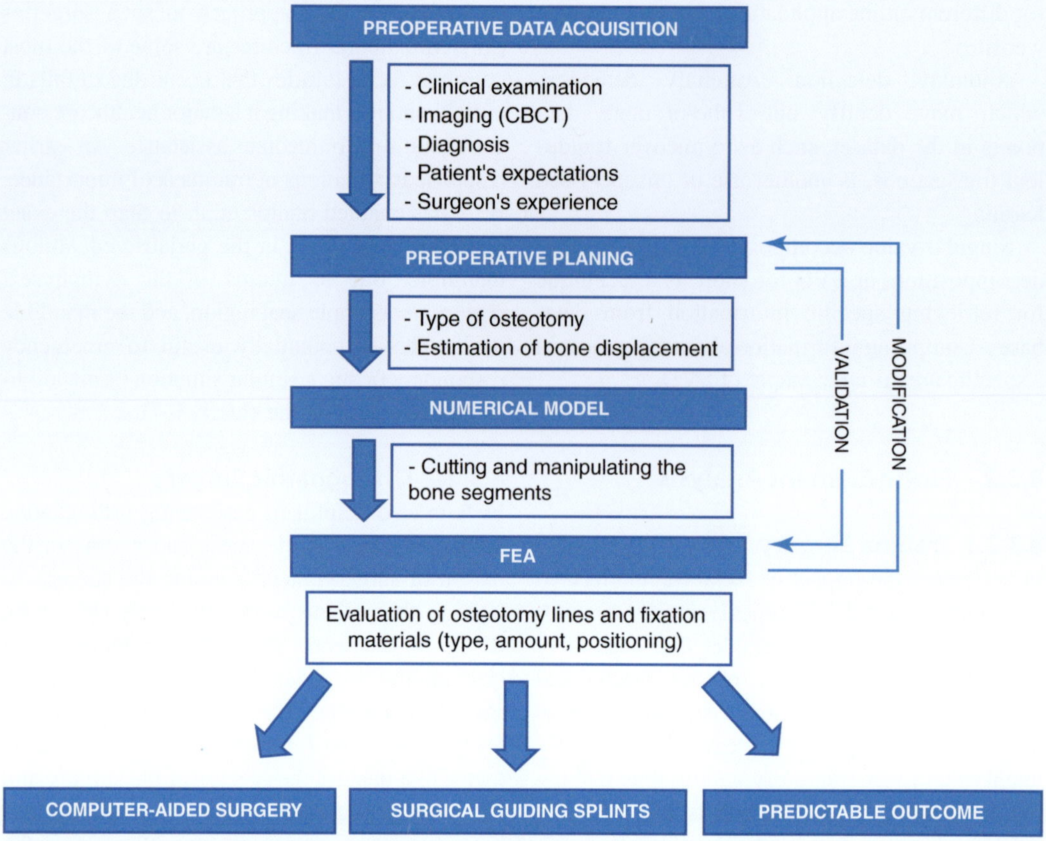

Fig. 8.6 Application of FEA in computer-aided planning of orthognathic surgeries. (This figure was reproduced with permission from (Lisiak-Myszke M et al. 2020) [13])

procedures in the surgery, thus enabling surgeons to better plan and assess the risks and benefits of selecting specific procedures during the osteotomy [42].

8.3.2.3 Orthodontics and Dentofacial Orthopedics

FEM makes it possible to foresee how the tissue will react to the use of orthodontic mechanics. Photoelastic models provide an alternative experimental model for analyzing the biomechanics of tooth movement [43]; however, they have the drawback of just studying the model's surface, leaving interior structures, like the periodontal ligament, unexplored. The FEM has transformed biomechanical research in orthodontics by eliminating the aforementioned drawbacks. It stands for a precise, noninvasive procedure that offers quantitative information about the physiological reactions taking place in tissues like the periodontal ligament and the alveolar bone [44]. It is challenging to accurately estimate the potential stress and tension that might emerge in oral tissues using any other experimental techniques because of the interplay between the surrounding tissues and the individual reaction. One advantage of FEM is that it makes it possible to evaluate all research factors and a homogenous sample at the same time [45]. It is critical to utilize resources in which anatomical data changes could be easily monitored and studied accurately for the creation of a geometrically accurate model for simulating the experiments in the CADD software. Image processing and digital reconstruction software, such as Mimics (Materialize, Leuven Belgium) or Simpleware 4, are used to create a virtual model for such purposes (Simpleware Ltd., Exeter, UK) [46]. The maxillomandibular complex is reconstructed using computed tomography. Cross sections that are at least 0.25 mm apart could be used to perform computed tomography at a higher resolution. After being recorded in the DICOM (Digital Imaging and Communications in Medicine) format, the sections are loaded into software for image processing and digital reconstruction. Nonetheless, it is well known that the clinical tomography's contrast and definition levels lead to inadequate reconstruction outcomes for the reconstruction software's automatic segmentation structures. Determining the boundaries of anatomical features such as the periodontal ligament, enamel, or even the medullary and cortical bone becomes difficult as a result. However, micro CTs enable the acquisition of gauge-scale information [47].

After FEM processing, the data makes it possible to examine how pressures between the periodontal ligament and the bone have distributed stress throughout the craniofacial region. This highlights the areas of tension and, in turn, the movements of the teeth. Because of it, we can also make judgments about areas that are more susceptible to root resorption. These results are illustrated with colors and arrows that indicate the direction of tooth displacement following force application. Together with the distribution of tension on the periodontal ligament, the deformation of the orthodontic wire and its areas of stress concentration are apparent.

8.3.3 Computational Fluid Dynamics

The upper airway must be analyzed using a geometrical model as part of the first step of a CFD simulation. The airway dimensions can be analyzed and described with the use of the geometric model. It is produced from the upper airway's CBCT or MRI-based scanned pictures. The fluid domain of interest is first identified before segmentation. Mesh generation in the fluid domain of interest refers to the process of further subdividing the domain into smaller portions through the use of grids and other features. Meshes can be created using commercial programs such as Gridgen, Tgrid, ANSYS Workbench, ANSYS ICEM CFD, and CFD-GEOM [48–50].

Preprocessor, solver (processor), and post-processor are the three primary categories into which all of the flow-related data and overall performance evaluations of CFD are divided (Fig. 8.7). The preprocessor, which is the input of the modeling element, solves problems and creates a computational model by discretization (meshing). The processing part, referred to as the solver, solves governing equations using algebraic and numerical techniques. To visualize the computational results, the post-processor is the output component that successfully converges the solved equations of state for each cell [15].

8.3.3.1 Preprocessing

Preprocessing, which includes domain interest identification, domain construction for the upper airway, and domain mesh development, is the first step of the CFD simulation analysis. Preprocessing is frequently used in the CFD study of numerous engineering challenges, not just upper airway-related ones. The defined upper airway problem must be amply highlighted by the modeling goals at this point, as well as the initial airflow assumptions (like steady and unsteady flow) and the model (like laminar and turbulent flow) that are used to characterize the

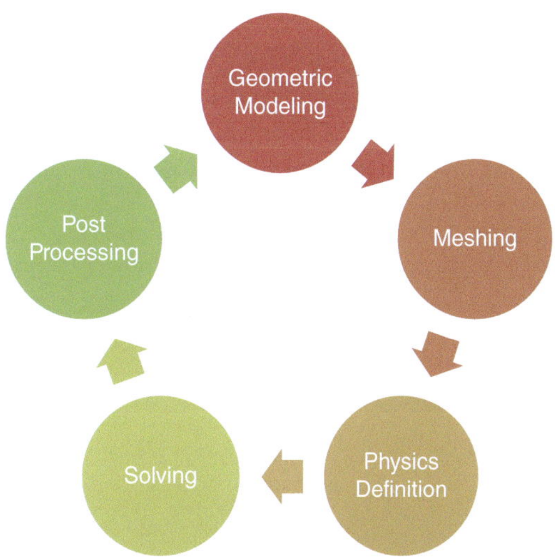

Fig. 8.7 Steps in CFD workflow

airflow. Moreover, the degree of accuracy, processing speed, and simplicity must all be taken into account at the beginning of the CFD simulation process.

The following is included in the preprocessing stage of the CFD analysis:

Identifying the domain of interest: Several cross sections are created from the nasal airway areas according to the terminology and airflow velocity (Fig. 8.8) [51, 52]. The region according to the study's interest is taken into account when choosing a certain segment.

Creating an upper airway model of the domain: Generally, 2D and 3D models are used to build the computational domain for the upper airway. The simplified upper airway model makes the simulation run more quickly. A 2D approximation is taken into consideration while working with continuous geometry, such as a model with chamfered ribs and several fundamental shapes (such as circular, semicircular, rectangular, and triangular). However, a 3D approximation is often used to depict complex geometries, such as arc-shaped roughness and V- and Z-shaped rib roughness. Computer-aided design (CAD) software is often used to generate the upper airway model before the fluid (the upper airway) or solid (the soft tissue) components of the model are defined. The upper airway's extraneous elements, including its form, margin, and image noise from the CT or MRI scan, will be removed at this point. By making the model simpler, the intricate process of creating a grid or mesh can be avoided [53]. The computational model views the soft palate as a movable plate that divides the nasal and oral inlets. The upper airway model can be built as either an accurate model or an approximation model in the computational research of the upper airway.

Mesh generation on the domain: Mesh generation or grid generation is used to split the airflow domain into numerous subdomains (elements or cells) after the domain is constructed. In the 3D realm, the hexahedron and tetrahedron elements are commonly utilized at this stage. However, in the 2D physical world, triangles and quadrilaterals are created. The accuracy of the simulation results, the rate of convergence, and the computation time are all significantly impacted by the meshing quality in CFD simulations. Moreover, appropriate boundary restrictions are defined at the meshing elements of the domain. It is anticipated that the boundary layer meshing will improve stability throughout the trial. It is anticipated that the

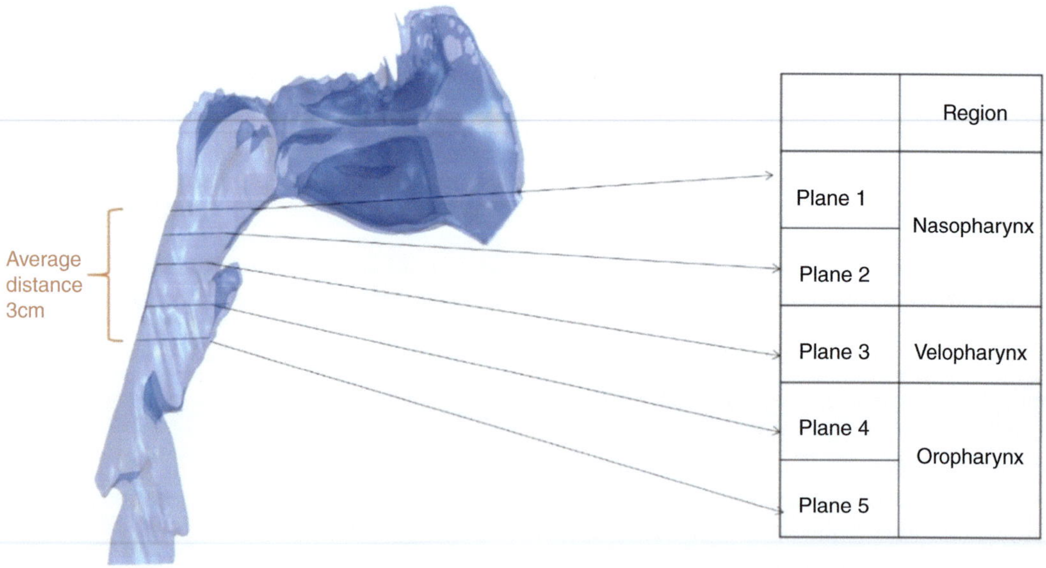

Fig. 8.8 Different planes for the cross-sectional measurement. (Source: Wadhwa, P et al. 2021) [52]

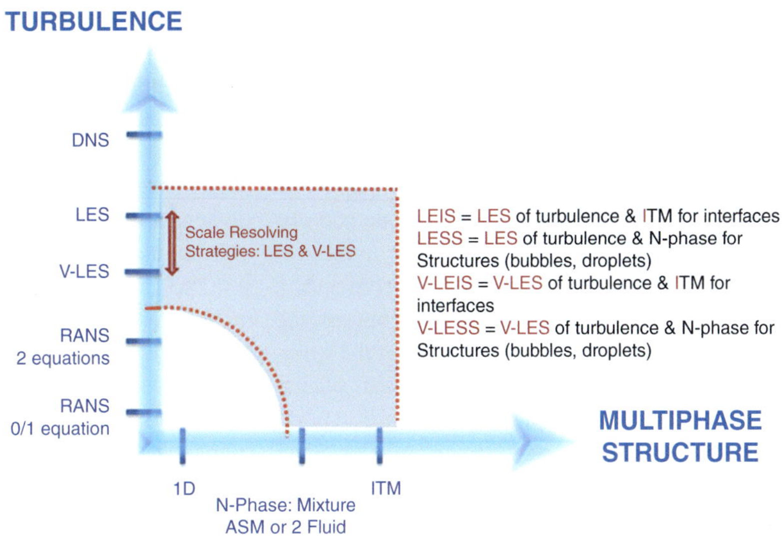

Fig. 8.9 Possible combinations of computational techniques and models. (Source: Faizal WM, et al. 2020) [56]

boundary layer meshing will improve stability throughout the trial. After the domain is constructed, mesh generation or grid generation is performed to divide the airflow domain into many subdomains (elements or cells). At this point, the hexahedron and tetrahedron elements are frequently used in the 3D world. However, in the 2D physical world, triangles and quadrilaterals are created. The accuracy of the simulation results, the rate of convergence, and the computation time are all significantly impacted by the meshing quality in CFD simulations. Additionally, suitable boundary constraints are established at the domain's meshing components. Eventually optimal, airflow can be precisely anticipated while using fewer computer resources, such as time. Different numbers of components are taken into account for the domain in the grid independence test [54].

8.3.3.2 Solver of Turbulence Model

The mean flow characteristics that could be representative of the actual flow state in a CFD simulation are determined by the flow model selected. The choice of flow model is also influenced by the applications and the nature of the problem. Three basic turbulence models—Reynolds-averaged Navier-Stokes (RANS), large-eddy simulation (LES), and direct numerical simulation—are among the six turbulence models that make up the CFD (Fig. 8.9) (DNS) [55]. The simulation models all of the flow's turbulent motions. The LES approach-based model only solves the filtered Navier-Stokes equations in large-scale flow variables; it does not directly anticipate smaller vortices. Finite computational elements might be used in a DNS-based model. While this is going on, DNS solves the entire set of unstable Navier-Stokes equations, which resolves the entire range of turbulent scales and makes precise but time-consuming turbulent flow prediction possible. It has long been acknowledged that a computation time-efficient method is one of the conditions for generating reliable CFD findings within a suitable study length. Therefore, in simulated research on the human upper airway, it is recommended to employ a two-equation RANS model or the standard k-(SKE) model [55].

8.3.3.3 Post-processing

To accurately conclude the CFD models, an accurate analysis of the simulated findings must be conducted, which is done as part of the post-processing of the simulated data [56]. A thorough representation of the flow's physics as well as other simulation results that act as decision-makers is also presented. In the CFD analysis of the human upper airway, post-processing is employed to visualize the airflow and examine desirable flow parameters including turbulent Reynolds number, pressure, and velocity. The bulk of post-processing software has features for visualizing data and producing numerical reports. To determine the values of temperature, pressure, velocity, and surface and integrated values, to mention a few quantitative outputs, one can utilize a numerical reporting tool. The numerical reporting tool can also be used to construct a graph of the quantitative findings. In contrast, the visualization tool presents the results of the simulation and extracts the flow properties in several plots, such as surface plots, 2D and 3D renderings, contour, vector, and streamline plots. The visualization tool can also be used to produce the animation of flow properties. Commercial software products such as ANSYS CFD-Post, Field View, Tecplot 360, and ANSYS EnSight are commonly used in post-processing. To improve the accuracy of the simulation model, these commercial programs make it simple to revise models for the computational domain, grid size, boundary conditions, beginning conditions, and relaxation parameters.

CFD offers a variety of benefits. In addition to being valued, the nasal airflow characteristic may also be researched in several biomedical science fields, including the analysis of postoperative outcomes, the facilitation of precision surgery, and the indication of a better understanding of the anatomical and physiological aspects of human biology with high efficacy and benign medical equipment. In geophysical and biological fluid dynamics, CFD can mimic flow circumstances that are not repeatable in experimental experiments, such as situations that are too large, too small, or too far away to replicate experimentally [56].

8.4 Limitations of Computational Techniques

Computational techniques such as machine learning and finite element analysis have analyzed medical images in the craniofacial region simpler. These computational analyses assist the doctor in making a quick diagnosis and help in the treatment processes as well. However, research on the applications of these techniques in craniofacial surgery and other diagnosis purposes needs to be supplemented in some aspects to ensure the long-term sustainability of the analysis methods involving these techniques [57].

The drawbacks of machine learning techniques for the analysis of images in the craniofacial region are as follows: The data in such analyses are mostly internal, thus necessitating extensive labeling by an expert, to enable comparisons objectively. Big data research involving images is challenging the medical field due to the existing disparity among the quality of the images and other medical records associated with them. The availability of data is another impediment to machine learning analyses. In some cases, the three-dimensional data of CBCT images are found to be insufficient to train a robust model for the analysis. More importantly, techniques such as deep learning and machine learning cannot be intellectualized completely due to the requirement of a large number of data samples for the training of an effective model that can evaluate and predict new data [58]. The reproducibility crisis is another challenge associated with the inclusion of ML in the decision-making processes in orthodontics. It has been noticed that the replication of experiments cannot be done by two different groups of scientists. This is mainly due to the lack of knowledge of the metrics and the workings of the algorithm. Furthermore, the sensitivity of the algorithm about hyperparameters such as initiation strategy, iteration times, and study rate is ignored by most researchers, thus contributing to the reproducibility crisis [59, 60].

The drawbacks of finite element analysis are as follows: Finite element analysis can be subject to bias because the parameters of the analysis are most often decided by the programmer. This may lead to false conclusions being drawn from the results. Initially, the simulation models lacked geometric precision which is crucial in the analysis of 3D images. This was due to the generalization of structures; for example, intricate anatomical details of some structures along with their morphological details were ignored during bone modeling stages, leading the reader to question the validity of the results [61]. Finally, an effective model requires more intricate details of the anatomical structures along with the morphological details to achieve greater precision and accuracy, thus necessitating the requirement for greater computational capacity, which further makes the construction of the model itself time-consuming and expensive [62, 63].

Cons: CFD has probably lagged in the medical field because of the intricacy of human anatomy and the behavior of bodily fluids inside the circulatory system. To determine the exact CFD solutions for phenomena such as compressibility, multiphase flow, and turbulence, CFD can only accurately depict physical models and the caliber of input data derived from actual processes. As a result, to correctly evaluate the calculated results, numerical results need to be carefully inspected and assessed. To get an efficient result, the mechanical engineer and the medical expert should collaborate. It is important to use an interdisciplinary method that will generate feedback on the outcomes of each stage of the entire process.

8.5 Summary

Time is a precious commodity. However, experimental research is tedious and requires time to perfect solutions to a problem. Thus, precise and less time-consuming experiments that aid in the decision-making process in the medical field are advantageous to everyone involved. Computational techniques such as machine learning and finite element analysis are instrumental in medical imaging and have gradually penetrated fields such as dentistry and craniofacial surgery. Discussion of the various applications and drawbacks of the computational techniques in craniofacial research will help researchers and doctors consider the advantages of computational analysis and make decisions keeping the pitfalls of each technique in mind.

Acknowledgments NM thanks the Global Innovation and Technology Alliance (GITA), Department of Science and Technology (DST) [project no. GITA/DST/TWN/P-95/2021], and Indian Council of Medical Research (ICMR) (project no. ITR/Ad-hoc/43/2020-21, ID no. 2020-3286), Government of India, India for financial support.

References

1. Bi WL, Hosny A, Schabath MB, Giger ML, Birkbak NJ, Mehrtash A, Allison T, Arnaout O, Abbosh C, Dunn IF, Mak RH. Artificial intelligence in cancer imaging: clinical challenges and applications. CA Cancer J Clin. 2019;69:127–57.
2. King BF Jr. Artificial intelligence and radiology: what will the future hold? J Am Coll Radiol. 2018;15:501–3.
3. Topol EJ. Deep medicine: how artificial intelligence can make healthcare human again. 1st ed. Basic Books; 2019.
4. Kiers HA, Rasson JP, Groenen PJ, Schader M, editors. Data analysis, classification, and related methods. Springer Science & Business Media; 2012.
5. Benke K, Benke G. Artificial intelligence and big data in public health. Int J Environ Res Public Health. 2018;15:2796.
6. Dhall D, Kaur R, Juneja M. Machine learning: a review of the algorithms and its applications. Proc ICRIC. 2019;2020:47–63.
7. Calamuneri A, Donato L, Scimone C, Costa A, D'Angelo R, Sidoti A. On machine learning in biomedicine. Life Safety Sec. 2017;5:96–9.
8. Akella B. Types of machine learning—supervised and unsupervised. 2023. https://intellipaat.com/blog/tutorial/machine-learning-tutorial/types-of-machine-learning/. Accessed 21 Feb 2023.
9. Sharma S, Aggarwal A, Choudhury T. Breast cancer detection using machine learning algorithms. In: 2018 international conference on computational techniques, electronics and mechanical systems (CTEMS) IEEE. 2018. pp. 114–8.
10. Mehta F, Joshi H. Finite element method: an overview. IOSR J Dental Med Sci. 2016;15:38–41.
11. Trivedi S. Finite element analysis: a boon to dentistry. J Oral Biol Craniof Res. 2014;4:200–3.
12. Soares CJ, Versluis A, Valdivia AD, Bicalho AA, Veríssimo C, Barreto BD, Roscoe MG. Finite element analysis in dentistry-improving the quality of oral health care. In: Finite element analysis from biomedical applications to industrial developments. Intech Open; 2012. p. 25–56.
13. Lisiak-Myszke M, Marciniak D, Bieliński M, Sobczak H, Garbacewicz Ł, Drogoszewska B. Application of finite element analysis in oral and maxillofacial surgery—a literature review. Materials. 2020;13:3063.
14. Lee BK. Computational fluid dynamics in cardiovascular disease. Korean Circ J. 2011;41:423–30.

15. Basri EI, Basri AA, Riazuddin VN, Farhana S, Zuber M, Ahmad KA. Computational fluid dynamics study in biomedical applications: a review. Int J Fluid Heat Transf. 2016;1:2–14.
16. Van Leer B, Powell KG. Introduction to computational fluid dynamics. Encycl Aerosp Eng. 2010:1–14.
17. Zubair M, Ahmad KA, Abdullah MZ, Sufian SF. Characteristic airflow patterns during inspiration and expiration: experimental and numerical investigation. J Med Biol Eng. 2015;35:387–94.
18. Cohen AM, Ip HS, Linney AD. A preliminary study of computer recognition and identification of skeletal landmarks as a new method of cephalometric analysis. Br J Orthod. 1984;11:143–54.
19. Arik SÖ, Ibragimov B, Xing L. Fully automated quantitative cephalometry using convolutional neural networks. J Med Imaging. 2017;4:014501.
20. Wang CW, Huang CT, Lee JH, Li CH, Chang SW, Siao MJ, Lai TM, Ibragimov B, Vrtovec T, Ronneberger O, Fischer P. A benchmark for comparison of dental radiography analysis algorithms. Med Image Anal. 2016;31:63–76.
21. Yue W, Yin D, Li C, Wang G, Xu T. Automated 2-D cephalometric analysis on X-ray images by a model-based approach. IEEE Trans Biomed Eng. 2006;53:1615–23.
22. Kunz F, Stellzig-Eisenhauer A, Zeman F, Boldt J. Artificial intelligence in orthodontics. J Orofac Orthop. 2020;81:52–68.
23. Hwang HW, Park JH, Moon JH, Yu Y, Kim H, Her SB, Srinivasan G, Aljanabi MN, Donatelli RE, Lee SJ. Automated identification of cephalometric landmarks: part 2-might it be better than human? Angle Orthod. 2020;90:69–76.
24. Park JH, Hwang HW, Moon JH, Yu Y, Kim H, Her SB, Srinivasan G, Aljanabi MN, Donatelli RE, Lee SJ. Automated identification of cephalometric landmarks: part 1—comparisons between the latest deep-learning methods YOLOV3 and SSD. Angle Orthod. 2019;89:903–9.
25. Dot G, Rafflenbeul F, Arbotto M, Gajny L, Rouch P, Schouman T. Accuracy and reliability of automatic three-dimensional cephalometric landmarking. Int J Oral Maxillofac Surg. 2020;49:1367–78.
26. Gupta A, Kharbanda OP, Sardana V, Balachandran R, Sardana HK. A knowledge-based algorithm for automatic detection of cephalometric landmarks on CBCT images. Int J Comput Assist Radiol Surg. 2015;10:1737–52.
27. Ma Q, Kobayashi E, Fan B, Nakagawa K, Sakuma I, Masamune K, Suenaga H. Automatic 3D landmarking model using patch-based deep neural networks for CT image of oral and maxillofacial surgery. Int J Med Robot Comput Assist Surg. 2020;16:e2093.
28. Lee SM, Kim HP, Jeon K, Lee SH, Seo JK. Automatic 3D cephalometric annotation system using shadowed 2D image-based machine learning. Phys Med Biol. 2019;64:055002.
29. Li P, Kong D, Tang T, Su D, Yang P, Wang H, Zhao Z, Liu Y. Orthodontic treatment planning based on artificial neural networks. Sci Rep. 2019;9:1–9.
30. Choi HI, Jung SK, Baek SH, Lim WH, Ahn SJ, Yang IH, Kim TW. Artificial intelligent model with neural network machine learning for the diagnosis of orthognathic surgery. J Craniofac Surg. 2019;30:1986–99.
31. Jeong SH, Yun JP, Yeom HG, Lim HJ, Lee J, Kim BC. Deep learning-based discrimination of soft tissue profiles requiring orthognathic surgery by facial photographs. Sci Rep. 2020;10:1–5.
32. Lin HH, Chiang WC, Yang CT, Cheng CT, Zhang T, Lo LJ. On construction of transfer learning for facial symmetry assessment before and after orthognathic surgery. Comput Methods Prog Biomed. 2021;200:105928.
33. Setzer FC, Shi KJ, Zhang Z, Yan H, Yoon H, Mupparapu M, Li J. Artificial intelligence for the computer-aided detection of periapical lesions in cone-beam computed tomographic images. J Endod. 2020;46:987–93.
34. Perestrelo PF, de Oliveira JA, Noritomi PY, da Silva JV. Application of a virtual cranial model in a trauma simulation. Procedia CIRP. 2016;49:19–22.
35. Bezerra TP, Junior FS, Scarparo HC, Costa FW, Studart-Soares EC. Do erupted third molars weaken the mandibular angle after trauma to the chin region? A 3D finite element study. Int J Oral Maxillofac Surg. 2013;42:474–80.
36. Szucs A, Bujtár P, Sándor GK, Barabás J. Finite element analysis of the human mandible to assess the effect of removing an impacted third molar. J Can Dent Assoc. 2010;76:a72.
37. Santos LS, Rossi AC, Freire AR, Matoso RI, Caria PH, Prado FB. Finite-element analysis of 3 situations of trauma in the human edentulous mandible. J Oral Maxillofac Surg. 2015;73:683–91.
38. Larson BE, Lee NK, Jang MJ, Jo DW, Yun PY, Kim YK. Comparative evaluation of the sliding plate technique for fixation of a sagittal split ramus osteotomy: finite element analysis. Oral Surg Oral Med Oral Pathol Oral Radiol. 2017;123:148–52.
39. Ghorashi SM, Keshavarzi MM, Damercheli S, Parhiz A. The comparison of three different fixation methods on bilateral sagittal split ramus osteotomy mandibular on a 3D of fully modelled mandible by the finite element method. J Craniomaxillofac Res. 2019:113–21.
40. Hassan MK, Ring M, Stassen LF. A finite element analysis study comparing 3 internal fixation techniques in mandibular sagittal Split osteotomy. Int J Otolaryngol Head Neck Surg. 2018;7:298–311.
41. Tamura N, Takaki T, Takano N, Shibahara T. Three-dimensional finite element analysis of bone fixation in bilateral sagittal split ramus osteotomy using individual models. Bull Tokyo Dent Coll. 2018;59:67–78.
42. Fujii H, Kuroyanagi N, Kanazawa T, Yamamoto S, Miyachi H, Shimozato K. Three-dimensional finite element model to predict patterns of pterygomaxillary dysjunction during Le fort I osteotomy. Int J Oral Maxillofac Surg. 2017;46:564–71.
43. Caputo A, Chaconis SJ, Hayashi RK. Photoelastic visualization of orthodontic forces during canine retraction. Am J Orthod. 1974;65:250–9.

44. Kamble RH, Lohkare S, Hararey PV, Mundada RD. Stress distribution pattern in a root of maxillary central incisor having various root morphologies: a finite element study. Angle Orthod. 2012;82:799805.
45. Viecilli RF. Self-corrective T-loop design for differential space closure. Am J Orthod Dentofacial Orthop. 2006;129:48–53.
46. Jones ML, Hickman J, Middleton J, Knox J, Volp C. A validated finite element method study of orthodontic tooth movement in the human subject. Am J Orthod. 2001;28:29–38.
47. Andreaus U, Colloca M, Iacoviello D. Coupling image processing and stress analysis for damage identification in a human premolar tooth. Comput Methods Prog Biomed. 2011;103:61–73.
48. Xiong GX, Zhan JM, Jiang HY, Li JF, Rong LW, Xu G. Computational fluid dynamics simulation of airflow in the normal nasal cavity and paranasal sinuses. Am J Rhinol. 2008;22:477–82.
49. Vos WD, De Backer J, Devolder A, Vanderveken O, Verhulst S, Salgado R, Germonpré P, Partoens B, Wuyts F, Parizel P, De Backer W. Correlation between severity of sleep apnea and upper airway morphology based on advanced anatomical and functional imaging. J Biomech. 2007;40:2207–13.
50. Cole P. Nasal airflow resistance: a survey of 2500 assessments. Am J Rhinol. 1997;11:415–20.
51. Jeong SJ, Kim WS, Sung SJ. Numerical investigation on the flow characteristics and aerodynamic force of the upper airway of patient with obstructive sleep apnea using computational fluid dynamics. Med Eng Phys. 2007;29:7–651.
52. Wadhwa P, Jang HS, Park SH, Kim HH, Lee ES. Computational fluid dynamic analysis of the pharyngeal airway after bimaxillary orthognathic surgery in patients with mandibular prognathism. PRO. 2021;9:152.
53. Khalili M, Larsson M, Müller B. Interaction between a simplified soft palate and compressible viscous flow. J Fluids Struct. 2016;67:85–105.
54. Yadav AS, Bhagoria JL. A CFD (computational fluid dynamics) based heat transfer and fluid flow analysis of a solar air heater provided with circular transverse wire rib roughness on the absorber plate. Energy. 2013;55:1127–42.
55. Launder BE, Spalding DB. The numerical computation of turbulent flows. Comput Methods Appl Mech Eng. 1974;3:269–89.
56. Faizal WM, Ghazali NNN, Khor CY, Badruddin IA, Zainon MZ, Yazid AA, Ibrahim NB, Razi RM. Computational fluid dynamics modelling of human upper airway: a review. Comput Methods Prog Biomed. 2020;196:105627. https://doi.org/10.1016/j.cmpb.2020.105627. Epub 2020 Jun 26.
57. Iwasaki T, Sato H, Suga H, Minami A, Yamamoto Y, Takemoto Y, Inada E, Saitoh I, Kakuno E, Kanomi R, Yamasaki Y. Herbst appliance effects on pharyngeal airway ventilation evaluated using computational fluid dynamics. Angle Orthod. 2017;87:397–403.
58. Schwendicke F, Golla T, Dreher M, Krois J. Convolutional neural networks for dental image diagnostics: a scoping review. J Dent. 2019;91:103226.
59. Cai L, Gao J, Zhao D. A review of the application of deep learning in medical image classification and segmentation. Ann Transl Med. 2020;8:713–28.
60. Liu J, Chen Y, Li S, Zhao Z, Wu Z. Machine learning in orthodontics: challenges and perspectives. Adv Clin Exp Med. 2021;30:1065–74.
61. Alsubai S. A critical review on the 3D cephalometric analysis using machine learning. Computers. 2022;11:154–70.
62. Oguz Y, Uckan S, Ozden AU, Uckan E, Eser A. Stability of locking and conventional 2.0-mm miniplate/screw systems after sagittal split ramus osteotomy: finite element analysis. Oral Surg Oral Med Oral Pathol Oral Radiol Endod. 2009;108:174–7.
63. Baeck K, Goffin J, Vander SJ. An investigation into the use and limitations of different spatial integration schemes and finite element software in head impact analyses. Comput Methods Biomech Biomed Engin. 2014;17:405–15.

9 Visualization Techniques for Craniofacial Anthropometry

Apurba Patra, Adil Asghar, K. S. Ravi, Priti Chaudhary, and Anjana Rajagopalan

9.1 Introduction

Using precise measurements and reference points, craniofacial anthropometry is a technique for determining the dimensions of the human head and face [1]. It depends on locating certain landmarks on the head and face that are then used to estimate distances between various points. While soft tissue markers may also be employed in rare circumstances, these landmarks are often bony sites on the skull. The metrics from facial anthropometry may be compared to norms or reference values to evaluate the individual's facial traits.

The surface topography of the facial architecture may be assessed quantitatively using this simplistic and noninvasive procedure to identify any alterations. For decades, this area of research has indeed been employed to comprehend the variety of human appearances and has evolved in relevance within dentistry and other areas of healthcare. Facial anthropometry measures may be used to evaluate face symmetry, balance, and proportion, critical elements in planning orthodontic treatment, prosthodontic rehabilitation, and facial reconstruction.

In dentistry, the value of face anthropometry is widely recognized since it offers crucial information for maxillofacial surgery, prosthodontic rehabilitation, orthodontic evaluation, and surgical preparation. The connection between the jaws and teeth may be evaluated in orthodontics using facial anthropometry, which can also assist in determining the degree of correction required to obtain the optimum occlusion. Facial anthropometry may help prosthodontists create restorations that are by the patient's natural facial characteristics.

Moreover, forensic investigations may make use of face anthropometry to help identify people based on their facial characteristics. It has also been explored in research on facial ageing and may provide useful data for creating anti-ageing remedies.

Since its debut, direct and indirect anthropometry have been the principal methods used in craniofacial anthropometry [2–8]. According to Farkas [2], direct anthropometry is the measuring process that necessitates direct bodily exchange with the individuals. As this measurement technique is manual, it requires a lot of time, accuracy from the doctor, and compliance from the patient.

A. Patra · P. Chaudhary (✉)
Department of Anatomy, All India Institute of Medical Sciences, Bathinda, Punjab, India

A. Asghar
Department of Anatomy, All India Institute of Medical Sciences, Patna, Bihar, India

K. S. Ravi
Department of Anatomy, All India Institute of Medical Sciences, Gorakhpur, Uttar Pradesh, India

A. Rajagopalan
Department of Dentistry, All India Institute of Medical Sciences, Bathinda, Punjab, India

S. S. Rana et al. (eds.), *Applications of Three-dimensional Imaging for Craniofacial Region*,
https://doi.org/10.1007/978-981-97-4608-8_9

An indirect anthropometry approach was subsequently created to mitigate the drawbacks of manual anthropometry. Using photographic imaging technology, the human face was captured in two dimensions (2D) or three dimensions (3D), and measurements were then taken on the 2D or 3D images. The vast majority of indirect anthropometry research [7] makes use of manually generated landmarks on 2D or 3D images. With 3D images, there is more information that may be viewed, including height, breadth, and depth. The library of 3D human face pictures has expanded greatly as a consequence of the tremendous popularity of 3D image capture techniques in craniofacial imaging [9, 10].

This chapter discusses various methods for visualizing the craniofacial region, from traditional analogue to three-dimensional photography to virtual and augmented reality and how they can be used for surgical planning and training.

9.2 Manual Anthropometry

Callipers, gauze, and measuring tapes are often used to get anthropometric data from patients themselves. The proportions were established by including these criteria. Traditional manual anthropometry is a labour-intensive process that sometimes involves the use of sharp equipment and demands proximity to the subject. Young children or adults who, for personal or cultural reasons, do not enjoy direct touch ought to avoid being subjected to this. The obligation to constantly locate landmarks may lengthen measurement time and contribute to mistakes. Moreover, since patients must stay motionless while the measures are obtained, compliance is an issue. Since this approach just captures the facial traits as a series of numbers and does not maintain the face's look, certain errors become perpetual [11].

The operator's expertise and experience will unavoidably affect how accurate the measurements are. There is a significant risk of error when performing anthropometry, particularly by amateurs. In studies, manual anthropometry has been most commonly utilized to evaluate abnormalities like craniosynostoses and cleft lip and palate [12–16]. Because of the aforementioned limitations, this approach is not often employed as a therapeutic tool.

Anthropometric Landmarks: Farkas [17] provided definitions for 47 maxillofacial landmarks for craniofacial anthropometry (Table 9.1). Although many of these landmarks are readily identified visually (Fig. 9.1), a few are easier to find by palpation of the underlying skeletal components [18].

Table 9.1 Frequently used anthropometric landmarks used in manual craniofacial anthropometry [1]

Region	Name	Abbreviation	Definitions
Head	Vertex	ver	The highest point on the head in the Frankfort horizontal plane
	Trichion	trich	A point on the hairline in the midline of the forehead
	Glabella	glab	The most prominent midline between eyebrows
Nose	Nasion	n	The midpoint on the nasal root at the level of the frontonasal suture
	Sellion	se	The most posterior point of the frontonasal soft Tissue contour in the midline of the base of the nasal root
	Pronasale	prn	The most anterior midpoint of the nasal tip
	Subnasale	sn	The midpoint on the nasolabial soft tissue contour between the columella crest and the upper lip
	Alare	al	The most lateral point on each alar contour
	Alar curvature (or alar crest) point	ac	The most lateral point in the curved baseline of each ala
	Columella apex	c'	The most anterior point the columella crest at the apex of the nostril
Eye	Exocanthion	ex	The soft tissue point located at the outer commissure of each eye fissure
	Endocanthion	en	The soft tissue point located at the inner commissure of each eye fissure
	Palpebrale superius	ps	The highest point in the mid portion of the free margin of each upper eyelid
	Palpebrale inferius	pi	The lowest point in the mid portion of the free margin of each lower eyelid

(continued)

Table 9.1 (continued)

Region	Name	Abbreviation	Definitions
Ears	Tragion	t	The notch at the upper margin of the tragus
	Otobasion inferius	obi	The point of attachment of the ear lobe to the cheek
	Otobasion superius	obs	The point of attachment of the helix in the temporal region
	Postaurale	pa	The most posterior point on the free margin of the Ear
	Preaurale	pra	The most anterior point of each ear, located just in front of the helix attachment to the head
	Superaurale	sa	The highest point of the free margin of the auricle
	Subaurale	sba	The lowest point of the free margin of the ear lobe
Chin	Sublabiale	sl	The midpoint of the labiomental sulcus
	Pogonion	pg	The most anterior midpoint of the chin
	Gnathion	gn	The lowest median landmark on the lower border of the mandible
Lips and mouth	Labiale superius	ls	The midpoint of the vermilion line of the upper lip
	Crista philtri	cph	The point at each elevated margin of the philtrum just above the vermilion line
	Cheilion	ch	The point located at each labial commissure
	Stomion	sto	The midpoint of the labial fissure when the lips are closed naturally
	Labiale inferioris	li	The midpoint of the lower vermilion line

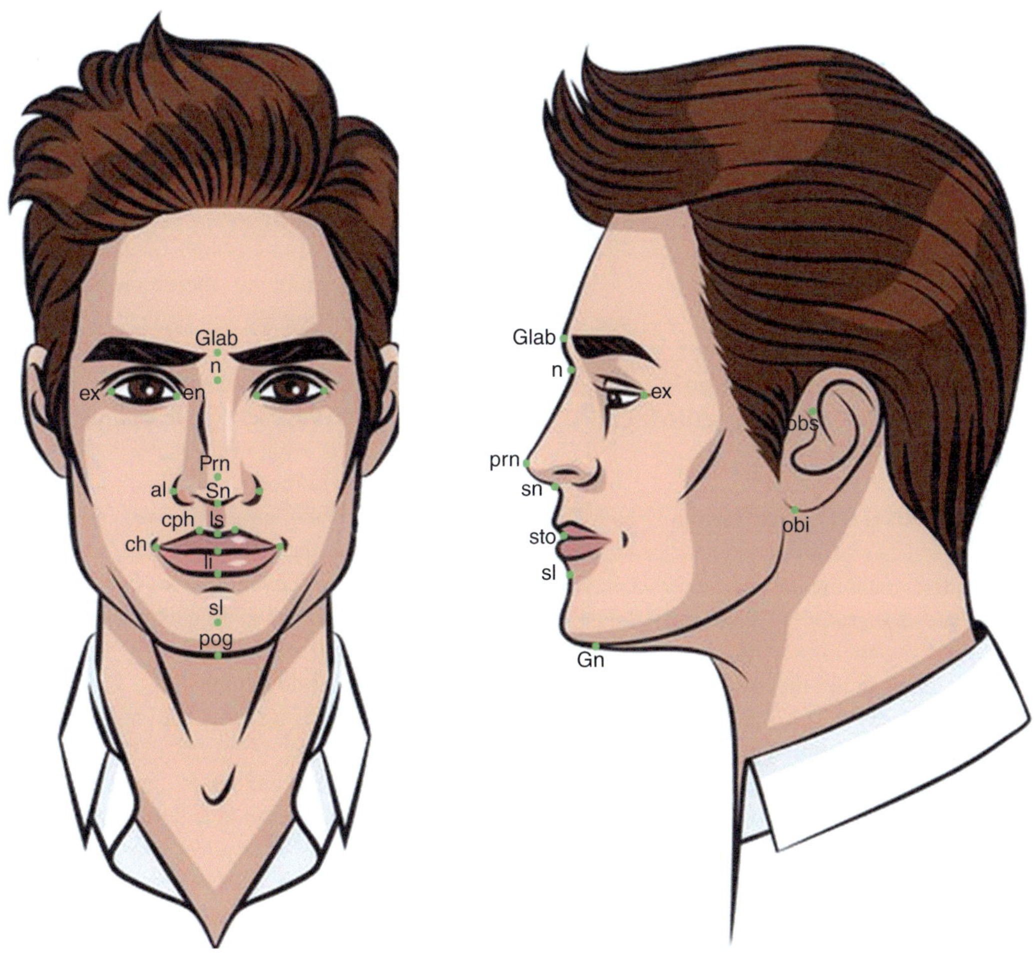

Fig. 9.1 Showing frequently used craniofacial anthropometric landmarks

9.3 Digital Anthropometry

Because of the discovery of stereo photography, it is now possible to create a realistic 3D picture of the face with true texture and colour. Stereo photography systems acquire three-dimensional surface data using multiple pairs of identical cameras positioned at particular points. Commercial systems can capture 180-degree facial pictures in about 2 ms [19]. Most modern software can recognize anthropometric markers on 3D imagery. Traditional anthropometric landmarks must be felt to be reliably distinguished; however, measurements for these landmarks cannot be included in a 3D application's performance.

As a result, with the required changes, standard anthropometric methods may be utilized to measure 3D imagery. Novel digital measures that traditional equipment cannot calculate can also be computed. To separate themselves from conventional manual anthropometry approaches, researchers using such technology have labelled their processes "3D anthropometry" and "digital anthropometry" [20–22].

9.4 Digital Anthropometry Techniques with Their Applications in Craniofacial Assessment

9.4.1 Virtual AYRA Software

Preoperative planning is critical in identifying appropriate allografts in face transplantation, particularly in obtaining an anatomically compatible graft that matches the recipient defect as precisely as practicable. The initial stage in capturing anthropometric measurements and producing such a suitable graft that accompanies the harvesting of face transplants involves employing virtual reality technologies. The cryopreserved donated human skulls undergo measurements for anthropometric elements, which include the assessment of hard and soft bone tissue. This compares the digital measurements from 3D reconstructions built using the AYRA software with the conventional analogue indicators. To ensure successful transplantation, it is crucial that the morphometric parameters of the potential donor closely align with those of the defect. The anthropometric data of the subjects and the findings produced using the VR program were found to be statistically comparable to those acquired using the standard analogue approach. The use of the 3D reconstructions in the virtual AYRA software is to describe the donor's facial features [23].

During the transplantation procedure, the morphometric parameters of the possible face donor must match the defect. The anthropometric measurements obtained from the virtual reality application showed a strong correlation with those obtained using the standard analogue technique. The virtual AYRA software's 3D reconstructions are potentially valuable for accurately depicting the donor's facial features [23].

9.4.2 3D Photographic System/Stereoscopy

3D photography combines the depth perception of two-dimensional photos to recreate the sensation of three-dimensional images acquired via binocular vision. Stereoscopy or stereoscopic imaging refers to the backdrop technique used to produce the 3D illusion in 2D pictures. By shifting the locations of the lenses linked to them, 3D cameras may capture numerous points of view of the same thing at the same time. The whole line of 3D LifeViz® devices is a photographic system that enables physicians to digitalize their consultations and speak more effectively with their patients using 3D photographs [24]. This system is designed to be tiny and portable, with each camera capable of capturing crisp 3D imagery of the face. The 3D depiction of the craniofacial area, reinforced with anatomical reference points or preset landmarks, is an ideal way to generate standardized and comparable photographs of this region for digitalized consultations and hassle-free surgical planning. Therefore, assessing cosmetic treatments for volume changes cannot be represented using standard 2D images. Yet, the

3D photographic system may compare morphometric parameters such as angles, length, breadth, and face ratio before and after surgery [25–27].

9.4.3 Three-Dimensional Craniofacial Stereophotogrammetry Imaging System (3dMDface)

The 3dMDface system has the potential to be the most helpful, verified, and precise method for facial aesthetics and reconstructive surgery planning, particularly in long-term or protracted craniofacial care [28]. It helps obtain precise measurements from clients' digitally stored 3D face pictures, and it might be a fantastic tool for discussing present problems with patients and obtaining greater precision [3]. The Vectra-M5 360 System, a 3D stereophotogrammetry system manufactured by Canfield Scientific Inc. in Fairfield, New Jersey, is composed of five separately calibrated cameras (Fig. 9.2).

To conceal hair, apply a head cap and position the subject in the centre of the camera system. In addition, men must shave since the camera is unable to retexture facial hair. The cameras are connected via a desktop PC and Mirror Software [29–32].

These solutions make it simple for hospitals and professionals to save and transfer images.

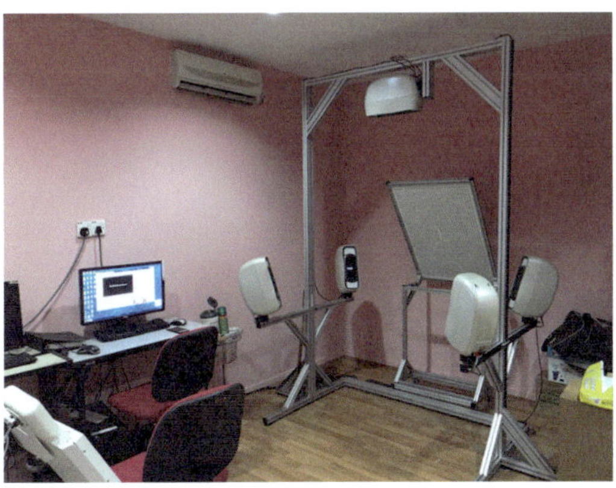

Fig. 9.2 The Vectra-M5 360 camera imaging system permitted under Creative Common License N.Y. 4.0. (Abu A et al., 2019) [48]

The data can also be used for research and auditing [33]. To create the 3D image, three separate stages are used [34, 35].

1. 3D surface capture using a laser or an optics-based technique.
2. Modelling: The surface pixels are placed within the polygonal mesh created by intricate algorithms to quantitatively represent the region's physical characteristics.
3. Rendering: Multicolour data is used to generate its texture, dimension, and realistically three-dimensional objects.

9.4.4 Craniofacial Measurements Based on 3D-CT Volume Rendering

Computed tomography (CT) of the head is frequently employed to detect and evaluate craniofacial anthropometric factors [36–40].

Three-dimensional computed tomography (3D-CT) may be utilized to analyse surgical outcomes, develop treatments, and define unique and complicated anatomy in cases involving craniofacial anomalies, dental implants, and fractures [36–41].

Several studies have used 3D-CT volume rendering methods to enhance visualization of the craniofacial area, cerebral aneurysms, vascular system, and internal organs, yielding long-term outcomes [42–46]. Prior research has shown the accuracy of several craniometric measures used in 3D surface rendering. A recent study executed assessments of both the precision and accuracy of craniometric data utilizing a specially designed computer system and the 3D-CT volume rendering technology. The study focused on the mental foramen and used a unique 3D-CT volume modelling approach for the evaluations. Nevertheless, a comprehensive evaluation of soft-tissue measurements' reliability has not been conducted.

Cavalcanti et al. [47] used 3D-CT volume simulation to compute the physical characteristics of cadaveric skulls. The specimens went through to a spiral CT scan from the vertex to the jaw. A 3.0 mm axial slices were used to capture high-resolution continuous pictures. The initial CT data was stored on a CD-ROM for further image analysis and manipulation. A supplementary workstation, equipped with a Precision running Windows, was used to generate 3D volumetric images for viewing, editing, and analysis. The software Vitreaw 2.3, developed by Vital Images Inc., may be employed for concurrent coronal and sagittal images for three-dimensional reconstructions of bones and soft tissues.

9.4.5 Craniofacial Landmark Recognition in Three-Dimensional (3D) Pictures Using Geometrical Properties

A specialized technique known as indirect anthropometry (IA) is utilized to quantify digitized facial photographs. A few defined areas or nodes on the structures of each face picture must be plotted as landmark points to create the linear measurements and nodes. Currently, most anthropometric research uses three-dimensional facial pictures with manually set landmarks. Measurement errors may result from process length and examiner bias, resulting in more measurement mistakes. Employing an automated technique to recognize landmarks may improve measurement accuracy. The automated craniofacial landmarks (ACL) are created upon a 3D facial imagery system by recognizing these nodes: pronase (prn), the nasion (n), alare (al), sub nasale (sn), stomion (sto), labiale superius (ls), chelion (ch), and labiale inferior (li). These markers are indicated in the .obj file format of the 3D face picture. Moreover, the IA is performed manually using Mirror software to map the craniofacial landmarks. When all landmarks have been identified, the eight linear measures are retrieved using either technique. Since it has been verified using the eight landmarks, ACL is suited for automated face recognition. ACL is a more reliable and helpful strategy to utilize instead of IA since it saves time and is free of human biases [48].

By using intricate geometric concepts and leveraging the development resources offered by the Qt framework version [49], ACL produces a graphical user interface technique. Qt is a costless and publicly available program technology that provides support for several platforms and operating systems. Visualization Toolkit (VTK) version 6.1.0 [50] identifies and constructs nodes for landmarks from 3D human face pictures. VTK, a cross-platform open-source 3D computer graphics and visualization software system, offers sophisticated modelling techniques such as Delaunay triangulation, implicit modelling, and polygon reduction. CMake 3.0.2 incorporates VTK and Qt framework libraries into workspaces and Makefiles [51]. CMake sets up and creates Makefiles and Visual Studio project files for VTK binary development. Qt Creator 3.1.2 supports code generation, operation compilation, and application code debugging [52].

9.4.6 Digital Craniofacial Measurements Using a Small-Format, Handheld, Three-Dimensional Facial Imaging Device: The Vectra H1

Three-dimensional (3D) facial imaging modalities are useful tools for assessing clinical outcomes in a variety of soft tissue craniofacial surgery procedures, in cluding orthodontics [53, 54], dental rehabilitation [55], craniofacial [56], maxillofacial [57–59], facial aesthetic surgery [8], and facial dermatology [60]. These technologies are based on the comparison of landmark locations, distances, surfaces, or volumes on a 3D numerical patient model before and after a surgical procedure. The conventional photogrammetric equipment is large and requires a particular room to be set up, but it produces a high-quality 3D model via a special acquisition employing a multi-angle camera system.

Vectra H1 is a device used for capturing three-dimensional images of face. Several surgical procedures involving the soft tissues of the head and face, such as orthodontics, dental rehabilitation, craniofacial surgery, maxillofacial surgery, facial cosmetic surgery, and facial dermatology, may be improved by using three-dimensional (3D) facial imaging techniques to assess the results of the treatment. These breakthroughs in technology rely on the comparison of 3D numerical models of patients before and after surgery, namely, in terms of the positioning of landmarks, distances, surfaces, and volumes. Although conventional photogrammetric equipment is large and requires a designated setup space, the use of a specific acquisition method that incorporates a multi-angle camera system yields high-quality 3D models, justifying the investment. The cost of Vectra H1 technology is lower compared to other 3D face imaging technologies since it does not use ionizing radiation, is portable, and has a versatile configuration. Employing a three-shot approach may lead to mistakes caused by patient motion during treatment or inadequate camera placement during consecutive images, while our double-lens reflex camera technology minimizes spatial requirements. Due to the need to construct a 3D model over three consecutive captures, this method may provide less accurate and consistent outcomes. Several investigations have been carried out to evaluate the consistency and dependability of virtual three-dimensional models generated using Vectra H1 [61–63]. Savoldelli et al. found that it exhibits high technical precision in identifying landmarks. Based on the test results, it seems that the Vectra H1 findings are consistent and do not vary over time. Unlike multi-pod devices, the Vectra H1 allows for a linear evaluation of clinical parameters utilizing face shape analysis, which is both space-saving and cost-effective [64].

9.4.7 DIVA: A 3D Virtual Reality Platform as an Educational Tool for Craniofacial Trauma

With the intricate nature of cranial anatomy, instructors may struggle to convey it to trainees in a manner that they will understand. A variety of cutting-edge technologies have recently aided in the process. The use of virtual realities, stereoscopy, motion tracking technology, and total 3D immersion simplifies the process of seeing three-dimensional architecture.

DIVA can automatically and accurately reconstruct CT images in three dimensions. DIVA generates avatars from DICOM CT166 raw scan images. DIVA employs a high refresh rate, which is 60 Hz or above, together with superior volume rendering quality to provide a seamless user experience. Virtual reality customers are oblivious to latency. The use of DIVA [65] might perhaps contribute to the advancement of cranial-facial trauma research.

This technology is precise for identifying specific points on the head and neck and for analysing their three-dimensional shape.

According to Alsabbagh et al., virtual reality (VR) models of craniofacial fractures may have superior accuracy than CT scans [66]. Our results show that 82% of students were able to discover previously unnoticed lesions in 3D representations while using virtual reality, confirming the technology's practical relevance. Virtual reality (VR) technologies, such as DIVA, may improve traditional teaching approaches for complex three-dimensional parts like the head, such as a two-dimensional sketch, three-dimensional renderings, and cadaveric dissections [67–71]. Virtual reality (VR) technologies, such as DIVA, have the potential to enhance contentment and tolerance. CT scans and MRI data may be used to provide comparable methodologies for evaluating craniofacial abnormalities, head and neck cancer, and traumatology.

9.4.8 Mixed Reality (Virtual Reality/Augmented Reality) in Preoperative Imaging in Maxillofacial Surgery

The management line has undergone substantial modification as a result of advances in imaging technology and their ability to gather images to see and interpret anatomical areas of interest. The usage of a virtual reality system allows for the creation of a virtual environment in which different anatomical regions of the body may be exam-

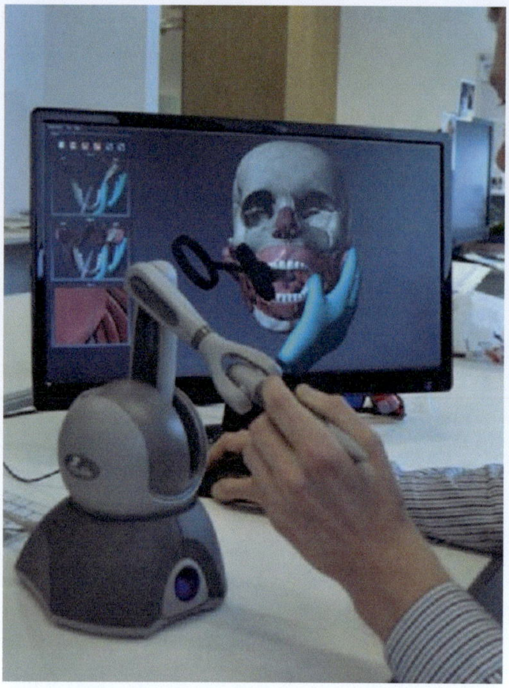

Fig. 9.3 Demonstration of haptic technology of injection of the inferior dental nerve. (Permitted under license 1349408-1 dated 27.04.2023)

ined topographically. This improves both the diagnosis and planning of surgical treatments. Augmented reality enables the display of a patient's three-dimensional actual pictures onto the operation field using partly see-through glasses (Fig. 9.3).

HMD visors can fully engage viewers in a three-dimensional world, enabling a more accurate evaluation of the restored anatomical components. VR goggles can enhance the assessment of three-dimensional imaging (CT, cone-beam CT, and MRI) in the field of oral and maxillofacial surgery. Technological advancements have made it possible to use surgical treatments like as orthognathic surgery, oral and maxillofacial surgery, and dental implantology [72]. Virtual reality (VR) facilitates precise alignment between virtual recommendations and the actual outcomes in mandibular and maxillary reconstruction. This includes the planes of resection, the diameter of the segmental defect, and the closeness of the transplanted zone to the surrounding bone [73]. Precise positioning of dental implants is crucial in the field of implantology to successfully meet both functional and aesthetic goals [74]. A preoperative CT scan (CBCT) is used in virtual reality to judge the dimensions, position, symmetry, and proximity of the implant to vital structures. A guide is produced with computer-aided design and computer-aided manufacturing (CAD/CAM) [75]. A surgical protocol was developed using a virtual template to assist in the placement of the implant.

9.5 Limitations and Challenges

Although face anthropometry is a useful technique in dentistry, it does have limits and obstacles. Some of the limits and constraints of face anthropometry in dentistry are as follows:

1. Individual variability: Individual variability in face characteristics might make developing consistent measurements and reference values difficult.
2. Two-dimensional imaging limitations: Most facial anthropometry is based on two-dimensional imaging, which may not offer an accurate representation of the three-dimensional structure of the face. As a consequence, measurements and evaluations may be inaccurate.
3. Soft tissue changes over time: Because of age, weight fluctuations, and other variables, soft tissue features such as the lips and cheeks may vary over time. This may make predicting the long-term effects of prosthodontic therapy based on facial anthropometric measures challenging.
4. Cultural and ethnic differences: Face characteristics may change greatly across cultural and ethnic groups, making it difficult to produce standardized assessments that are relevant across populations.
5. Intra- and interobserver variability: Intra- and interobserver variability may impair the accuracy and reliability of face anthropometric measures. As a result, various examiners may receive different measures, resulting in discrepancies in diagnosis and treatment planning.

6. Equipment limitations: The quality of the imaging equipment employed may also impact the accuracy of face anthropometric measures. Lower-quality equipment may create photos that are blurry or contain distortions, resulting in erroneous measurements.

9.6 Future Scope

Several intriguing potential avenues for face anthropometry in dentistry emerge as technology evolves and our knowledge of facial anatomy and physiology improves. Some possible growth opportunities include the following:

1. Three-dimensional imaging: Improvements in imaging techniques enable more detailed and precise three-dimensional pictures of the face to be obtained. This would enable more exact measurements and analyses of facial anatomy, perhaps leading to better treatment results.
2. Computer-assisted diagnosis and treatment planning: Computer software can evaluate face anthropometric measures and produce personalized treatment programs for specific patients. As these instruments evolve, they may become an even more important tool for dentists.
3. Integration with genetics and genomics: As our knowledge of genetics and genomics develops, individualized treatment strategies based on a patient's genetic profile may be conceivable. Facial anthropometry, which provides information on an individual's face shape and proportions, might play a crucial role in this process.
4. Artificial intelligence and machine learning: AI and machine learning algorithms may be taught to spot patterns in face anthropometric data, which might aid in the identification of risk factors for particular dental problems and the development of more effective treatment strategies.
5. Telemedicine: The COVID-19 epidemic has hastened the use of telemedicine in dentistry, and face anthropometry has the potential to play a major role in remote diagnosis and treatment planning. Dentists may examine patients remotely and design treatment programs using digital imaging and analytic technologies, eliminating the necessity for in-person consultations.

9.7 Summary

Between the two strategies, there are some general parallels and differences. Both strategies need qualified individuals to carry out the measurements. Examiners' assessments of correctness may differ when a huge dataset is involved. Both strategies need time: interacting with patients and charting landmarks. Nevertheless, indirect anthropometry is preferable to direct anthropometry, which first takes a picture of the subject's face using a camera imaging system before measuring it. It is also more useful than direct anthropometry. After the capture of the face picture, measurements may be conducted whenever and by anyone. For direct anthropometry, the patient and the operator must agree on a time to do the evaluation. You cannot alter any dimensions.

References

1. Jayaratne YS, Zwahlen RA. Application of digital anthropometry for craniofacial assessment. Craniomaxillofac Trauma Reconstr. 2014;7(2):101–7.
2. Farkas LG. Anthropometry of the head and face in medicine. New York: Elsevier; 1981.
3. Bagic I, Verzak Z. Craniofacial anthropometric analysis in Down's syndrome patients. Coll Antropol. 2003;27(Suppl 2):23–30.
4. Fakhroddin M, Ahmad G, Imran S. Morphometric characteristics of craniofacial features in patients with schizophrenia. J Psychiatry. 2014;17:514–9.
5. Kolar JC, Munro IR, Farkas LG. Patterns of dysmorphology in Crouzon syndrome: an anthropometric study. Cleft Palate J. 1988;25(3):235–44.
6. Kolar JC, Farkas LG, Munro IR. Surface morphology in Treacher Collins syndrome: an anthropometric study. Cleft Palate J. 1985;22(4):266–74.
7. Edler R, Agarwal P, Wertheim D, Greenhill D. The use of anthropometric proportion indices in the measurement of facial attractiveness. Eur J Orthod. 2006;28(3):274–81.

8. Enciso R, Shaw AM, Neumann U, Mah J. Three-dimensional head anthropometric analysis. In: Medical imaging. SPIE; 2003. p. 8.
9. Cao C, Weng Y, Zhou S, Tong Y, Zhou K. FaceWarehouse: a 3D facial expression database for visual computing. IEEE Trans Vis Comput Graph. 2014;20(3):413–25.
10. Kairos Human Analytics Blogs https://www.kairos.com/blog/. Accessed 18 Apr 2023.
11. Allanson JE. Objective techniques for craniofacial assessment: what are the choices? Am J Med Genet. 1997;70(1):1–5.
12. Farkas LG, Hajniš K, Posnick JC. Anthropometric and anthroposcopic findings of the nasal and facial region in cleft patients before and after primary lip and palate repair. Cleft Palate Craniofac J. 1993;30(1):1–12.
13. Mulliken JB, Burvin R, Farkas LG. Repair of bilateral complete cleft lip: intraoperative nasolabial anthropometry. Plast Reconstr Surg. 2001;107(2):307–14.
14. Kolar JC, Salter EM. Preoperative anthropometric dysmorphology in metopic synostosis. Am J Phys Anthropol. 1997;103(3):341–51.
15. Kolar JC, Salter EM, Weinberg SM. Preoperative craniofacial dysmorphology in isolated sagittal synostosis: a comprehensive anthropometric evaluation. J Craniofac Surg. 2010;21(5):1404–10.
16. Ridgway EB, Wu JK, Sullivan SR, et al. Craniofacial growth in patients with FGFR3Pro250Arg mutation after fronto-orbital advancement in infancy. J Craniofac Surg. 2011;22(2):455–61.
17. Farkas LG. Anthropometry of the head and face. 2nd ed. New York, NY: Raven Press; 1994.
18. Farkas LG, Deutsch CK. Anthropometric determination of craniofacial morphology. Am J Med Genet. 1996;65(1):1–4.
19. Jayaratne YS, Zwahlen RA, Lo J, Tam SC, Cheung LK. Computeraided maxillofacial surgery: an update. Surg Innov. 2010;17(3):217–25.
20. Azouz ZB, Rioux M, Shu C, Lepage R. Characterizing human shape variation using 3D anthropometric data. Vis Comput. 2006;22:302–14.
21. Landes CA, Bitsakis J, Diehl T, Bitter K. Introduction of a threedimensional anthropometry of the viscerocranium. Part I: measurement of craniofacial development and establishment of standard values and growth functions. J Craniomaxillofac Surg. 2002;30(1):18–24.
22. Bush K, Antonyshyn O. Three-dimensional facial anthropometry using a laser surface scanner: validation of the technique. Plast Reconstr Surg. 1996;98(2):226–35.
23. Fernandez-Alvarez JA, Infante-Cossio P, Barrera-Pulido F, Gacto-Sanchez P, Suarez-Mejias C, Gomez-Ciriza G, Sicilia-Castro D, Gomez-Cia T. Virtual reality AYRA software for preoperative planning in facial allotransplantation. J Craniofac Surg. 2014;25(5):1805–9. https://doi.org/10.1097/SCS.0000000000000989.
24. LifeViz® infinity: all in one system for face, body & breast. https://www.quantificare.com/3d-photography-systems_old/lifeviz-infinity/. Accessed 18 Apr 2023.
25. Wong JY, Oh AK, Ohta E, et al. Validity and reliability of craniofacial anthropometric measurement of 3D digital photogrammetric images. Cleft Palate Craniofac J. 2008;45(3):232–9. https://doi.org/10.1597/06-175.
26. Aldridge K, Boyadjiev SA, Capone GT, DeLeon VB, Richtsmeir JT. Precision and error of three-dimensional phenotypic measures acquired from 3dMD photogrammetric images. Am J Med Genet. 2005;138:247–53.
27. Ayoub A, Garrahy A, Hood C, White J, Bock M, Sibert JP, Spencer R, Ray A. Validation of a vision-based, three-dimensional facial imaging system. Cleft Palate Craniofac J. 2003;40:523–9.
28. Naini FB, Akram S, Kepinska J, et al. Validation of a new three-dimensional imaging system using comparative craniofacial anthropometry. Maxillofac Plast Reconstr Surg. 2017;39:23. https://doi.org/10.1186/s40902-017-0123-3.
29. Aynechi N, Larson BE, Leon-Salazar V, Beiraghi S. Accuracy and precision of a 3D anthropometric facial analysis with and without landmark labelling before image acquisition. Angle Orthod. 2011;81:245–52.
30. Heike CL, Upson K, Stuhag E, Weinberg SM. 3D digital stereophotogrammetry: a practical guide to facial image acquisition. Head Face Med. 2010;6:18.
31. Ireland AJ, McNamara C, Clover MJ, et al. 3D surface imaging in dentistry—what we are looking at. Br Dent J. 2008;205:387–92.
32. Kau HC, Richmond S, Zhurov AI, Hunter L. The investigation of changing facial appearance of identical twins employing a three-dimensional laser imaging system. Orthod Craniofac Res. 2004;8:85–70.
33. Yamada T, Mori Y, Katsuhiro M, Katsuaki M, Tsukamoto Y. Three-dimensional analysis of facial morphology in normal Japanese children as control data for cleft surgery. Cleft Palate Craniofac J. 2002;39:517–26.
34. Hajeer MY, Ayoub AF, Millet DT, Siebert JP. Application of 3D imaging in orthodontics: part I. J Orthod. 2004;31:62–70.
35. Schendel AC, Duncan KS, Lane C. Image fusion in preoperative planning. Facial Plast Surg Clin North Am. 2011;19:577–90.
36. Hildebolt C, Vannier MW. Three-dimensional measurement accuracy of skull surface landmarks. Am J Phys Anthropol. 1988;76:498–503.
37. Hildelbolt C, Vannier MW, Knapp R. Validation study of skull threedimensional computerized tomography measurements. Am J Phys Anthropol. 1990;82:283–94.
38. Richtsmeier JT, Paik CH, Elfert PC, Cole TM III, Dahlman HR. Precision, repeatability, and validation

of the localization of cranial landmarks using computed tomography scans. Cleft Palate Craniofac J. 1995;32:217–27.
39. Cavalcanti MGP, Vannier MW. Quantitative analysis of spiral computed tomography for craniofacial clinical applications. Dentomaxillofac Radiol. 1998;27:344–50.
40. Dufresne C, Richtsmeier JT. The interaction of craniofacial dysmorphology, growth and the prediction of surgical outcome. J Craniofac Surg. 1995;6:270–81.
41. Kim DO, Kim HJ, Jung H, Jeong HK, Hong SI, Kim KD. Quantitative evaluation of acquisition parameters in threedimensional imaging with multidetector computed tomography using human skull phantom. J Digit Imaging. 2002;15(Suppl 1):254–7.
42. Carls FR, Schuknecht B, Sailer HF. Value of three-dimensional computed tomography in craniomaxillofacial surgery. J Craniofac Surg. 1994;5:282–8.
43. Cavalcanti MGP, Vannier MW. Measurement of the volume of oral tumors by three-dimensional spiral computed tomography. Dentomaxillofac Radiol. 2000;29:35–40.
44. Jani AB, Pelizzari CA, Chen GTY, Roeske J, Hamilton RJ, Macdonald RL, et al. Volume rendering quantification algorithm for reconstruction of CT volume-rendered structures: part I: cerebral arteriovenous malformations. IEEE Trans Med Imaging. 2000;19:12–24.
45. Johnson PT, Fishman EK, Duckwall JR, Calhoum PS, Heath DG. Interactive three-dimensional volume rendering of spiral CT data: current applications in the thorax. Radiographics. 1998;18:165–87.
46. Pretorius ES, Fishman EK. Volume-rendered three-dimensional spiral CT: musculoskeletal applications. Radiographics. 1999;19:1143–60.
47. Shimizu T, Yoshikawa S, Uesugi Y, Tabuchi K, Nakata Y, Matsui R, et al. Three-dimensional computed tomographic angiography and pulmonary vessels. Radiat Med. 1999;17:151–4.
48. Cavalcanti MGP, Rocha SS, Vannier MW. Craniofacial measurements based on 3D-CT volume rendering: implications for clinical applications. Dentomaxillofac Radiol. 2004;33(3):170–6.
49. Abu A, Ngo CG, Abu-Hassan NIA, et al. Automated craniofacial landmarks detection on 3D image using geometry characteristics information. BMC Bioinform. 2019;19(Suppl 13):548. https://doi.org/10.1186/s12859-018-2548-9.
50. Qt 5.3 Release—Qt Wiki. https://wiki.qt.io/Qt_5.3_Release. Accessed 16 Apr 2023.
51. VTK—The Visualization Toolkit. https://www.vtk.org/. Accessed 16 Apr 2023.
52. Download | CMake. https://cmake.org/download/. Accessed 16 Apr. 23 2023.
53. Download Qt: choose commercial or open source. https://www.qt.io/download. Accessed 16 Apr 2023.
54. Masoud MI, Bansal N, Castillo C, Manosudprasit A, Allareddy V, Haghi A, et al. 3D dentofacial photogrammetry reference values: a novel approach to orthodontic diagnosis. Eur J Orthod. 2017;39:cjw055. https://doi.org/10.1093/ejo/cjw055.
55. Manosudprasit A, Haghi A, Allareddy V, Masoud MI. Diagnosis and treatment planning of orthodontic patients with 3-dimensional dentofacial records. Am J Orthod Dentofacial Orthop. 2017;151:1083. https://doi.org/10.1016/j.ajodo.2016.10.037.
56. Hanawa S, Kitaoka A, Koyama S, Sasaki K. Influence of maxillary obturator prostheses on facial morphology in patients with unilateral maxillary defects. J Prosthet Dent. 2015;113:62. https://doi.org/10.1016/j.prosdent.2014.06.016.
57. Mertens C, Wessel E, Berger M, Ristow O, Hoffmann J, Kansy K, et al. The value of three-dimensional photogrammetry in isolated sagittal synostosis: impact of age and surgical technique on intracranial volume and cephalic index—a retrospective cohort study. J Cranio-Maxillofacial Surg. 2017;45:2010. https://doi.org/10.1016/j.jcms.2017.09.019.
58. Choi JW, Lee JY, Oh TS, Kwon SM, Yang SJ, Koh KS. Frontal soft tissue analysis using a 3 dimensional camera following two-jaw rotational orthognathic surgery in skeletal class III patients. J Cranio-Maxillofacial Surg. 2014;42:220. https://doi.org/10.1016/j.jcms.2013.05.004.
59. Jung J, Lee C-H, Lee J-W, Choi B-J. Three dimensional evaluation of soft tissue after orthognathic surgery. Head Face Med. 2018;14:21.
60. Terzic A, Schouman T, Scolozzi P. Accuracy of morphological simulation for orthognatic surgery. Assessment of a 3D image fusion software. Rev Stomatol Chir Maxillofac Chir Orale. 2013.
61. Verhulst A, Hol M, Vreeken R, Becking A, Ulrich D, Maal T. Three-dimensional imaging of the face: a comparison between three different imaging modalities. Aesthetic Surg J. 2018;38:579. https://doi.org/10.1093/asj/sjx227.
62. Camison L, Bykowski M, Lee WW, Carlson JC, Roosenboom J, Goldstein JA, et al. Validation of the Vectra H1 portable three-dimensional photogrammetry system for facial imaging. Int J Oral Maxillofac Surg. 2017;47:403. https://doi.org/10.1016/j.ijom.2017.08.008.
63. Gibelli D, Pucciarelli V, Cappella A, Dolci C, Sforza C. Are portable Stereophotogrammetric devices reliable in facial imaging? A validation study of VECTRA H1 device. J Oral Maxillofac Surg. 2018;76:1772. https://doi.org/10.1016/j.joms.2018.01.021.
64. Kim AJ, Gu D, Chandiramani R, Linjawi I, Deutsch ICK, Allareddy V, et al. Accuracy and reliability of digital craniofacial measurements using a small-format, handheld 3D camera. Orthod Craniofacial Res. 2018;21:132. https://doi.org/10.1111/ocr.12228.
65. Savoldelli C, Benat G, Castillo L, Chamorey E, Lutz JC. Accuracy, repeatability and reproducibility of a handheld threedimensional facial imaging device: the Vectra H1. J Stomatol Oral Maxillofac Surg. 2019;120(4):289–96.

66. El Beheiry M, Godard C, Caporal C, Marcon V, Ostertag Ć, Sliti O, et al. DIVA: natural navigation inside 3D images using virtual reality. J Mol Biol. 2020;432:4745. https://doi.org/10.1016/j.jmb.2020.05.026.
67. Alsabbagh AY, Watt-Smith S, Leeson R. Comparison of CT, 3D reconstruction, and virtual reality in the interpretation of maxillofacial fractures. Br J Oral Maxillofac Surg. 2019;57:e69. https://doi.org/10.1016/j.bjoms.2019.10.205.
68. Bartella AK, Kamal M, Scholl I, Schiffer S, Steegmann J, Ketelsen D, et al. Virtual reality in preoperative imaging in maxillofacial surgery: implementation of "the next 258 level"? Br J Oral Maxillofac Surg. 2019;57:644–8. https://doi.org/10.1016/j.bjoms.2019.02.014.
69. Pulijala Y, Ma M, Ayoub A. VR surgery: interactive virtual reality application for training oral and maxillofacial surgeons using oculus rift and leap motion. In: Ma M, Oikonomou A, editors. Serious games edutainment Appl, vol. II. Cham: Springer International Publishing; 2017. p. 187–202. https://doi.org/10.1007/978-3-319-51645-5_8.
70. Estai M, Bunt S. Best teaching practices in anatomy education: a critical review. Ann Anat - Anat Anz. 2016;208:151–7. https://doi.org/10.1016/j.aanat.2016.02.010.
71. Pulijala Y, Ma M, Pears M, Peebles D, Ayoub A. Effectiveness of immersive virtual reality in surgical training-a randomized control trial. J Oral Maxillofac Surg. 2018;76:1065–72. https://doi.org/10.1016/j.joms.2017.10.002.
72. Kwon HB, Park YS, Han JS. Augmented reality in dentistry; a current perspective. Acta Odontol Scand. 2018;76(7):497–503.
73. Hanken H, Schablowsky C, Smeets R, Heiland M, Riecke B, Nourwali I, Vorwig O, Grobe A, Al-Dam A. Virtual planning complex head and neck reconstruction results in satisfactory match between real outcomes and virtual models. Clin Oral Investig. 2015;19(3):647–56.
74. Jemt T. A retro-prospective effectiveness study on 3448 implant operations at one referral clinic: a multifactorial analysis. Part II: clinical factors associated to peri-implantitis surgery and late implant failures. Clin Implant Dent Res. 2017;19(6):972–9.
75. Ayoub A, Pulijala Y. The application of virtual reality and augmented reality in Oral & Maxillofacial Surgery. BMC Oral Health. 2019;19:238. https://doi.org/10.1186/s12903-019-0937-8.

Segmentation of 3D Craniofacial Imaging and Volumetric Measurement

10

Nalla Maheswara Rao
and Bala Chakravarthy Neelapu

10.1 Introduction

Craniofacial imaging is the process of visualizing the bones and tissues of the skull and face using various imaging technologies. In the early 1980s, x-rays were used for imaging and then came computed tomography, which gave much more detailed images than x-rays; CT is used as a tool for craniofacial images till the 1990s; later magnetic resonance imaging became popular for craniofacial imaging which used magnetic field and radio waves for construction of detailed tissues of the body, which includes hard and soft tissues of the face and skull.

In recent years, several techniques came into existence, one of which is cone beam computed tomography (CBCT) [1], which uses an x-ray beam to give highly detailed images of the face and skull.

10.2 Importance of 3D Craniofacial Imaging

3D craniofacial imaging is a noninvasive way of acquiring accurate images of the head and face with the help of different imaging modalities, which is used in different medical fields, including orthodontics, plastic surgery, dentistry, and maxillofacial reconstruction [2]. One of the most important benefits of 3D craniofacial imaging is that it gives a more detailed diagnosis. With the help of 3D imaging, radiologists can view maxillofacial and craniofacial structures from any point of view, i.e., axial, coronal, and sagittal, which enables clinicians to understand the breakages or wrecks in the facial structures and better identify the surgical regions of interest, which can also be used to identify tumors, cysts, and other abnormalities [3]. 3D craniofacial image analysis is also important for the planning and execution of surgical procedures. By creating 3D models of skull and mandibular structures, doctors can accurately plan the placement of implants, determine the optimal surgical approach, and stimulate the outcome of the surgery. With the help of 3D imaging, clinicians can create accurate treatment plans as per the patient's requirement.

This kind of imaging analysis reduces the risk associated with invasive surgical procedures by accurately locating the structures and abnormalities. Which can improve satisfaction and overall experience [4]. The treatment plan is at its best, which in turn reduces the cost associated with the treatment as compared to the traditional imaging methods. This kind of procedure can save time and money for doctors and patients, respectively.

N. M. Rao · B. C. Neelapu (✉)
Biotechnology and Medical Engineering, National Institute of Technology, Rourkela, Odisha, India
e-mail: neelapubc@nitrkl.ac.in

S. S. Rana et al. (eds.), *Applications of Three-dimensional Imaging for Craniofacial Region*,
https://doi.org/10.1007/978-981-97-4608-8_10

10.3 Significance of Image Segmentation and Volumetric Analysis

Three-dimensional (3D) imaging and volumetric measurement are essential tools in craniofacial analysis. The craniofacial region is a complex structure consisting of bones, muscles, and soft tissue that interact to determine the shape and function of the face and head. Precise measurement and analysis of the craniofacial region are important in diagnosing and treating craniofacial abnormalities, such as cleft lip and palate, craniosynostosis, and other developmental disorders [5]. Image segmentation is the process of separating an image into multiple segments, each segment representing a different region of the original image. In the case of 3D craniofacial imaging, segmentation is used to identify and isolate different anatomical structures such as the skull, maxilla, inferior alveolar canal, and teeth. The significance of image segmentation lies in its ability to produce accurate and reliable measurements of the various anatomical structures. This information is vital for surgical planning and treatment. For example, image segmentation can be used to determine the volume of the upper airway, which is essential in the treatment of sleep apnea. Figure 10.1 depicts the anatomical structure

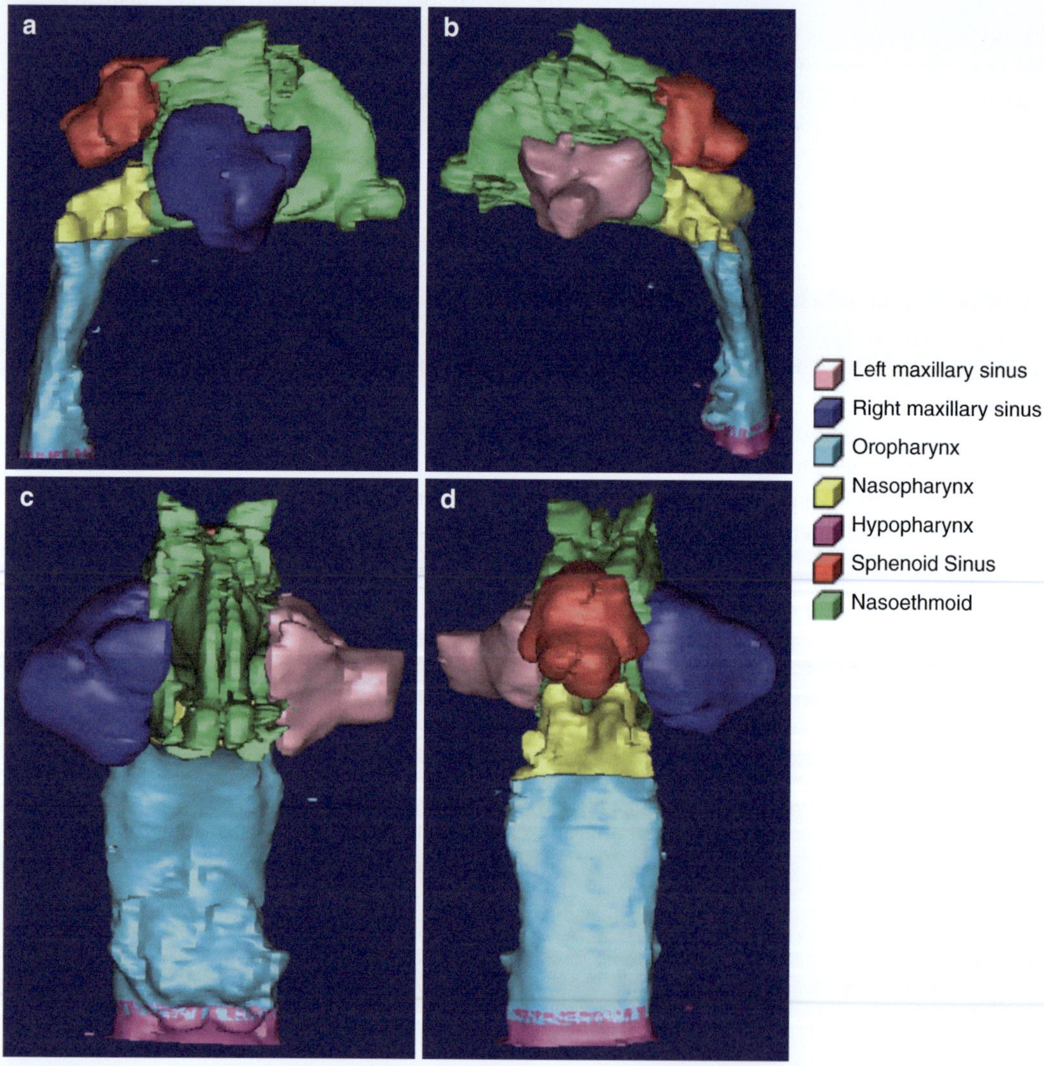

Fig. 10.1 Anatomy of upper airway (**a** and **b**) Lateral views, (**c**) Posterior view, (**d**) Anterior view

of the upper airway and maxillary sinus, where each part can be segmented separately and volume can be calculated. It can also be used to identify the exact location and extent of dental abnormalities, which in turn can help the clinicians to better treatment.

Volumetric measurement is the process of calculating the volume of an object or an extracted region. In the case of 3D craniofacial imaging, volumetric measurement is used to quantify the size and shape of the anatomical structures such as the cranial vault, maxilla, etc. The significance of volumetric measurement is that it can provide a more complete and accurate assessment of the craniofacial region than traditional 2D imaging techniques. For example, volumetric measurement can be used to calculate the volume of the cranial vault in patients with craniosynostosis, a condition where the structures between the bones of the skull fuse prematurely [6].

10.4 Segmentation Techniques

10.4.1 Manual Segmentation

Manual segmentation is a process in which a radiology expert manually identifies and outlines the boundaries of structures of interest in 3D craniofacial image data. Manual segmentation can be used to identify the maxillary sinus, inferior alveolar canal, and upper airway tract from the 3D craniofacial image data. Manual segmentation can be a time and labor-intensive process, but often times it is required for accuracy and detailed analysis [7]. It is particularly important for surgical planning, orthodontic treatment, etc.

The manual segmentation process typically involves the following steps:

1. Image Segmentation: In this step, clinicians obtain high-quality image data from cone beam computed tomography or magnetic resonance imaging scans. The data must be carefully inspected and prepared for segmentation by an experienced radiologist to ensure that the images are clear and accurate.
2. Selection of Region of Interest: The selected region of interest will be segmented. In craniofacial imaging, this may include the entire skull or specific parts like the mandible or maxilla.
3. Segmentation: Once the region of interest is selected, the expert will manually draw the boundaries of the structure of interest using specialized software tools. This process involves carefully tracing the region interest slice by slice through the 3D imaging data.
4. Quality Control: After the completion of segmentation, the expert will inspect the results to ensure accuracy and completeness. This may involve a comparison of segmented structures with anatomical references or other imaging data.
5. Analysis and Interpretation: Finally, the segmented images can be used for further analysis and interpretation, which may include measuring the size and shape of specific structures, comparing the data to a reference population, or using the data for surgical planning.

Even though manual segmentation is useful, it has its own drawbacks. First of all, it is a time-consuming and labor-intensive process, that is, it may take hours sometimes to complete if it is complicated, resulting to treatment delay. Moreover, manual segmentation is a subjective process, i.e., results can vary depending on the expertise and experience of the radiologist. There can be differences between different individuals segmenting the same structures, leading to various results and affecting reliability. Also, it is difficult to reproduce if the segmentation is performed by a single expert. This can limit the ability to replicate segmentation. Manual segmentation is a hectic procedure that requires high levels of concentration, which may lead to fatigue and human error.

10.4.2 Semiautomatic Segmentation

Semiautomatic segmentation is a technique in which a clinician interacts with a computer algorithm to segment an image into a required region of interest. In 3D craniofacial imaging, this technique is used to separate the skull and facial structures from surrounding soft tissues. Initially, the radiologist has to obtain the 3D images from different imaging modalities such as CBCT or MRI, and then the radiologist uses the software to select a seed point within the image. The seed point will act as a starting point for the segmentation algorithm. The computer uses mathematical algorithms to identify similar structures in the surrounding area. Then, it can adjust the segmentation boundaries as per the patient's requirement [8].

The most used mathematical algorithms are the following:

1. Region-based segmentation
2. Threshold-based segmentation
3. Contour-based segmentation

Region-based segmentation [9] is a simple technique that groups pixels or voxels into regions based on their properties such as intensity, texture, or shape. One common method is region growing, which starts with a seed point or voxel and grows by adding neighboring pixels with certain criteria, such as similar intensity values or gradients. Another one is clustering, which groups pixels based on the similarity in a feature space, such as color or texture, but if the seed point is not set properly by the clinician, then a false region may grow. Clustering can be used to segment craniofacial anatomical structures like the upper airway, mandibular, maxillary, etc.

Threshold-based segmentation [10] is an another widely used technique, which involves setting a threshold value to distinguish two or more classes of voxels. The threshold can be selected manually or automatically determined by statistical methods. Once the threshold is set, then all the pixels with intensity values below the threshold are assigned to another class. It is used when there are intensity differences in the medical image, such as separating bone from soft tissues or separating blood vessels from surrounding tissues in angiography.

In the contour-based segmentation technique [11], the boundary or contour of the region of interest in an image is identified, and segmentation is then performed based on this shape. Another one is a level set, which is a function that evolves over time to represent the boundary of an object. Contour-based segmentation is often used to segment irregularly shaped objects, such as tumors or lesions.

The above segmentation techniques are incorporated into some of the software. The most widely used ones are Invesalius, Seg3D which uses a binary threshold algorithm, Dolphin-3D, 3D slicer which uses the region growing method, and ITK-SANP which uses the active contour method for the segmentation.

Invesalius is an open-source software [12] that can be used for the visualization and analysis of medical images, which includes CT and MRI scans. Once the data is loaded into the software and the radiologist selects the ROI, Invesalius uses a Binary threshold algorithm to segment the relevant structures from the surrounding tissues, and a 3D model is created. This model allows clinicians to analyze the segmented anatomical structure, rotate and view from different angles and even adjust the transparency to see the inside of the skull, and use different color schemes to highlight different structures. They can also measure the distance between two points or calculate the volume of a particular anatomical structure.

Seg3D is another segmentation software [13] that uses the same principle as Invesalius 3D, i.e., threshold-based segmentation. It can also be used to create a 3D model of the anatomical structures which can be analyzed and manipulated. One of the strengths of Seg3D is its user-friendly interface, which allows the user to interact with the data in an intuitive way. The user can easily switch between the different models such as axial, sagittal, and coronal slices. Seg3D has a variety of segmentation tools that allow the user to separate different structures from each other based on their intensity, texture, or shape.

Dolphin 3D is designed to facilitate the diagnosis and treatment planning of craniofacial deformities. In contrast to Invesalius and Seg3D, Dolphin 3D uses the region-growing method to segment the interested anatomical structures. One of the key features of Dolphin 3D is its ability to simulate treatment outcomes using virtual orthodontic appliances, such as braces and aligners [14]. The clinician can adjust the position and orientation of the teeth in real-time, and the software will automatically calculate the changes in tooth position and occlusion. Another important feature is that it can generate surgical templates for orthognathic surgery. It can plan the precise location and orientation of the osteotomies required to reposition the jaws and can generate a 3D-printed surgical guide to facilitate the surgical procedure.

ITK-SNAP is another semiautomatic segmentation tool that uses the active contour method. It is used for seamless 3D navigation; it has a modern graphical user interface (GUI) for supporting different 3D image formats. It allows users to view concurrently, it provides automatic and manual image registration, and it has a 3D cutplane tool for quick post-processing through the distributed segmentation service.

10.4.3 Automatic Segmentation

Manual and semiautomatic segmentation needs human intervention and they have intra-observer variability problems. Automatic segmentation eliminates such kind of problems and promises to give outstanding precision and accuracy when we use artificial intelligence (AI). Automatic segmentation using AI refers to the use of machine learning algorithms to analyze 3D images of the face and skull to identify and segment different structures like the mandibular canal, upper airway, maxillary sinus, etc. This AI-based segmentation also reduces postoperative complications.

There are various approaches to automatic segmentation using AI, including supervised and unsupervised learning. In supervised learning, a machine learning algorithm is trained on a large dataset of annotated images, where each structure of interest has been labeled by a human expert. The algorithm can then use this training data to segment new images. In contrast, unsupervised learning involves using clustering algorithms to group similar structures together without the need for human annotation.

AI-based automatic segmentation offers several benefits, including increased accuracy and efficiency compared to manual segmentation methods, which can be time-consuming and prone to errors. Furthermore, AI-based segmentation can provide objective and standardized measurements that can be used for diagnosis, treatment planning, and research.

This automatic segmentation starts with acquiring the DICOM image dataset from cone-beam computed tomography or any other imaging modality. Then we can annotate different anatomical structures if required. Depending on the dataset and requirement, we can select either a machine learning model or a deep learning model; after selection, we have to train the model and then evaluate the results of the model; for the evaluation of the model, we can consider parameters like Intersection over Union (IoU), Dice Similarity Coefficient (DSC), accuracy, precision, and confusion matrix [15]. If the results are not satisfactory, then we have to tune the parameters (hyperparameter tuning) in such a way that we get the desired results. Once the training is completed, then we can go for validation and testing by feeding a new set of images to the already trained model. The efficiency of the model is then compared with the manual or semi-automatic methods for a better understanding of the performance of the model. Figure 10.1 depicts the flow chart.

The IoU and DSC are two commonly used metrics for evaluating the performance of image segmentation models.

The IoU is defined as the ratio of the intersection of the predicted segmentation and the ground truth segmentation to the union of these two sets. It is a measure of how well the predicted segmentation overlaps with the ground truth segmentation. A perfect segmentation would have an IoU score of 1, while a completely incorrect segmentation would have an IoU score of 0.

The Dice Similarity Coefficient, also known as the F1 score, is another measure of how well the predicted segmentation overlaps with the ground truth segmentation. It is defined as twice the intersection of the predicted segmentation and the ground truth segmentation divided by the sum of the areas of these two sets. A perfect segmentation would have a DSC score of 1, while a

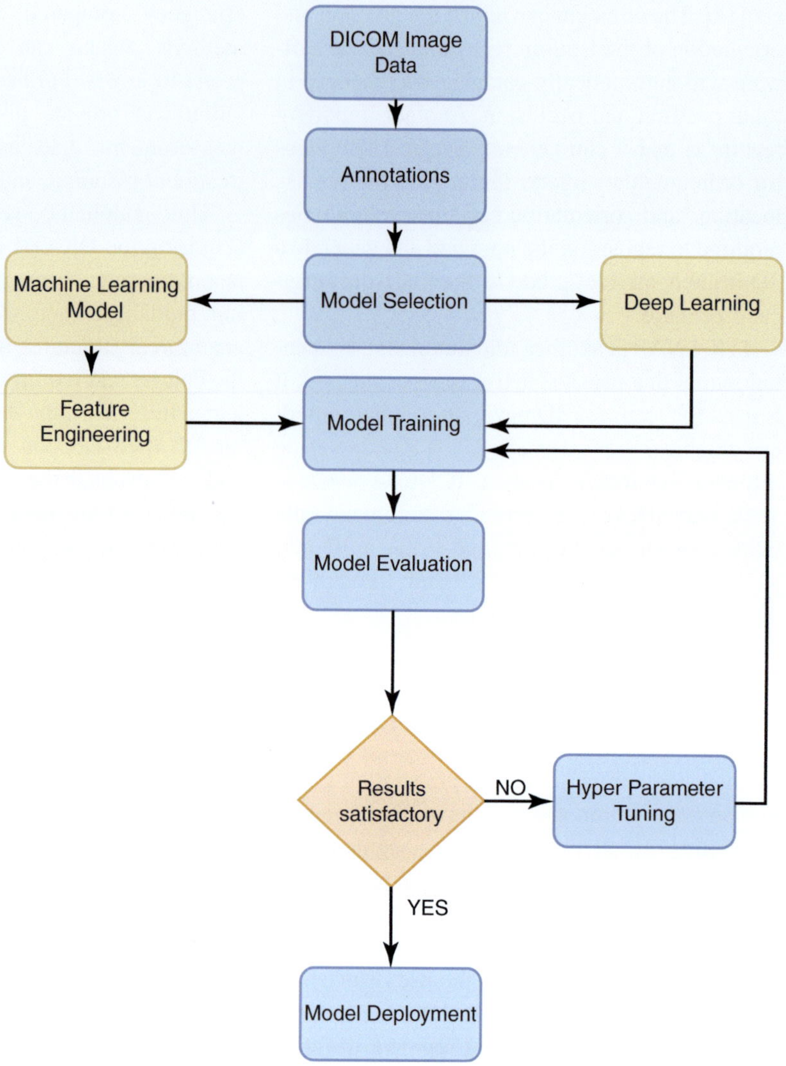

Fig. 10.2 Flow chart for AI segmentation

completely incorrect segmentation would have a DSC score of 0.

Figure 10.2 shows the flow chart for automatic image segmentation using machine learning or deep learning algorithms.

10.5 3D U-Net

Convolutional neural network (CNN) technology improves upon traditional manual or semiautomatic segmentation methods for CBCT images by providing a time-efficient, precise, and consistent automatic segmentation. Segmentation of the maxillary sinus poses a considerable challenge due to its close proximity to the nasal passages and the roots of the teeth. Furthermore, the presence of anatomical variations and frequent sinus thickening further complicates the segmentation process CNNs have proven to provide excellent performance in the field of 3D image analysis. CNN model can provide an accurate generation of 3D models for diagnosis and virtual treatment planning.

The 3D U-Net architecture [16] is a CNN-based deep neural network that has been widely used in medical image segmentation tasks, including craniofacial image segmentation. The architecture consists of an encoder path, a decoder path, and skip connections that connect

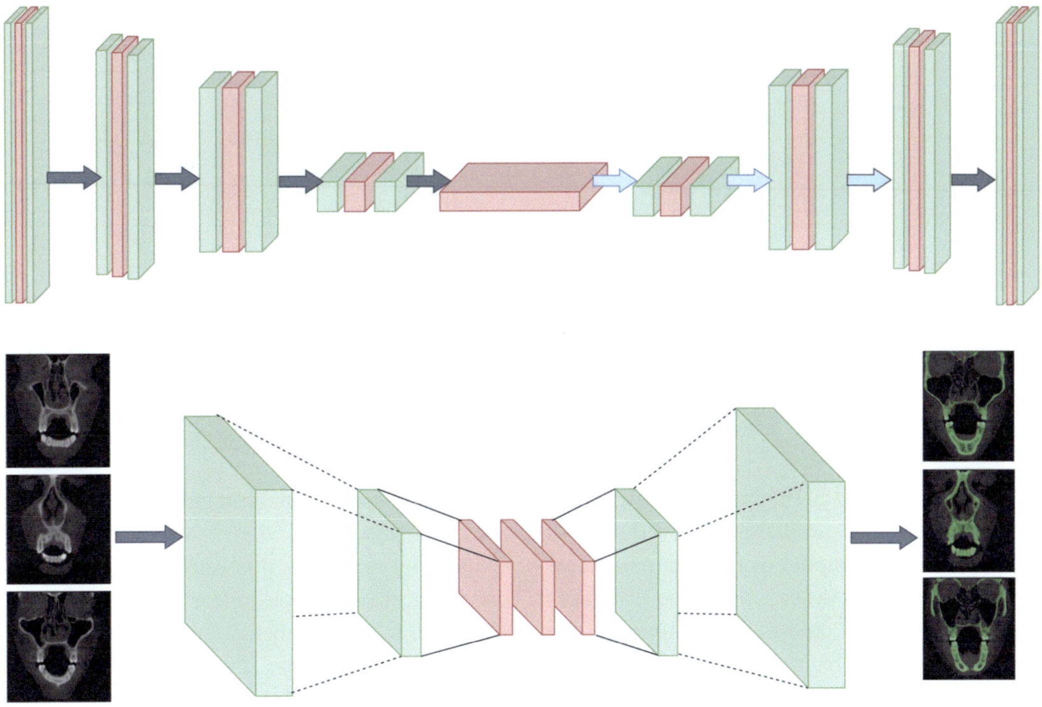

Fig. 10.3 Flowchart for AI segmentation

the corresponding layers in the encoder and decoder paths.

The encoder path in the 3D U-Net architecture employs a series of convolutional and max-pooling layers to progressively decrease the spatial resolution of the input volume while increasing the number of feature maps. This step-by-step reduction facilitates the network in capturing intricate features and abstract representations of the input volume.

Conversely, the decoder path in the 3D U-Net architecture comprises convolutional and up-sampling layers that gradually enhance the spatial resolution of the feature maps while decreasing the number of feature maps. This gradual increment enables the network to generate a segmentation map with high resolution, aligning it spatially with the input volume.

The incorporation of skip connections in the 3D U-Net architecture facilitates the fusion of feature maps from the encoder path with corresponding layers in the decoder path. This integration ensures the preservation of fine-grained spatial information from the input volume and mitigates information loss during the encoding process. Figure 10.3 provides the broad U-Net architecture used in many automated segmentation algorithms.

10.6 Maxillary Sinus Segmentation

The maxillary sinus is the largest of the paranasal sinuses and is located within the body of the maxilla, which is one of the facial bones. In dentistry, the maxillary sinus is important because the roots of the maxillary molars can sometimes extend into the sinus. This can complicate dental procedures such as extractions or implants, and special care must be taken to avoid damaging the sinus during these procedures. Figure 10.4 depicts the maxillary sinus segmentation.

Morgan et al. [17] introduced an innovative automated methodology based on convolutional neural networks (CNN) for segmenting the maxillary sinus using CBCT images. The researchers developed a CNN-based deep learn-

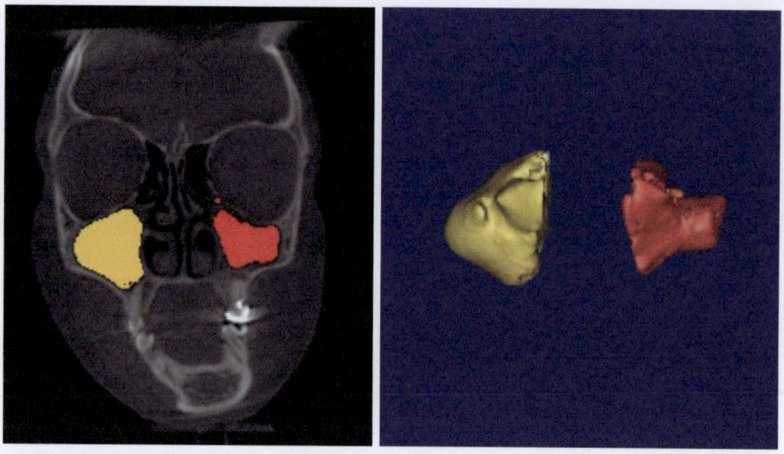

Fig. 10.4 Maxillary sinus segmentation

ing algorithm called 3D U-Net and compared its performance with semiautomatic models in terms of different model evaluation parameters like accuracy, consistency, and time efficiency. They collected a dataset consisting of 264 sinuses obtained from two different CBCT devices; the data is randomly subdivided for training the algorithm and then for validation and testing purposes.

The results demonstrated that the proposed CNN algorithm accurately pin-pointed the segmented region with a 98.4% dice similarity value. Furthermore, the automated segmentation significantly reduced the average time required to segment a sinus, taking only 0.4 min, in contrast to the 60.8 min consumed by the semiautomatic approach. When evaluating the interobserver reliability of minor adjustments made to the automatic segmentation, the CNN model demonstrated exceptional performance with a DSC of 99.6%.

The presented CNN algorithm not only provided a time-efficient and precise automatic segmentation but also ensured consistency across different observers. This enhanced segmentation technique enables the accurate generation of 3D models, which can be utilized for proper diagnosis and treatment planning. The study emphasizes the significance of precise 3D segmentation of the maxillary sinus in various diagnostic and treatment applications, highlighting the superiority of CNN technology over traditional manual or semiautomatic segmentation methods for CBCT images.

Another research published by [15] introduced an innovative deep-learning approach for fully automated segmentation of the maxillary sinus on CBCT images. Precise segmentation of the maxillary sinus is crucial for treatment planning and diagnosis including implant surgery, tooth extraction, and odontogenic disease diagnosis. The proposed model employed a CNN-based U-Net algorithm and utilized a dataset of 19,350 images extracted from 90 maxillary sinuses of two different classes: clear sinus and hazy sinus.

To enhance the accuracy of the U-Net segmentation results, the researchers applied post-processing techniques aimed at eliminating prediction errors. The initial average prediction outcomes of the U-Net model produced 0.9090 ± 0.1921 dice similarity (DSC) and 2.7013 ± 4.6154 Hausdorff distance (HD). However, after implementing the post-processing step, the average results improved to 0.9099 ± 0.1914 of DSC and 2.1470 ± 2.2790 of HD.

Accurate segmentation serves as a fundamental component in the development of automated diagnosis and treatment planning models, specifically for segmenting the area of mucosal thickening. The maxillary sinus holds great significance in dentistry, and its evaluation and analysis are of paramount importance. The proposed model, along with the post-processing techniques, exhibited promising outcomes in segmenting clear and hazy maxillary sinuses. This method has the prospect to assist dental clinicians in accurately segmenting the maxillary sinus, providing comparable accuracy across various cases.

10.7 Upper Airway Segmentation

The anatomy of the upper airway [18] is a complex and interconnected system that plays a vital role in breathing, speech, and the protection of the lower respiratory tract. Upper airway segmentation can be used to identify and isolate various structures within the respiratory system, such as the nasal cavity, pharynx, larynx, and trachea.

The nasal cavity is located at the uppermost part of the respiratory tract and is responsible for filtering, warming, and moistening incoming air. It is composed of a series of interconnected bones and cartilage, with a mucous membrane lining that contains tiny hairs called cilia. The pharynx, a muscular tube that connects the nasal cavity and mouth to the larynx and esophagus, is divided into three regions: the nasopharynx, oropharynx, and laryngopharynx. The larynx, or voice box, is located at the top of the trachea and is responsible for producing sound and protecting the lower respiratory tract from aspiration. The trachea, a flexible tube that connects the larynx to the lungs, is lined with ciliated epithelium and contains cartilage rings that help keep the airway open.

Segmentation of these structures can be useful in a variety of clinical applications, such as surgical planning, radiation therapy planning, and the assessment of upper airway obstructions or abnormalities. By isolating specific structures within the upper airway, medical professionals can gain a better understanding of their anatomical relationships and identify potential issues that may require treatment. Furthermore, segmentation can aid in the development of personalized treatment plans that are tailored to the unique needs of each patient. Orhan et al. [19] proposed an AI-based solution for the automatic segmentation of pharyngeal airway evaluations in patients with obstructive sleep apnea (OSA). The study developed and validated an automatic detection algorithm using AI software named Diagnocat for measuring the pharyngeal airway on CBCT image data. A CNN-based deep learning algorithm was employed for segmenting the pharyngeal airways for the classification of OSA and non-OSA patients. To compare the performance of the AI algorithm, they compared the manual results against results generated by AI.

The study classified and compared the airway volumes of different OSA patients into minimal, mild, moderate, and severe groups. Additionally, the narrowest points, field, and volume of the airway in both OSA and non-OSA patients were also compared. The research conducted did not reveal any statistically significant distinction between the total airway volume measurements obtained through manual measurements, automatic measurements, and DC measurements in both non-OSA and OSA patients. However, a thorough examination of the output images was conducted to investigate the reason behind the higher mean value observed in the DC measurement for the total airway. It was observed that the DC algorithm includes the volume of the epiglottis and the posterior nasal aperture in its measurements due to the limited contrast of soft tissue in CBCT images. This inclusion of additional structures ultimately leads to higher values in the measurement of airway volume. Figure 10.5 shows the pharyngeal airway region of interest for the segmentation in mimics software.

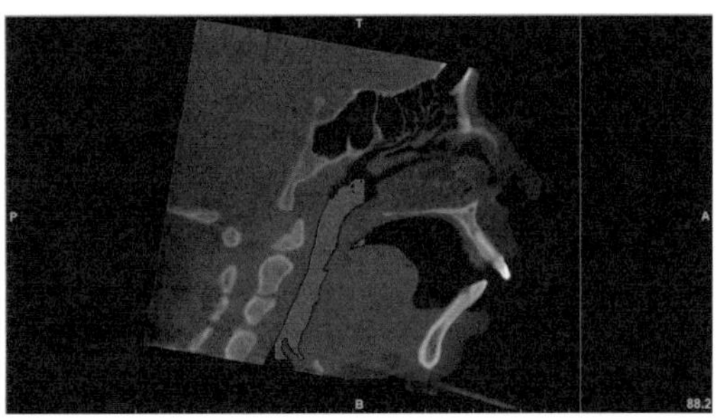

Fig. 10.5 Pharyngeal air way

10.8 Volumetric Measurement

Volumetric measurement [20] of craniofacial imaging, encompassing the maxillary sinus and upper airway, plays a pivotal role in assessing anatomical structures and their dimensions. This advanced technique offers a comprehensive evaluation of the three-dimensional characteristics, providing valuable insights for clinical diagnosis and treatment planning. When comparing the automatic measurement method with manual and semiautomatic approaches, notable distinctions arise.

Manual measurement, traditionally employed, involves meticulous analysis of radiographic images by skilled professionals. This method demands a significant amount of time and effort, relying on the expertise and subjective judgment of the operator. Conversely, automatic measurement utilizes sophisticated algorithms and machine learning techniques to extract quantitative data from imaging data sets. This approach significantly reduces human error and bias, offering consistent and reliable measurements. Moreover, automatic measurements have the advantage of processing large volumes of data rapidly, enhancing efficiency and productivity in a clinical setting.

On the other hand, semiautomatic measurement techniques combine the strengths of both manual and automatic approaches. They typically involve a preliminary automated extraction of anatomical landmarks, followed by manual refinement by the operator. This hybrid method offers an optimal balance between accuracy and efficiency, as it benefits from the precision of automated algorithms while also accounting for the expertise and judgment of the operator. Each measurement technique has its merits and limitations. Manual measurements allow for a detailed assessment, but they are time-consuming and subject to individual interpretation. Automatic measurements offer speed, objectivity, and consistency, but they may lack the nuanced evaluation possible through manual inspection. Semiautomatic measurements strike a balance by combining the strengths of both approaches. Consequently, the choice of measurement method should be based on the specific clinical requirements, available resources, and desired level of detail for craniofacial imaging analysis.

10.9 Summary

In conclusion, craniofacial segmentation and volumetric measurement have been a really important factor for particular disease detection and surgeries. Manual segmentation has been the gold standard till now, but it is also susceptible to observable errors. Semiautomatic segmentation reduced human intervention in the segmentation processes, but it is also prone to inter and intra-observable errors. For the semiautomatic segmentation, seed point plays a major role and might differ from clinician to clinician. Finally, automatic segmentation has been the new technology in the field of medical image segmentation; because of its prediction accuracy and less time requirement, it became the go choice for segmentation; and yet it is far from implementation. A lot of research is currently focused on implementing artificial intelligence in medical imaging and segmentation, with powerful AI-based algorithms expected to soon assist clinicians.

References

1. Scarfe WC, Farman AG, Levin MD, Gane D. Essentials of maxillofacial cone beam computed tomography. Alpha Omegan. 2010;103(2):62–7.
2. Jyothikiran H, Shanthara JR, Subbiah P, Thomas M. Craniofacial imaging in orthodontics—past present and future. Int J Orthodontics (Milwaukee, Wis). 2014;25(1):21–6.
3. Henneman WJ, Postma AA, Treumann T. Radiology of craniofacial trauma. In: Craniofacial trauma: diagnosis and management; 2019. p. 35–54.
4. Mercan E, Atmosukarto I, Wu J, Liang S, Shapiro LG. Craniofacial image analysis. In: Health monitoring and personalized feedback using multimedia data. Springer; 2015. p. 9–29.
5. Mian M, Tan J, Yong R, Williams R, Labrinidis A, Anderson PJ, et al. Craniofacial phenomics: three-dimensional assessment of the size and shape of cranial and dentofacial structures. In: Craniofacial development: methods and protocols. Springer; 2021. p. 107–27.

6. Eley KA, Delso G. Automated 3D MRI rendering of the craniofacial skeleton: using ZTE to drive the segmentation of black bone and FIESTA-C images. Neuroradiology. 2021;63:91–8.
7. Andersen TN, Darvann TA, Murakami S, Larsen P, Senda Y, Bilde A, et al. Accuracy and precision of manual segmentation of the maxillary sinus in MR images—a method study. Br J Radiol. 2018;91(1085):20170663.
8. Wallner J, Schwaiger M, Hochegger K, Gsaxner C, Zemann W, Egger J. A review on multiplatform evaluations of semi-automatic open-source based image segmentation for cranio-maxillofacial surgery. Comput Methods Prog Biomed. 2019;182:105102.
9. Ansari M, Anand RS. Region based segmentation and image analysis with application to medical imaging. 2007.
10. Jardim S, António J, Mora C. Image thresholding approaches for medical image segmentation-short literature review. Procedia Comput Sci. 2023;219:1485–92.
11. Chen X, Williams BM, Vallabhaneni SR, Czanner G, Williams R, Zheng Y, editors. Learning active contour models for medical image segmentation. In: Proceedings of the IEEE/CVF conference on computer vision and pattern recognition; 2019.
12. Amorim P, Moraes T, Silva J, Pedrini H, editors. InVesalius: an interactive rendering framework for health care support. In: Advances in visual computing: 11th international symposium, ISVC 2015, Las Vegas, NV, USA, December 14–16, 2015, Proceedings, Part I 11; 2015. Springer.
13. Maleike D, Nolden M, Meinzer H-P, Wolf I. Interactive segmentation framework of the medical imaging interaction toolkit. Comput Methods Prog Biomed. 2009;96(1):72–83.
14. Lo Giudice A, Ronsivalle V, Grippaudo C, Lucchese A, Muraglie S, Lagravère MO, et al. One step before 3D printing—evaluation of imaging software accuracy for 3-dimensional analysis of the mandible: a comparative study using a surface-to-surface matching technique. Materials. 2020;13(12):2798.
15. Choi H, Jeon KJ, Kim YH, Ha E-G, Lee C, Han S-S. Deep learning-based fully automatic segmentation of the maxillary sinus on cone-beam computed tomographic images. Sci Rep. 2022;12(1):1–9.
16. Jung S-K, Lim H-K, Lee S, Cho Y, Song I-S. Deep active learning for automatic segmentation of maxillary sinus lesions using a convolutional neural network. Diagnostics. 2021;11(4):688.
17. Morgan N, Van Gerven A, Smolders A, de Faria VK, Willems H, Jacobs R. Convolutional neural network for automatic maxillary sinus segmentation on cone-beam computed tomographic images. Sci Rep. 2022;12(1):7523.
18. Ball M, Hossain M, Padalia D. Anatomy, airway. 2017.
19. Orhan K, Shamshiev M, Ezhov M, Plaksin A, Kurbanova A, Ünsal G, et al. AI-based automatic segmentation of craniomaxillofacial anatomy from CBCT scans for automatic detection of pharyngeal airway evaluations in OSA patients. Sci Rep. 2022;12(1):1–9.
20. Chousangsuntorn K, Bhongmakapat T, Apirakkittikul N, Sungkarat W, Supakul N, Laothamatas J. Upper airway areas, volumes, and linear measurements determined on computed tomography during different phases of respiration predict the presence of severe obstructive sleep apnea. J Oral Maxillofac Surg. 2018;76(7):1524–31.

Cephalometric Analysis Using Three-Dimensional Imaging System

11

Karthik Sennimalai, Sharvari Vichare, Shailendra Singh Rana, Babu Lal, and Madhanraj Selvaraj

11.1 Introduction

The importance of data collection and record-keeping in orthodontics cannot be overstated. The human face is a complex and harmonious system, comprising the craniofacial complex and overlying soft tissue. In addition, most craniofacial abnormalities are asymmetric and conform to three-dimensional (3D) deformations. Therefore, the routine two-dimensional (2D) assessment is inadequate in understanding the craniofacial complex, necessitating 3D data acquisition [1, 2]. 3D cephalometry, performed using 3D imaging data, is useful in various fields, such as orthodontics, maxillofacial surgery, and craniomaxillofacial imaging. In orthodontics, it is used to diagnose and plan treatment for skeletal malocclusions or in a complex condition such as multiple impacted teeth (Fig. 11.1). In maxillofacial surgery, it can help to plan complex surgical procedures, such as jaw reconstruction or maxillofacial trauma surgery. It is also used in craniomaxillofacial imaging to diagnose and monitor various craniofacial conditions, such as sleep apnea, congenital deformities, temporomandibular joint disorders, and facial asymmetries (Fig. 11.2).

Overall, 3D cephalometry provides a more precise and comprehensive analysis of the craniofacial structures than traditional 2D radiographs, enabling more accurate diagnosis and treatment planning [3, 4]. Like 2D cephalometry, 3D cephalometry has evolved over the years as technology has advanced, and the need for more accurate and comprehensive analysis of craniofacial structures has increased [5–7]. Various 3D cephalometric analyses, including automation, have been recently developed [8, 9]. This chapter will provide an overview of the evolution, current state of knowledge, and potential recent advancements of 3D cephalometry.

K. Sennimalai
Department of Orthodontics, All India Institute of Medical Sciences, Vijaypur, Jammu, India

S. Vichare
All India Institute of Medical Sciences, Bathinda, Punjab, India

S. S. Rana (✉)
Department of Dentistry, All India Institute of Medical Sciences, Bathinda, Punjab, India

B. Lal
Department of Trauma and Emergency Medicine, All India Institute of Medical Sciences, Bhopal, Madhya Pradesh, India

M. Selvaraj
Division of Orthodontics and Dentofacial Orthopedics, Department of Dentistry, Jawaharlal Institute of Postgraduate Medical Education and Research, Puducherry, India

S. S. Rana et al. (eds.), *Applications of Three-dimensional Imaging for Craniofacial Region*, https://doi.org/10.1007/978-981-97-4608-8_11

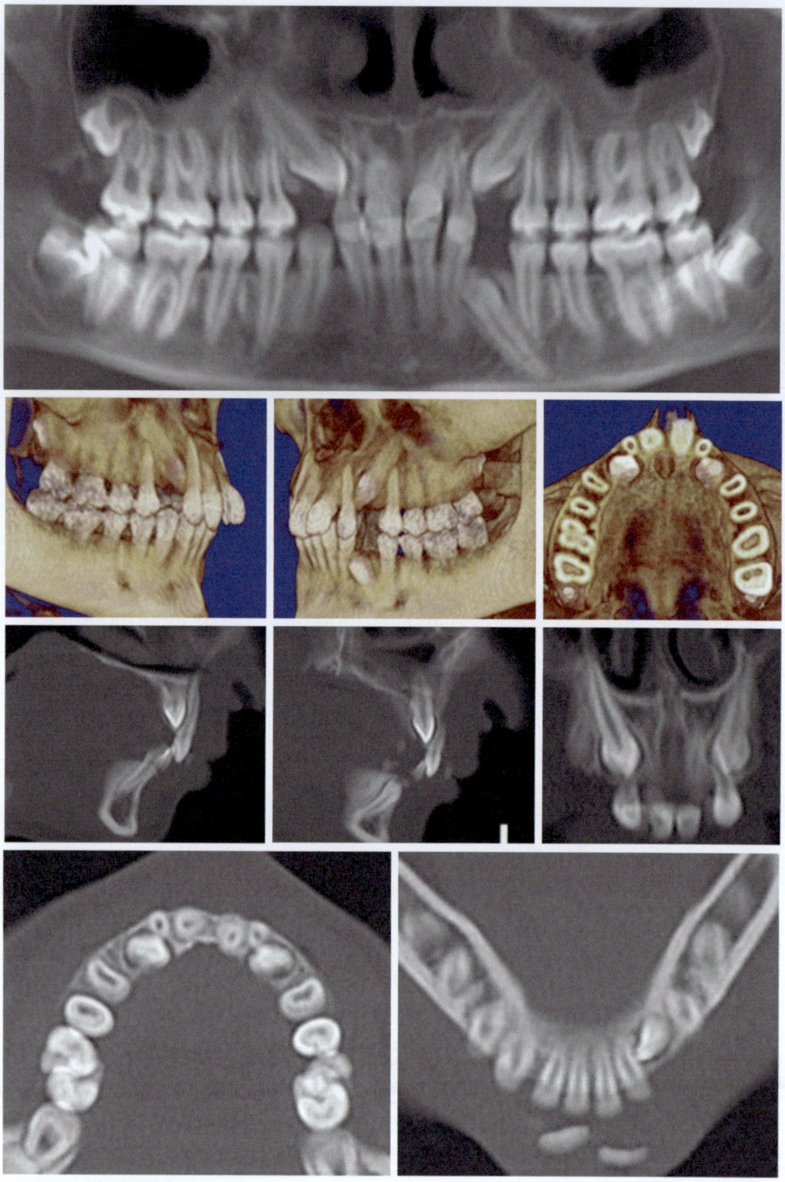

Fig. 11.1 Cone beam computed tomography has emerged as a valuable diagnostic tool in orthodontics, especially in managing impacted canines. By providing detailed three-dimensional images of the impacted tooth and surrounding structures, CBCT imaging can help guide treatment planning and improve treatment outcomes such as accurate visualization of the impacted tooth and adjacent structures, identification of anatomical variations, evaluation of eruption pathway, and biomechanics

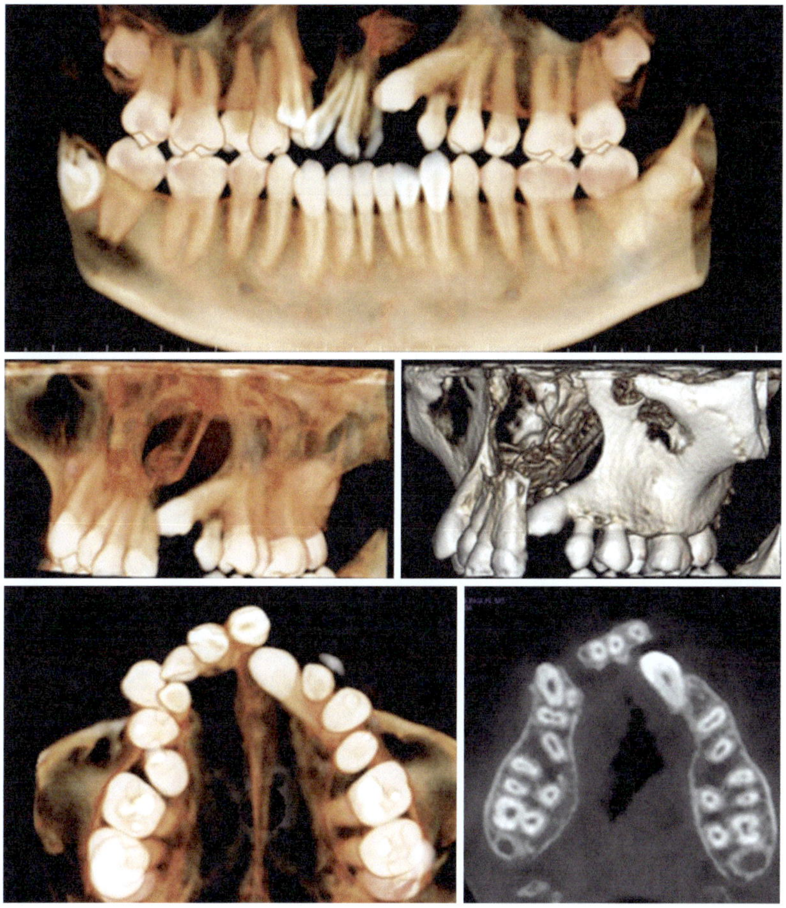

Fig. 11.2 CBCT helps to visualize the three-dimensional structure of the cleft and surrounding structures, including teeth, bone, and soft tissues. This information is useful for assessing the severity of the cleft, identifying any associated anomalies, and planning surgical and orthodontic treatment

11.2 History of Cephalometry

There has always been a fascination with measuring the dimensions of the human body (anthropometry) and skull (craniometry), dating back to ancient Egyptian and Greek times. The terms cephalometry and craniometry are often used interchangeably, but cephalometry refers to the radiographic measurement of the skull, while craniometry is the direct measurement of the skull of living or dead [10].

Roentgen's discovery of X-rays in 1895 led to the emergence of the dental radiology [11]. Two weeks after the publication of the discovery of X-rays, German dentist Otto Walkhoff acquired a radiograph of his teeth with an exposure time of 25 min [12]. In 1922, A.J. Pacini took the first standardized lateral radiograph, which is credited as a landmark in the field of orthodontics [13]. Broadbent established reproducible head positioning of the cephalostat in 1930, which set a precedent for using lateral cephalometric radiographs in orthodontics [14]. Holly Broadbent and Todd Wingate from the United States and Herbert Hofrath from Germany simultaneously developed the first cephalostat in 1931 [12, 13].

In 1948, Dr. Downs developed the first and most widely used cephalometric analysis. This was followed by the establishment of multiple analyses, and lateral cephalograms became the standard tool for diagnosis and treatment planning in the orthodontics [15]. Some notable contributions to cephalometric analysis in routine orthodontic diagnosis include Steiner [16], Tweed [17], Sassouni [18], Ricketts [19, 20], Jarabak and Fizzell [21], Holdaway [22], Burstone et al. [23], Legan and Burstone [24], McNamara [25], and Arnett et al. [26].

11.3 Limitations of 2D Cephalometry

Cephalograms are a two-dimensional representation of the three-dimensional structures, therefore leading to a limited understanding of the true anatomic structures of the craniofacial complex. The lateral cephalogram provides a sagittal and vertical evaluation of the craniofacial morphology but cannot accurately quantify features related to the transverse plane, such as paranasal and infraorbital deficiencies [6]. On the other hand, the frontal cephalogram is useful for evaluating facial asymmetry in the transverse plane but ignores the sagittal dimension. Several errors in 2D cephalometry can be categorized as follows:

- Projection errors: These are errors related to the superimposed (midline and bilateral structures) two-dimensional (2D) shadow of a three-dimensional (3D) structure [27–29].
- Magnification errors: These are errors occurring due to the enlargement between a distance that is displayed on an image of an object and the distance measured on the actual object [30, 31].
- Patient positioning errors: These are errors that arise due to the difficulty of reliably positioning patients in the cephalostat. These errors may affect the angular measurements during cephalometric analysis [30, 32].
- Landmark identification errors: These are errors caused by incorrect identification of landmarks in cephalometry, resulting in a characteristic pattern [33–35]. Landmarks located on curves tend to have poorer validity, for example, measurements that contain landmarks A-point, condylion, and gonion. Superimposition of adjacent structures may lead to confusion in the identification of some landmarks, such as condylion, orbitale, and porion [36]. The extent of error depends on the landmark's susceptibility to the particular axis, and the overall error ranges from 0.15 to 1.99 mm for the x-axis and 0.23 mm to 2.63 mm for the y-axis [37]. Poor definition of soft tissues can also affect landmark plotting. All these limitations with two-dimensional radiography undoubtedly affect the measurements and can, therefore, affect the clinician's diagnosis [38].

11.4 Transition from 2D to 3D Cephalometry

The process of cephalometry has undergone various advancements over time, with each step contributing to improvements in speed, accuracy, and efficiency of analysis. Initially, manual tracing of cephalograms onto acetate paper was the primary method, but the use of digital radiographs soon replaced it [39]. The digital radiographs improved the quality of the images and allowed for easy storage and image sharing [40, 41]. It also paved the way for computer software to be used for analysis. This greatly improved the speed and accuracy of the analysis process [42, 43]. In recent years, automated landmark identification and measurement software has become widely available [44, 45]. These algorithms are designed to identify landmarks and perform measurements, reducing the potential for human error and providing more accurate results in a real-time [46–48].

While three-dimensional imaging techniques like computed tomography (CT) and magnetic resonance imaging (MRI) offer higher accuracy levels for analyzing the craniofacial complex, they are not commonly used in routine orthodontic practice due to their high equipment costs [49], lengthy acquisition times for MRI [50], and high radiation exposure levels for CT [51]. In contrast, cone beam computed tomography (CBCT) has grown in popularity and has various applications in dentistry, including the assessment of impacted teeth, facial asymmetry, root resorption, alveolar bone morphology, and temporomandibular joint (TMJ) complex [52–54]. Software applications have further enhanced the role of CBCT, such as 3D cephalometric analysis [29], computing volumetric changes [55], and virtual planning for orthognathic surgery (Table 11.1) [56]. Apart from 3D analysis, rendering of two-dimensional images from a three-dimensional dataset has helped in the transition of paradigm from the 2D to the 3D diagnosis so that the comparison with traditional cephalometric norms is possible [57, 58] (Fig. 11.3).

Table 11.1 A list of 3D cephalometric software

S. No.	Software	Applications	Link
1.	Romexis 3D cephalometry	– Placing anatomical landmarks in 3D view or on 2D slice views – Head orientation tool for manual adjustment – Dynamic measurements and analyses – Measurement table for comparisons against the norms – Landmark, plane, and measurement visualization in 2D views and 3D – Analysis types: TFA Perrotti analysis, Orthognathic Surgery analysis	https://www.planmeca.com/software/software-modules/planmeca-romexis-3d-cephalometry/
2.	Dolphin [58]	• Fast 3D rendering • 3D airway analysis • Precise volume orientation • Volume stitching, etc.	https://www.dolphinimaging.com/
3.	Anotomage	• Assisted landmark plotting • Custom 3D analysis • Automatic 3D surgical cuts • Compatible with traditional 2D analysis • Photo wrapping and soft tissue simulation	https://anatomage.com/3d-analysis/
4.	NemoFAB [60]	• Image analysis • Cephalometric analysis • Treatment, management • Visualization • Diagnostic • Treatment planning, etc.	https://www.nemotec.com/en/software/nemofab
5.	CephX by Orca Dental	• Tracing landmarks • Scale calibration • Accuracy estimation • Conventional 2D analysis • Superimpositions	https://cephx.com/cephalometric-analysis/
6.	Invivo 6 [62]	• Volume rendering • Implant planning • Orthodontic applications • Anatomage cloud • Endodontic visualization • Airway analysis • Case sharing • Accurate planning and many other	https://anatomage.com/invivo/ https://dexis.com/en-us/software-invivo-6

(continued)

Table 11.1 (continued)

S. No.	Software	Applications	Link
7.	OrisCeph RX CE	• Convert DICOM to STL • Create a mesh model from the CT image • Create a mesh model from an MRI image • 3D surface rendering • Volume calculation	https://www.solidworks.com/partner-product/3d-doctor
8.	Trident dental facial and orthopedics (DFO)	• Differential analysis • Orthodontic analysis • Images stored in DICOM format • Interactive tutor • User setup • Analysis in different colors • Automatic zoom and filters	https://www.trident-dental.com/en/software/#!/dfo

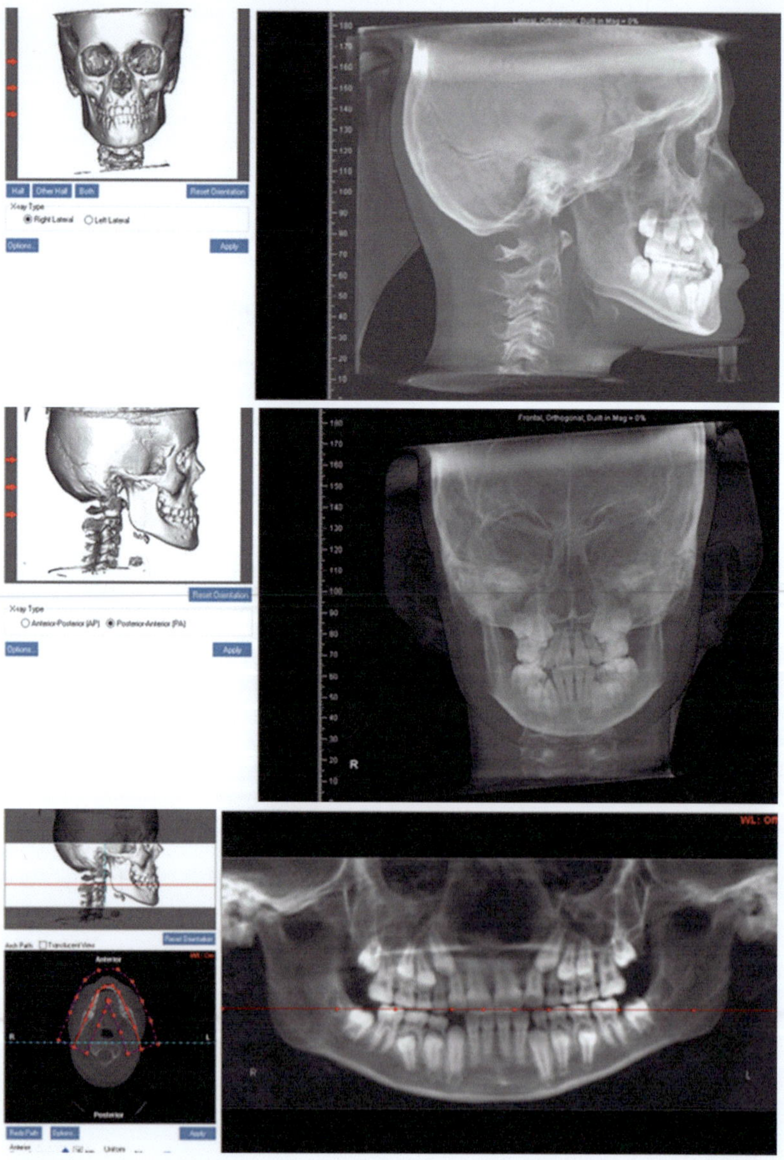

Fig. 11.3 3D volumetric CBCT data can be transformed into two-dimensional (2D) images, such as panoramic or cephalometric radiographs, using the inbuilt program in various software. The figure shows 2D X-rays derived from large FOV CBCT using the inbuilt option in Dolphin 3D™ imaging software

The amount of radiation associated with CBCT is a major concern, and it cannot be considered a standard method of diagnosis due to its higher radiation dose than a conventional 2D cephalogram [59]. Although the effective radiation dose of the CBCT is lower than the CT, it is still higher than that of a conventional 2D cephalogram [60]. However, there are indications where CBCT should replace 2D radiographs as part of the initial diagnostic records collection or as soon as possible after a problem is suspected [61]. To minimize radiation dose, the imaging should be limited to the area of interest. Besides research purpose, the CBCT data taken with a large FOV, such as for orthognathic surgical planning, are only the ideal situation where 3D cephalometry can be explored to the maximum [62]. Despite the potential benefits of 3D cephalometry, factors like radiation exposure and cost are holding back its wider adoption in routine orthodontic practice.

11.5 Evolution of 3D Cephalometry

The origins of 3D cephalometry can be traced back to 1975 when Broadbent et al. introduced the Broadbent orientator, a tool utilized for acquiring standardized lateral and anteroposterior planar radiographs of the human skull. The assumption was made that the beams of the posterior and lateral tube head intersect orthogonally at the center of the head. The orientator was specifically designed to convert the information gathered from biorthogonal plain film radiographs into 3D data points [63]. Nevertheless, the manual operation of the Broadbent orientator was deemed cumbersome, leading to limited attempts at 3D data collection during the early stages. Consequently, orthodontists worldwide primarily emphasized the use of lateral head films, largely overlooking the posteroanterior and submental vertex views [13].

Since the mid-1970s, various methods were attempted to perform 3D analyses and measurements. Earlier, the term "3D cephalometric analysis" referred to analyses primarily based on the lateral, frontal, and transverse planes produced by 2D X-rays; for instance, Grayson's technique introduced in 1983 employed this method [64]. However, this method did not provide an accurate 3D representation of the skull.

In 2006, Swennen et al. developed and validated a voxel-based 3D cephalometry method using spiral multi-slice CT data. The method involved several steps, including the acquisition and orientation of a 3D data set, extracting high-quality virtual lateral and frontal cephalograms using orthogonal projections, identifying landmarks such as nasion and sella, establishing the anterior cranial base plane, and establishing a precise and dependable anatomical Cartesian 3D cephalometric reference system. Additionally, the method required accurately defining 3D cephalometric landmarks for both hard and soft tissues, setting up 3D cephalometric planes, and conducting a valid and reliable analysis of both hard and soft tissues in three dimensions [65, 66].

In 2009 a study was conducted that involved digitizing directly onto the 3D rendered view. They assessed the reliability and reproducibility of their approach by comparing it to the traditional 2D Steiner cephalometry method, utilizing both lateral and posteroanterior cephalograms [67].

However, due to the non-availability of standardized protocols for 3D analysis, several studies have been conducted on cephalometric images derived from CBCTs. There are two primary methods for generating 2D images from CBCT data: orthogonal projection and perspective projection. In orthogonal projection, the focus is positioned at an infinite distance from the projection plane, resulting in parallel rays and no introduction of magnification factor in the derived 2D X-rays. On the other hand, perspective projection emulates the geometry of conventional cephalometric radiographs by placing the focus at a finite distance from the projection plane. As a result, perspective images derived from CBCT data closely replicate the inherent magnification observed in conventional 2D cephalograms. The orthogonal CBCT projections yielded images that were in closer proximity to the skull and demonstrated higher precision compared to the perspective projections, as measured by the absolute differences. The perspective projection images can be effectively utilized for comparisons of CBCT-derived cephalograms with 2D normative data or serial records from conventional 2D X-rays [57]. These derived lateral cephalometric images are shown to be accurate and comparable with direct measurements on skulls and conventional cephalograms of patients [57, 58]. However, it is important to note that while this approach utilizes a 2D technique, its results may not be applicable for validating 3D cephalometric analyses.

11.6 3D Cephalometric Techniques

The main steps in the 3D cephalometric analysis include the following:

- Define the reference frame and orientation of 3D dataset.
- Identify the 3D landmarks and their coordinates.
- Calculate the linear and angular measurements.

11.6.1 Defining Reference Planes and Orientation of 3D Dataset

The importance of standardized head positioning is emphasized in 2D cephalometry, but it is not as critical during 3D image acquisition. Several studies have suggested that minor differences in head positioning do not result in clinically significant inaccuracies in 3D measurements [68]. This is because the spatial relationships between various points remain unchanged despite variations in head positioning. However, the effect of head positioning on airway parameters needs to be taken into consideration [69, 70]. To address this issue, Hsung et al. developed a method that utilizes the patient's natural head position (NHP), which is obtained from the scout images of CBCT scans, to correct the orientation of the regular CBCT scan by aligning the scout image with the CBCT scan [71].

Any investigation, including 3D cephalometric analysis, requires an accurate, repeatable reference system that can be transferred reliably to enable cross-sectional and longitudinal comparison of craniofacial morphology. These are crucial when comparing the patient's pre- and posttreatment outcomes. Various anatomic reference systems for traditional 2D cephalometry have been proposed. The Frankfort horizontal or anterior cranial base (S-N) is the most commonly used reference plane. In addition, a reference system with a horizontal plane 6° below the S-N line was recommended. Numerous researches have suggested various planes for the 3D dataset's orientation that are similar to 2D lateral cephalogram when viewed from a sagittal perspective. A widely adopted method involves constructing a midsagittal plane (MSP) by utilizing three reference points: nasion, sella turcica, and basion. Alternatively, two midline structure points can be used and oriented perpendicular to a plane such as the Frankfort horizontal plane (Fig. 11.4).

A combination of different midline structures can also be employed to construct the MSP, such as the crista galli and anterior nasal spine; nasion, sella, and anterior nasal spine or the most superior edge of the crista galli; and the midpoint of the anterior clinoid processes. However, these approaches may have limitations and biases, making them unsuitable for patients with asymmetrical skeletal structures involving these landmarks. Another method involves the morphometric approach, which utilizes visible facial anatomical landmarks in the supraorbital and nasal bridge regions as references for partial ordinary Procrustes analysis. However, constructing the MSP for patients with orbital malformation may result in inaccuracies. To address these limitations, a 3D external reference system known as the "global coordinate system" was proposed. This system relies on external planes that are easy to define and are not influenced by facial deformities or asymmetry. However, the reliability of these planes depends on the orientation of the head in a natural posture [5].

Most methods have traditionally involved modifying standard 2D planes, such as the Frankfort horizontal (FH) plane, primarily focusing on orienting the head in the sagittal plane (pitch) only. However, a comprehensive study

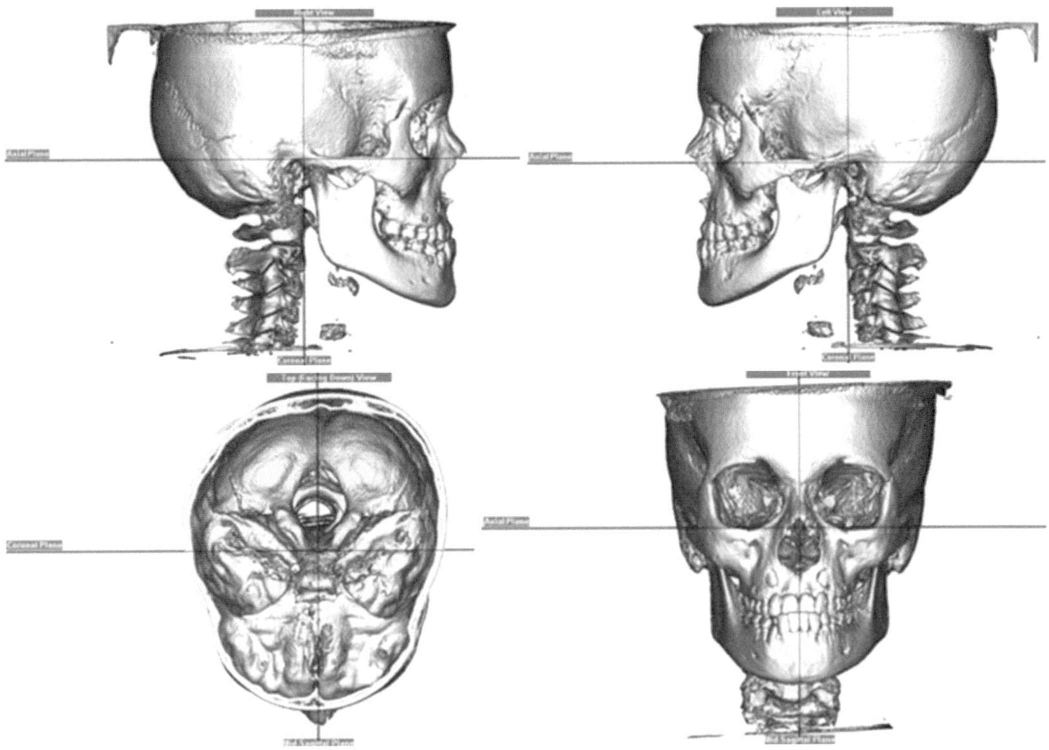

Fig. 11.4 The accurate orientation of 3D CBCT images is critical for accurate diagnosis and treatment planning. The orientation of 3D CBCT images involves importing the images, selecting a reference point, adjusting the orientation, and confirming the accuracy of the orientation. The CBCT dataset shown in this figure is oriented using the Frankfurt horizontal plane, transorbital plane, and midsagittal structures

was undertaken to assess the reproducibility of nine reference planes used in orienting CBCT images across all three axes. These planes comprised five for the sagittal plane, two for the coronal plane, and two for the axial plane to correct head posture. Five orientation methods were devised, each incorporating a reference plane in the sagittal, axial, and coronal axes. Among the five planes evaluated for pitch correction, the Opisthion–ANS plane exhibited the least variation, followed by the FH plane. For roll and yaw alignment, the transzygomatic suture plane and the anterior margin of the external acoustic meatus (AMEAM) line showed minimal variation, respectively [72].

Few software applications allow the user to orient the CBCT manually by identifying two or more landmarks and defining the plane. The planes are set using reproducible anatomical landmarks that could be easily identified and reproduced [73]. The commonly used method is described below.

- In the lateral view, the z-axis is aligned with the Frankfort horizontal plane, and a plane passing through the right porion, right orbitale, and left orbitale can be utilized. Subsequently, the y-axis is established perpendicular to the FH plane and passes through the porion bilaterally.
- In the frontal view, the x-axis is determined by a plane that traverses the right and left orbitales, while the y-axis extends through nasion and anterior nasal spine.
- In the superior view, the z-axis is defined by a plane that intersects crista galli, sella, and basion, and it is perpendicular to the transporionic plane.

The x-y plane corresponds to the coronal plane, which intersects the transporionic landmarks. The x-z plane represents the axial plane, which passes through the right porion and right and left orbitale. Finally, the y-z plane is the midsagittal plane, intersecting mid-sella and crista galli, nasion, and anterior nasal spine. The center of the coordinate system, or origin (0, 0, 0), is determined by the intersection of the transporionic (x-y) plane and the midsagittal plane (y-z) at the level of the Frankfurt horizontal plane (Fig. 11.4).

11.6.2 3D Cephalometric Landmarks

Orthodontic diagnosis using a 3D dataset is reliable and accurate, providing a clear basis for treatment planning. However, a significant barrier to 3D cephalometry is the time and skill required for manual landmark identification on 3D data. Unlike 2D cephalometric analysis, which uses the landmarks conceived with the sagittal plane view, 3D cephalometric analysis requires the identification of landmarks on complex curved structures along the three planes of space (Fig. 11.5).

Transitioning from 2D to 3D cephalometry presents several challenges in landmark identification. Some landmarks require redefinition, such as porion, while certain 2D landmarks cannot be utilized as they do not exist in 3D, like Articulare, being the product of 2D projections of 3D structures. Additionally, some anatomical structures not visible in 2D radiographs, such as mental foramina and infraorbital foramina, can be easily identified in 3D imaging with greater reliability and reproducibility. Furthermore, different structures exhibit distinct features, thus placing a landmark at the central part of a concave structure (e.g., sella turcica) differs significantly from positioning a landmark on a region of maximum curvature (e.g., gonion) or at the outermost point of a projection (e.g., anterior nasal spine).

The landmarks in the 3D cephalometric analysis are identified on 3D surface-rendered volumes

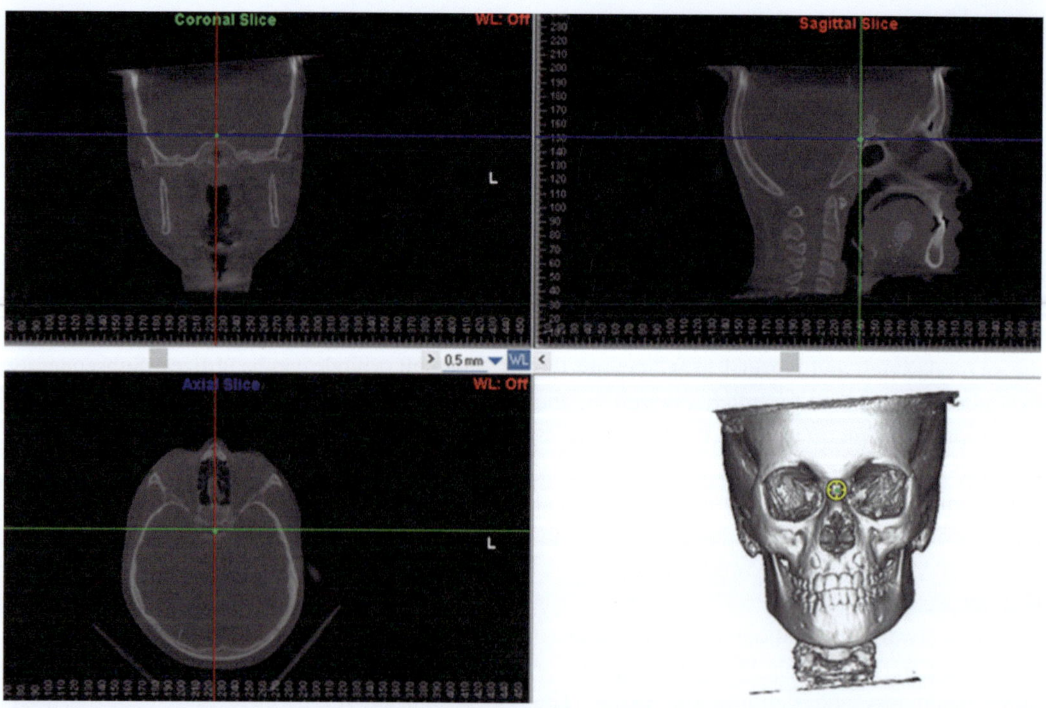

Fig. 11.5 Identifying 3D landmarks in CBCT images is an essential step in treatment planning. It involves importing the 3D images, selecting the area of interest, navigating in 3D space, identifying the landmarks, and verifying them in all MPR slices and volumetric images

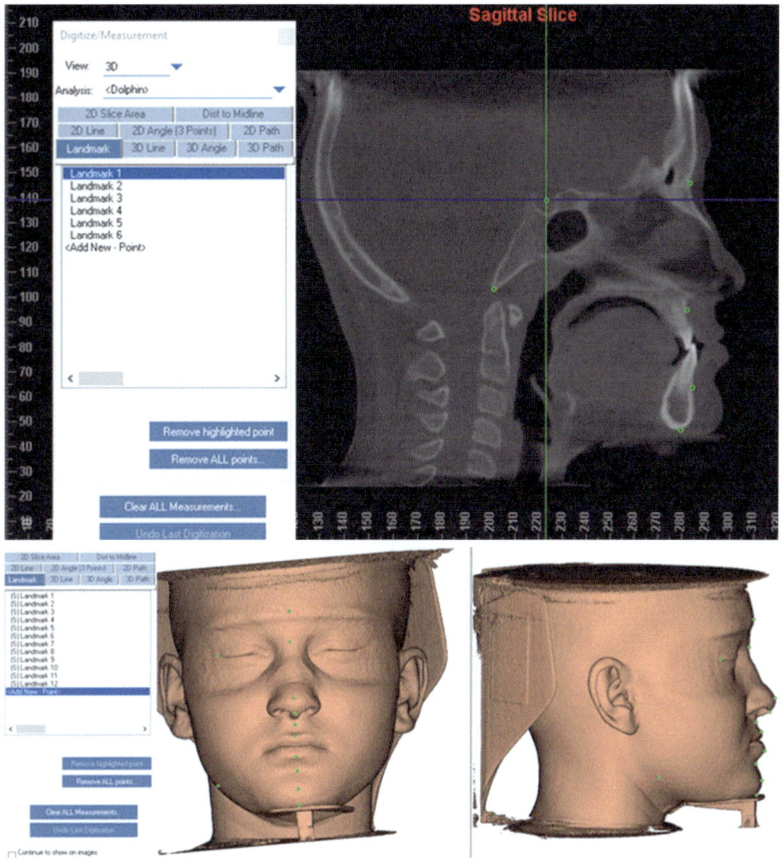

Fig. 11.6 Dolphin imaging software allows the clinician to navigate in 3D space to identify landmarks accurately. Various views such as MPR, hard tissue, and soft tissue volumetric images can be used for plotting and verifying the 3D landmarks. The software provides tools for rotating, zooming, and panning images to view the structures from different angles

or multiplanar reconstructed (MPR) views [74] (Fig. 11.6). The MPR images (i.e., sagittal, axial, and coronal views) improve the accuracy of landmark selection when compared to the 3D volumetric model because the segmentation threshold (i.e., the levels of Hounsfield units) used to construct the 3D model may vary every time resulting in unreliable landmark identification. While the accuracy is mainly influenced by imaging and rendering resolution, the reproducibility depends on the judgement and experience of the examiners' [75]. As far as the reliability and accuracy is concerned, the linear measurements on MPR images of 0.2 and 0.4 voxels were found to be reliable and accurate. However, the measurements performed on volume rendering images were reliable but inaccurate for all variables. Hence, it is recommended to utilize MPR images, which are typically available in most 3D software analysis programs, instead of relying solely on rendered or segmented 3D volumes [76]. Furthermore, for accurate reproducibility, it is crucial to precisely define the location of each point in all three planes of space using MPR images [77].

11.6.3 Analysis and Calculations

Few software has an inbuilt module to perform 3D cephalometric analysis like that of 2D cephalometric analysis. The landmarks are plotted using 3D volumes or MPR views, and the corresponding 2D measurements are obtained. At times measurements can be performed on the MPR views using the inbuilt tool. These are referred to as direct measurements (Fig. 11.7).

Another method that is used to evaluate the three-dimensional changes is through the Cartesian coordinate system. Using the Cartesian coordinates (X, Y and Z), any point on CBCT can be identified uniquely in three-dimensional space with respect to the origin or reference plane (Fig. 11.8). The distance and angle between the

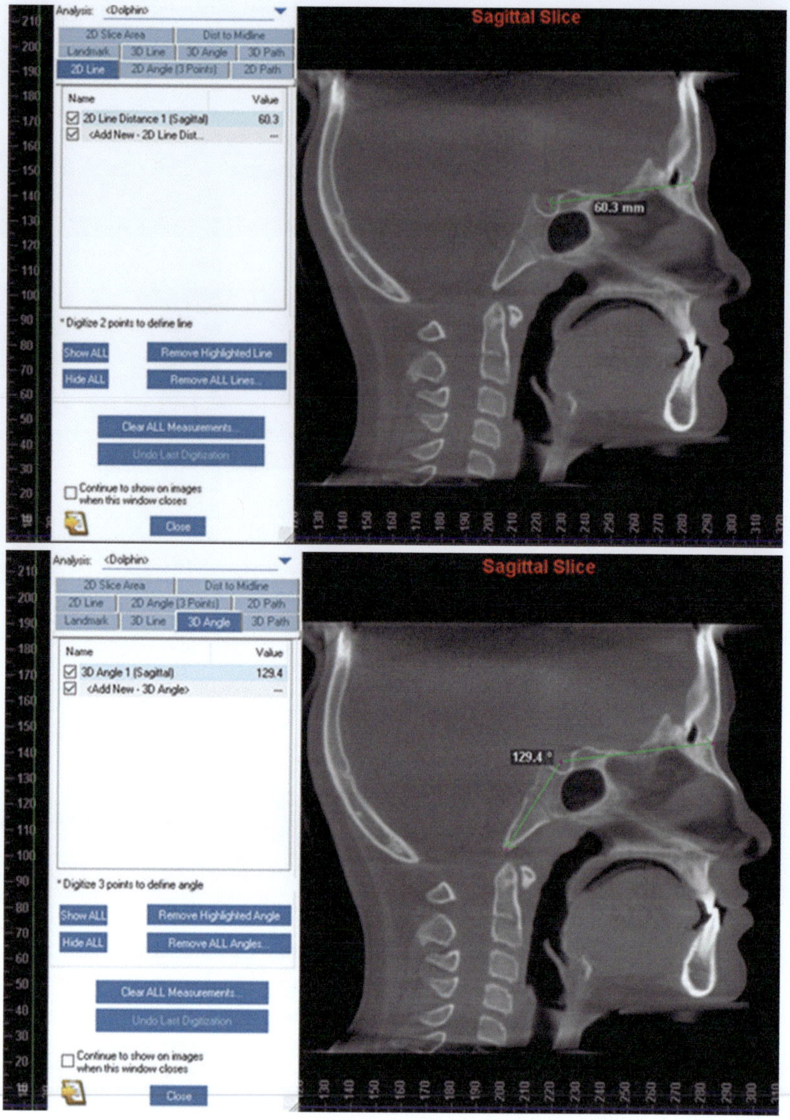

Fig. 11.7 Many software has built-in functions that allow direct linear and angular measurements to be taken between landmarks of interest. These measurements are displayed on the screen in real time, allowing clinicians to assess the data immediately

Landmark Name	--X--	--Y--	--Z--
Landmark 1	-40.6	-48.9	11.7
Landmark 2	-51.9	-0.4	-3.8
Landmark 3	-16.2	2.4	65.6
Landmark 4	-0.0	18.6	14.9
Landmark 5	-0.0	-14.5	-5.0
Landmark 6	-0.0	-24.1	73.7
Landmark 7	-0.0	-13.1	100.2
Landmark 8	-0.0	23.7	76.7
Landmark 9	-0.0	-71.9	71.5

Fig. 11.8 The format of 3D coordinates exported from Dolphin imaging software. The software allows users to export the coordinates of 3D landmarks in different file formats. It is a useful feature for researchers and clinicians who want to analyze the data further

landmarks (Table 11.2) can be calculated using a mathematical formula [78].

For instance, in three-dimensional space, the distance between points *A* (*x*1, *y*1, *z*1) and *B* (*x*2, *y*2, *z*2) is

$$d = \sqrt{(x2 - x1)^2 + (y2 - y1)^2 + (z2 - z1)^2}$$

Angular measurement between three points *A* (*x*1, *y*1, *z*1), *B* (*x*2, *y*2, *z*2), and *C* (*x*3, *y*3, *z*3) is calculated by

$$\theta = \text{arcos} \times \frac{a.b}{|a||b|}$$

Table 11.2 Sample 3D cephalometric analysis

Cranial base changes	
S-N	Anterior cranial base length
N-S-Ba	Cranial base angle
Maxillary base changes	
S-ANS	Distance between sella and anterior nasal spine
ANS-PNS	Maxillary anteroposterior dimension
ANS-rTb	Right maxillary anteroposterior dimension
ANS-lTb	Right maxillary anteroposterior dimension
S-rZS	Distance between sella to right zygomaticomaxillary suture
S-lZS	Distance between sella to left zygomaticomaxillary suture
rJ-lJ	Maxillary width
SNA	Anteroposterior position of maxilla in relation to cranial base
Mandibular base changes	
rGo-Me	Right mandibular body length
lGo-Me	Left mandibular body length
rCo-Gn	Total right mandibular length
lCo-Gn	Total left mandibular length
SNB	Anteroposterior position of mandible in relation to cranial base
rCo-rGo-Me	Right gonial angle
lCo-lGo-Me	Left gonial angle
Vertical facial changes	
N-Me	Total anterior facial height
ANS-Me	Lower Anterior facial height
rCo-Go	Right posterior facial height
lCo-Go	Left posterior facial height
N-A-Pg	Facial convexity angle (Skeletal)
Dental changes	
PNS-ANS-rUIE	Inclination of right upper incisor to palatal plane
rGo-Me-rLIE	Inclination of right lower incisor to mandibular plane

Sella (S): the center of the hypophyseal fossa, Nasion (N): Midpoint of the frontonasal sutures, Basion (Ba): most anterior point of the Foramen Magnum, Porion (Po): Most superior point of the external acoustic meatus, Orbitale (Or): most inferior point on the infraorbital rim, Zygonion (Zy): The most lateral point on the outline of the zygomatic arch: Frontozygomatic Suture (FZS): The point on the orbital rim showing the frontozygomatic suture, Zygomatic Maxillary Suture (ZMS): The anterior, lateral, inferior most point on the Zygomaticomaxillary suture, Infraorbital Foramen (IOF): The opening in the maxillary bone of the skull located below the infraorbital margin of the orbit, Lateral Piriform Aperture (LPA): The most lateral margin of the piriform aperture, Jugale point (J): The intersection of the lateral contour of the maxillary alveolar process and the lower contour of the maxillozygomatic (jugal) process of the maxilla, Posterior maxillary point (PMP): The point of maximum concavity of the posterior border of the palatine bone in the horizontal plane, Maxillary tuberosity (Tb): The most inferior and lateral point on the maxillary tuberosity, Anterior nasal spine (ANS): The most anterior midpoint of the anterior nasal spine of the maxilla, Posterior nasal spine (PNS): The most posterior midpoint of the posterior nasal spine of the palatine bone, A point (A): The point of maximum concavity in the mid-line of the alveolar process of the maxilla, B point (B): The point of maximum concavity in the mid-line of the alveolar process of the mandible, Pogonion (Pog): The most anterior midpoint of the chin on the outline of the mandibular symphysis, Gnathion (Gn): The most anterior and inferior point on the contour of the mandibular symphysis, Menton (Me): The most inferior midpoint of the chin on the outline of the mandibular symphysis, Gonion (Go): Angle of the mandibular body, Antegonion (Ag): The highest point of the notch or concavity of the lower border of mandibular body, Condylion (Co): The most posterosuperior point of the mandibular condyle in the sagittal plane, U1 incisal tip (U1T): The incisal tip of the crown of upper central incisor, U1 incisal apex (U1A): The incisor apex of the upper central incisor, L1 incisal tip (L1T): The incisal tip of the crown of lower central incisor, L1 incisor apex (L1A): The incisor apex of the lower central incisor, U6 cusp (U6C): The most inferior point of the mesial cusp of the crown of first upper molar, L6 cusp (L6C): The most superior point of the mesial cusp of the crown of first lower molar, Soft tissue Glabella (G'): The most anterior midpoint on the fronto-orbital soft tissue contour, Soft tissue Nasion (N′): The midpoint on the soft tissue contour of the base of the nasal root at the level of the frontonasal suture, Pronasale (Pn'): The most protruded point of the apex nasi, identified in lateral view, Subnasale (Sn′): The midpoint of the angle at the columella base where the lower border of the nasal septum and the surface of the upper lip meet, Labiale superius (Ls'): The midpoint of the upper vermilion line, Stomion (Stm'): The imaginary point at the center line between gently closed lips: Labiale inferius (Li′): The midpoint of the lower vermilion line, Soft tissue pogonion (Pog'): The most anterior point of the soft tissue chin in the centerline, Soft tissue menton (Gn'): The most inferior point of the soft tissue chin in the centerline where,

$$a=\sqrt{(x2-x1)^2++(y2-y1)^2+(z2-z1)^2} \text{ and}$$

$$\boldsymbol{b}=\sqrt{(\boldsymbol{x3}-\boldsymbol{x2})^2++(\boldsymbol{y3}-\boldsymbol{y2})^2+(\boldsymbol{z3}-\boldsymbol{z2})^2}$$

Alternatively, a composite analysis is proposed which takes three planes for reference perpendicular to one another, and measurement of the distances and angles from these planes to the landmarks can serve as a method of analyzing the craniofacial complex in three dimensions. These are referred to as projected measurements since the reference planes do not rely on any anatomic landmarks (Table 11.3).

Table 11.3 A composite analysis for assessment of the maxillofacial complex three dimensionally

Sr. No.	Parameter	Description	Reference analysis
Vertical skeletal measurements			
Linear:			
1.	HP-Or	Perpendicular distance from R and L orbitale to horizontal reference plane	–
2.	HP-ANS	Perpendicular distance from anterior nasal spine to horizontal reference plane	Swennen analysis, analysis of vertical heights
3.	HP-PNS	Perpendicular distance from posterior nasal spine to horizontal reference plane	Swennen analysis, analysis of vertical heights
4.	HP-Go	Perpendicular distance from R and L gonion to the horizontal reference plane	Jarabak analysis, analysis of vertical heights
5.	HP-Co	Perpendicular distance from R and L condylion to the horizontal reference plane	Swennen analysis, analysis of vertical heights
6.	HP-Fzs	Perpendicular distance from R and L frontozygomatic suture to the horizontal reference plane	Swennen analysis, analysis of vertical heights
Angular:			
1.	HP-OrP	Angle measured between the orbital plane (lines joining R and L orbitale) and the horizontal reference plane	–
2.	HP-FzP	Angle measured between the frontozygomatic plane (lines joining R and L frontozygomatic suture) and the horizontal reference plane	–
3.	HP-CoP	Angle measured between the condylion plane (lines joining R and L condylion) and the horizontal reference plane	–
4.	HP-GoP	Angle measured between the gonial plane (lines joining R and L gonion) and the horizontal reference plane	–
5.	HP-PP	Angle measured between the palatal plane (lines joining anterior and posterior nasal spine) and the horizontal reference plane	–
6.	HP-MP	Angle measured between the mandibular plane (plane formed by joining R and L gonion to menton) and the horizontal reference plane	–
Sagittal skeletal measurements			
Linear:			
1.	CP-OrP	Perpendicular distance from R and L orbitale to coronal reference plane	–
2.	CP-ANS	Perpendicular distance from anterior nasal spine to coronal reference plan	–

(continued)

Table 11.3 (continued)

Sr. No.	Parameter	Description	Reference analysis
3.	CP-PNS	Perpendicular distance from posterior nasal spine to coronal reference plan	–
4.	CP-Go	Perpendicular distance from R and L gonion to the coronal reference plane	Swennen analysis
5.	CP-Co	Perpendicular distance from R and L condylion to the coronal reference plane	Swennen analysis
6.	CP-Fzs	Perpendicular distance from R and L frontozygomatic suture to coronal reference plane	–
7.	CP-Pt. A	Perpendicular distance from point A to coronal reference plane	–
8.	CP-Pt. B	Perpendicular distance from point B to coronal reference plane	–
9.	CP-Pog	Perpendicular distance from pogonion to coronal reference plane	–
Transverse skeletal measurements			
1.	MSR-ROr	Perpendicular distance from R and L roof of orbit to midsagittal reference plane	PA Grummon's analysis, PA Rickett's analysis
2.	MSR-Fzs	Perpendicular distance from R and L frontozygomatic suture to midsagittal reference plane	PA Grummon's analysis, PA Rickett's analysis
3.	MSR-Or	Perpendicular distance from R and L orbitale to midsagittal reference plane	PA Grummon's analysis, PA Rickett's analysis
4.	MSR-Co	Perpendicular distance from R and L condylion to midsagittal reference plane	PA Grummon's analysis, PA Rickett's analysis
5.	MSR-Go	Perpendicular distance from R and L gonion to midsagittal reference plane	PA Grummon's analysis, PA Rickett's analysis
6.	MSR-Me	Perpendicular distance from menton to midsagittal reference plane	PA Grummon's analysis, PA Rickett's analysis
Vertical dental measurements			
Linear:			
1.	HP-UMcusp	Perpendicular distance from R and L mesiobuccal cusp of maxillary first molar to horizontal reference plane	–
2.	HP-Ctip	Perpendicular distance from R and L cuspid tip to horizontal reference plane	–
3.	HP Pr	Perpendicular distance from prosthion to the horizontal reference plane	–
4.	HP-Id	Perpendicular distance from infradentale to the horizontal reference plane	–
Angular:			
1.	HP-OP	Angle measured between the occlusal plane (plane formed by joining R and L UMcusp and UC1) and the horizontal reference plane	–
Sagittal dental measurements			
1.	CP-UMcusp	Perpendicular distance from R and L mesiobuccal cusp of maxillary first molar to the coronal reference plane	–
2.	CP-Ctip	Perpendicular distance from R and L cuspid tip to the coronal reference plane	–
3.	CP-UC1	Perpendicular distance from upper central incisor tip to the coronal reference plane	–

(continued)

Table 11.3 (continued)

Sr. No.	Parameter	Description	Reference analysis
4.	CP-LC1	Perpendicular distance from lower central incisor tip to the coronal reference plane	–
Transverse dental measurements			
1.	MSR-UMcusp	Perpendicular distance from R and L mesiobuccal cusp of maxillary first molar to the midsagittal reference plane	–
2.	MSR-Ctip	Perpendicular distance from R and L cuspid tips to the midsagittal reference plane	–
3.	MSR-UC1	Perpendicular distance from upper central incisor tip to the midsagittal reference plane	–
4.	MSR-LC1	Perpendicular distance from lower central incisor tip to the midsagittal reference plane	–
5.	MSR-Pr	Perpendicular distance from prosthion to the midsagittal reference plane	–
6.	MSR-Id	Perpendicular distance from infradentale to the midsagittal reference plane	–

11.7 3D Cephalometric Norms

From a clinical perspective, cephalometric norms are crucial because they offer practitioners helpful recommendations for planning orthodontic treatment and surgical procedures [79]. However, the linear and angular measurements obtained from 3D cephalometric analysis vary compared to 2D cephalometric measurements. Therefore, the 3D cephalometric measurements cannot be directly compared to the traditional 2D norms [80]. Furthermore, due to ethical concerns involving radiation exposures to untreated healthy individuals, only limited studies proposed a few ethnic-based 3D cephalometric norms. This limitation could impede the realization of the full potential benefits and advantages of 3D digital imaging modalities in orthodontics and orthognathic surgery. Without comprehensive datasets representing diverse ethnic populations, there may be challenges in accurately applying 3D imaging techniques across different patient demographics, potentially impacting diagnostic precision and treatment outcomes. Even though a precise landmark identification can be performed, the 3D cephalometric measurements are currently used only for asymmetry evaluation where the values of contralateral sides can be compared [81]. The longitudinal growth and treatment outcome at different time points are also compared when the 3D dataset is available [82, 83].

There is a clinically relevant difference between angular measurements taken from 2D cephalograms and radiographs or 3D models constructed from CBCT scans [27]. Gribel et al. found that correction of image magnification in the conventional 2D cephalogram was valid only for the landmarks located on the midsagittal plane. Using the algorithm proposed in the study, landmarks on and off the midsagittal plane of the 2D cephalogram were corrected into a 3D CBCT measurement. It was suggested that by using this algorithm and data from longitudinal growth studies, 3D norms could be established without exposing the untreated subjects to radiation [84].

Various ethnic-based 3D cephalometric norms have been in literature; Cheung et al. created a normative database of 3D cephalometric measurements for adult Chinese individuals using CBCT and stereophotogrammetry images. 3D virtual models were generated from imaging data, and cephalometric analysis was performed using specialized software. The 3D measurements were compared with the previously existing 2D cephalometric norms of Chinese individuals [37]. Bayome et al. introduced novel three-dimensional (3D) cephalometric variables namely the maxillary and mandibular curve length. These measurements were proposed alongside an evaluation of new variables and an assessment of the relationships between skeletal and dentoalveolar variables derived from 3D cephalometric analysis. Their study was conducted on a sample of individuals with normal occlusion, specifically of Korean origin [85].

Lee et al. conducted an evaluation of 3D cephalometry by comparing data obtained from normal Korean subjects with 2D data. They employed Delaire's approach to 3D architectural and structural craniofacial cephalometric analysis. The study revealed that while some parameters showed similar results between 2D and 3D analyses, significant differences were observed in certain parameters directly linked to the magnification of 2D cephalometric images [86]. Liang et al. built preliminary data using McNamara's cephalometric analysis on the lateral view of 3D CT of the population from northeast China [87]. Vahdettin et al. created a database of 3D cephalometric measurements of Turkish Cypriot patients using a 3D rendering software program [88]. Similarly, Santos et al. established CBCT cephalometric norms of McNamara analysis on Brazilian adults and assessed sexual dimorphism [89]. Ho et al. established a normative database of 3D Burstone cephalometric measurements for adult male and female Chinese-Taiwan individuals. They compared these measurements with 2D norms of Caucasians and subsequently utilized the 3D norms to evaluate the outcomes of computer-aided simulations of orthognathic surgery [90].

Similarly, Wang et al. developed a normative database of 3D cephalometric measurements for adult Chinese in Taiwan to understand the specific features and provide information for orthognathic surgery planning. On CBCT, 51 landmarks were digitized, and 3D cephalometric measurements of overall facial features, midface, maxilla, mandible, dentoalveolus, and soft tissue, were performed and analyzed. Therefore, establishing the 3D norms for different ethnic groups can help in accurate diagnosis and treatment planning and for evaluation of treatment outcomes of orthodontics or orthognathic surgery [91].

11.8 MRI-Based 3D Cephalometric Analysis

CBCT is justified only when conventional radiography cannot offer an accurate diagnosis or if it provides treatment optimization. Due to ethical concerns, the large Field of View (FOV) CBCT cannot be solely advised for 3D cephalometry or synthesizing 2D cephalograms for routine orthodontic diagnosis and treatment planning [92]. Any radiograph should strictly adhere to the ALARA (as low as reasonably achievable) and ALADA (as low as diagnostically achievable) principles [93]. It is worth noting that substantial efforts have been made to reduce radiation doses, such as introducing an ultra-low-dose CBCT imaging system [94] and a biplanar low-dose X-ray imaging system [95]. However, there are risks of radiation exposure, particularly in pediatric patients. With the possibility of acquiring high-resolution isotropic datasets in recent times, the use of MRI as a cephalometric tool has been explored widely (Figs. 11.9 and 11.10). Studies investigating the effectiveness of MRI for cephalometric analysis have yielded promising outcomes [96].

A short scanning time MRI system and post-processing algorithm were developed to transform the isotropic T1-weighted 3D MRI datasets into 2D cephalograms. However, it was time-consuming as the required slices had to be selected and cropped manually; moreover, trained expertise is warranted [97]. Another novel scan protocol was introduced, wherein an orthogonal MRI cephalometric projection (MCP) was obtained in a single shot without the need for post-processing or cropping. However, the findings were based on the observation of a single patient, and the intra-observer reliability was not assessed [98].

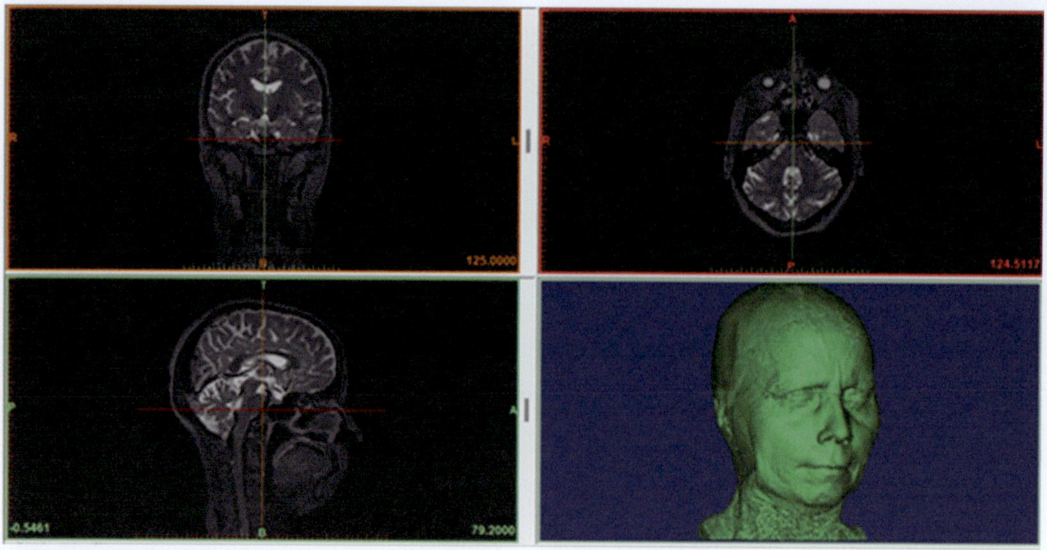

Fig. 11.9 With the possibility of acquiring a high-resolution isotropic MRI dataset, MRI-based 3D cephalometric analysis has become a reality. MPR and volumetric views can be reconstructed from the isotropic MRI dataset and used for cephalometric analysis. (Image shown here is the T2-weighted MRI dataset)

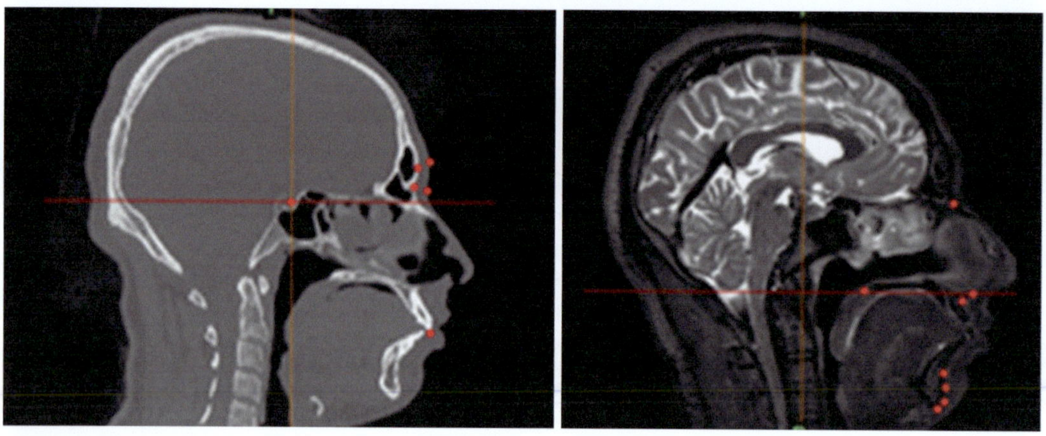

Fig. 11.10 Demonstration of landmark identification in the midsagittal slice of CBCT and T2-weighted MRI dataset of the same patient

The previous algorithms' limitations were addressed by Juerchott et al., who validated the geometric accuracy and reproducibility of a prototype sequence, specifically optimized for craniofacial MRI—a T1-weighted 3D MSVAT-SPACE. Their study demonstrated the potential of high-resolution MRI for accurate 3D cephalometric analysis. In vitro experiments confirmed the high concordance between landmark-based MRI measurements and corresponding actual values obtained from the phantom. Furthermore, in vivo studies demonstrated the landmark-based 3D cephalometric measurement's high reproducibility, independent of head positions [99]. The 3D MRI cephalometric analysis was compared with CBCT, which is currently considered the gold standard in 3D cephalometric analysis. The results revealed that MRI measurements had excellent reliability comparable to CBCT and high intermodal agreement levels for angular and linear 3D measurements [100].

According to Maspero et al., the T2-weighted sequence demonstrated superior contrast between hard and soft tissues, alongside high spatial resolution, and a short scanning duration of less than 6 min. The landmarks were identified in an axial, coronal, and sagittal section of both CBCT and 3 T-MRI and confirmed on corresponding 3D volumetric rendering images. The result demonstrated that 3 T-MRI with T2-weighted sequence had adequate reliability, repeatability, and satisfying agreement with values measured on CBCTs [101].

The main limitation of conventional MRI systems is the presence of metal artefacts, which may be caused by orthodontic appliances or fixed lingual retainers and impede MRI scanning [102]. However, recent MRI sequences have emerged that can mitigate the disadvantage of metal artefacts. In addition to this, there are drawbacks such as costs, machine availability, post-processing time, software availability for reconstruction, and expertise for interpreting MRI data and reporting incidental findings. Nevertheless, further investigations into different MRI sequences may lead to better image quality, faster post-processing, and a viable non-invasive alternative to ionizing radiation methods. This approach can be particularly beneficial for young orthodontic patients and patients requiring serial radiographs.

11.9 Role of Artificial Intelligence in 3D Cephalometry

Artificial Intelligence (AI) has primarily been used in medicine and dentistry for precise diagnosis and prediction of outcomes [103]. In 3D cephalometry, AI plays a role in automating and enhancing the analysis and interpretation of 3D images of the head and neck. This involves carrying out tasks such as image segmentation, feature extraction, measurements, and diagnosis [104]. The application of AI algorithms in these tasks can lessen the amount of time and effort required and also enhance accuracy and consistency in comparison to manual techniques [105].

AI's primary goal is to provide machines with the ability to exhibit intelligence. In other words, AI aims to enable machines to learn from data and solve problems on their own. To understand how AI is applied to real-world problems, it is essential to be familiar with several key terms:

- Machine learning (ML) is the main backbone of AI. It depends on algorithms to predict outcomes based on datasets and draws influence from many research disciplines. Its purpose is to facilitate machine learning from data to resolve issues without human input. Common ML techniques include support vector machine (SVM), logistic regression (LR), naive Bayesian classifier, decision tree (DT), random forest (RF), extreme learning machine (ELM), fuzzy k-nearest neighbor (FKNN), and convolution neural network (CNN).
- Deep learning (DL) is a subset of machine learning that uses networks with multiple layers to analyze input data. It requires a model to be fed a large amount of data to learn features about the data with abstractions from multiple processing layers, with the privilege that it does not require much effort to preprocess the data. Its purpose is to build a neural network that can automatically recognize patterns to improve feature detection. It has been notably used in visual object recognition and object detection.
- Neural networks, also known as artificial neural networks (ANNs) or simulated neural networks (SNNs), are a subset of machine learning and are at the heart of deep learning algorithms. Their name and structure are inspired by the human brain, mimicking the way that biological neurons signal to one another.

Knowledge-based methods for landmark detection in CBCT images use mathematical, anatomical, or geometrical descriptions. However, they face challenges in detecting landmarks due to difficulties in the edge detection of 3D anatomical contours or landmark localization onto an edge or contour [106]. Learning-based approaches were proposed to overcome these challenges by training algorithms on a diverse sample of images. Supervised learning is a type of ML where the algorithm is trained using pre-annotated training data, and based on that data, machines analyze/predict the output [107]. It is the optimal choice for developing an AI-based cephalometric system. Several authors have developed algorithms for automatically detecting landmarks on CBCT images. These learning-based methods are more robust in handling variations in the structures. For instance, Shahidi et al. combined feature-based and voxel similarity-based methods for image registration to develop an approach for automated localization of craniofacial landmarks on CBCT images with a mean error of 3.40 mm in detecting 14 landmarks [108]. Gupta et al. developed a knowledge-based algorithm for automatic detection of landmarks on 3D CBCT images, which had an overall mean error of 2.01 mm with a standard deviation of 1.23 mm in detecting 20 landmarks [109]. Neelapu et al. proposed an algorithm that used template matching algorithm on the midsagittal plane to identify the region of interest, and edge features were extracted, to form contours in the individual regions. This method had a mean error of 1.88 mm with a standard deviation of 1.10 mm in detecting landmarks that were used for both cephalometric and upper airway volumetric analysis [110].

In recent studies, the deep learning approach has been used for automatic 3D landmark identification, which has the advantage of properly addressing ambiguity in landmark plotting due to its enhanced efficiency, adaptation capability, and low sensitivity to noise [106]. However, a major challenge in this approach is the need for large training datasets to overcome anatomical variation. Although Zhang et al. [111] and Lee et al. [112] reported good mean errors of less than 1.5 mm using deep learning, they used a limited number of landmarks due to memory constraints or lack of expansibility. To overcome the limitation of high dimensionality of the input data, Yun et al. developed a semi-supervised learning approach using a variational autoencoder to obtain low-dimensional representations of a large, anonymized dataset, achieving a mean error of 2.88 mm for 90 landmarks [113].

In recent times, deep reinforcement learning (DRL) has gained attention for its effectiveness in 3D landmark localization. Ghesu et al. applied DRL to 3D landmark detection, achieving a remarkable detection accuracy of 3 mm or less [114, 115]. Similarly, Alansary et al. utilized various deep Q-network (DQN)-based models to detect multiple landmarks across three different medical imaging datasets, including fetal head ultrasound, adult brain, and cardiac MRI. Their findings revealed that the DQN-based model outperformed existing state-of-the-art supervised and deep reinforcement learning methods [116]. Additionally, Kang et al. proposed an automatic 3D cephalometric annotation system employing a multi-stage DRL [106]. This system takes into account the geometrical characteristics of landmarks and mimics human landmarking patterns, resulting in minimal detection errors and low inter-individual variation. Notably, the system does not require additional steps for segmentation and 3D mesh-object construction, rendering it suitable for rapid cephalometric analysis and planning.

Another aspect to consider is the ethical implications of AI. As with any application of AI, there are concerns about data privacy, algorithmic bias, and transparency [105, 117]. It is important to ensure that the algorithms are trained on diverse and representative data, that their decision-making processes are transparent and auditable, and that they adhere to establish ethical principles and regulations. There is also the need to integrate AI systems within the clinical workflow, ensuring that they are user-friendly, accessible, and compatible with existing tools and systems. The future of AI in 3D cephalometry looks promising, with the potential for real-time image analysis, personalized treatment planning, and improved patient outcomes. However, caution and responsible, ethical use are necessary.

11.10 Summary

The shift from traditional 2D cephalometric analysis to 3D cephalometry represents more than just an extension; it entails a fundamentally different approach. Analyzing cephalometry in 3D is inherently more intricate than traditional 2D methods, and 2D cephalometric norms cannot be directly applied to 3D analysis due to disparities in technique and accuracy. Transitioning to 3D analysis necessitates proper validation of landmarks, planes, and measurements, as well as accurate orientation in 3D space and access to 3D cephalometric norms. Achieving this requires a comprehensive understanding of the fundamental differences between 2D and 3D cephalometric techniques.

When taking radiographs, it is important to follow the ALARA and ALADA principles, especially in younger patients who are more sensitive to radiation. It is not recommended to take a large field CBCT scan solely for the purpose of synthesizing a 2D cephalometric image. Assessing cranial proportions and developing 3D cephalometric norms using 3D MRI datasets may open new avenues of research and increase the use of 3D cephalometry in clinical practice. As an orthodontist, it is vital to stay up to date on imaging techniques and AI-based methods. The integration of AI in 3D cephalometry is a fast-growing field that has the potential to enhance the efficiency, accuracy, and consistency of image analysis and interpretation. However, it is crucial to recognize that AI is not a replacement for human expertise and judgment; rather, it is a tool that can support and complement the work of clinicians.

References

1. Francisco I, Ribeiro MP, Marques F, Travassos R, Nunes C, Pereira F, Caramelo F, Paula AB, Vale F. Application of three-dimensional digital Technology in Orthodontics: the state of the art. Biomimetics (Basel). 2022;7(1):23.
2. Erten O, Yılmaz BN. Three-dimensional imaging in orthodontics. Turk J Orthod. 2018;31:86–94.
3. Ozsoy U, Demirel BM, Yildirim FB, Tosun O, Sarikcioglu L. Method selection in craniofacial measurements: advantages and disadvantages of 3D digitization method. J Craniofac Surg. 2009;37:285–90.
4. Day KM, Gabrick KS, Sargent LA. Applications of Computer Technology in Complex Craniofacial Reconstruction. Plast Reconstr Surg Glob Open. 2018;6:e1655.
5. Gateno J, Xia JJ, Teichgraeber JF. A new three-dimensional cephalometric analysis for orthognathic surgery. J Oral Maxillofac Surg. 2011;69:606–22.
6. Rossini G, Cavallini C, Cassetta M, Barbato E. 3D cephalometric analysis obtained from computed tomography. Review of the literature. Ann Stomatol (Roma). 2011;2:31–9.
7. Kogou T, Takaki T, Shibahara T. Three-dimensional analysis and evaluation in orthognathic surgical cases with facial asymmetry. Bull Tokyo Dent Coll. 2018;59:147–61.
8. Kim M-J, Liu Y, Oh SH, Ahn H-W, Kim S-H, Nelson G. Automatic cephalometric landmark identification system based on the multi-stage convolutional neural networks with CBCT combination images. Sensors. 2021;21:505.
9. Dot G, Schouman T, Chang S, Rafflenbeul F, Kerbrat A, Rouch P, et al. Automatic 3-dimensional cephalometric landmarking via deep learning. J Dent Res. 2022;101:1380–7.
10. Wahl N. Orthodontics in 3 millennia. Chapter 7: facial analysis before the advent of the cephalometer. Am J Orthod Dentofacial Orthop. 2006;129:293–8.
11. Goodman PC. The new light: discovery and introduction of the X-ray. AJR Am J Roentgenol. 1995;165:1041–5.
12. Keim RG. The evolution of orthodontic radiography. J Clin Orthod JCO. 2021;55:326.
13. Hans MG, Palomo JM, Valiathan M. History of imaging in orthodontics from Broadbent to cone-beam computed tomography. Am J Orthod Dentofacial Orthop. 2015;148:914–21.
14. Broadbent BH. A NEW X-RAY TECHNIQUE and ITS APPLICATION TO ORTHODONTIA. Angle Orthod. 1931;1:45–66.
15. Downs WB. Variations in facial relationships: their significance in treatment and prognosis. Am J Orthod. 1948;34:812–40.
16. Steiner CC. Cephalometrics for you and me. Am J Orthod. 1953;39:729–55.
17. Tweed CH. The diagnostic facial triangle in the control of treatment objectives. Am J Orthod. 1969;55:651–7.
18. Sassouni V. A roentgenographic cephalometric analysis of cephalo-facio-dental relationships. Am J Orthod. 1955;41:735–64.
19. Ricketts RM. Cephalometric synthesis: an exercise in stating objectives and planning treatment with tracings of the head roentgenogram. Am J Orthod. 1960;46:647–73.
20. Ricketts. Introducing computerized cephalometrics. Denver, CO: Rocky Mountain Data systems Inc.; 1969.

21. Jarabak JR, Fizzell JA. Technique and treatment with light-wire edgewise appliances. C. V. Mosby Company; 1972.
22. Holdaway RA. A soft-tissue cephalometric analysis and its use in orthodontic treatment planning. Part I. Am J Orthod. 1983;84:1–28.
23. Burstone CJ, James RB, Legan H, Murphy GA, Norton LA. Cephalometrics for orthognathic surgery. J Oral Surg. 1978;36:269–77.
24. Legan HL, Burstone CJ. Soft tissue cephalometric analysis for orthognathic surgery. J Oral Surg. 1980;38:744–51.
25. McNamara JA. A method of cephalometric evaluation. Am J Orthod. 1984;86:449–69.
26. Arnett GW, Jelic JS, Kim J, Cummings DR, Beress A, Worley CM, et al. Soft tissue cephalometric analysis: diagnosis and treatment planning of dentofacial deformity. Am J Orthod Dentofacial Orthop. 1999;116:239–53.
27. van Vlijmen OJC, Maal T, Bergé SJ, Bronkhorst EM, Katsaros C, Kuijpers-Jagtman AM. A comparison between 2D and 3D cephalometry on CBCT scans of human skulls. Int J Oral Maxillofac Surg. 2010;39:156–60.
28. Park C-S, Park J-K, Kim H, Han S-S, Jeong H-G, Park H. Comparison of conventional lateral cephalograms with corresponding CBCT radiographs. Imaging Sci Dent. 2012;42:201–5.
29. Pittayapat P, Limchaichana-Bolstad N, Willems G, Jacobs R. Three-dimensional cephalometric analysis in orthodontics: a systematic review. Orthod Craniofac Res. 2014;17:69–91.
30. Chadwick JW, Prentice RN, Major PW, Lam EWN. Image distortion and magnification of 3 digital CCD cephalometric systems. Oral Surg Oral Med Oral Pathol Oral Radiol Endod. 2009;107:105–12.
31. de Paula LK, Solon-de-Mello PA, Mattos CT, Ruellas ACO, Sant'Anna EF. Influence of magnification and superimposition of structures on cephalometric diagnosis. Dent press. J Orthod. 2015;20:29–34.
32. Schulze RKW, Gloede MB, Doll GM. Landmark identification on direct digital versus film-based cephalometric radiographs: a human skull study. Am J Orthod Dentofacial Orthop. 2002;122:635–42.
33. Houston WJ, Maher RE, McElroy D, Sherriff M. Sources of error in measurements from cephalometric radiographs. Eur J Orthod. 1986;8:149–51.
34. Baumrind S, Frantz RC. The reliability of head film measurements: 1. Landmark identification. Am J Orthod. 1971;60:111–27.
35. Leonardi R, Annunziata A, Caltabiano M. Landmark identification error in Posteroanterior cephalometric radiography: a systematic review. Angle Orthod. 2008;78:761–5.
36. Durão AR, Bolstad N, Pittayapat P, Lambrichts I, Ferreira AP, Jacobs R. Accuracy and reliability of 2D cephalometric analysis in orthodontics. Rev Port Estomatol Med Dentária E Cir Maxilofac. 2014;55:135–41.
37. Cheung LK, Chan YM, Jayaratne YSN, Lo J. Three-dimensional cephalometric norms of Chinese adults in Hong Kong with balanced facial profile. Oral Surg Oral Med Oral Pathol Oral Radiol Endod. 2011;112:e56–73.
38. Kharbanda OP. Orthodontics: diagnosis and management of malocclusion and dentofacial deformities, E-Book. Elsevier Health Sciences; 2019.
39. Tanna NK, AlMuzaini AAAY, Mupparapu M. Imaging in orthodontics. Dent Clin N Am. 2021;65:623–41.
40. Forsyth DB, Shaw WC, Richmond S. Digital imaging of cephalometric radiography, part 1: advantages and limitations of digital imaging. Angle Orthod. 1996;66:37–42.
41. Forsyth DB, Shaw WC, Richmond S, Roberts CT. Digital imaging of cephalometric radiographs, part 2: image quality. Angle Orthod. 1996;66:43–50.
42. Chen S-K, Chen Y-J, Yao C-CJ, Chang H-F. Enhanced speed and precision of measurement in a computer-assisted digital cephalometric analysis system. Angle Orthod. 2004;74:501–7.
43. Uysal T, Baysal A, Yagci A. Evaluation of speed, repeatability, and reproducibility of digital radiography with manual versus computer-assisted cephalometric analyses. Eur J Orthod. 2009;31(5):523–8.
44. Vucinić P, Trpovski Z, Sćepan I. Automatic landmarking of cephalograms using active appearance models. Eur J Orthod. 2010;32:233–41.
45. Rueda S, Alcañiz M. An approach for the automatic cephalometric landmark detection using mathematical morphology and active appearance models. Med Image Comput Comput-Assist Interv MICCAI Int Conf Med Image Comput Comput-Assist Interv. 2006;9:159–66.
46. Schwendicke F, Chaurasia A, Arsiwala L, Lee J-H, Elhennawy K, Jost-Brinkmann P-G, et al. Deep learning for cephalometric landmark detection: systematic review and meta-analysis. Clin Oral Investig. 2021;25:4299–309.
47. Junaid N, Khan N, Ahmed N, Abbasi MS, Das G, Maqsood A, et al. Development, application, and performance of artificial intelligence in cephalometric landmark identification and diagnosis: a systematic review. Healthc Basel Switz. 2022;10:2454.
48. de Queiroz Tavares Borges Mesquita G, Vieira WA, Vidigal MTC, Travençolo BAN, Beaini TL, Spin-Neto R, et al. Artificial intelligence for detecting cephalometric landmarks: a systematic review and meta-analysis. J Digit Imaging. 2023;36:1158. https://doi.org/10.1007/s10278-022-00766-w.
49. Ibrahim R, Samian S, Mazli M, Amrizal M, Aljunid SM. Cost of magnetic resonance imaging (MRI) and computed tomography (CT) scan in UKMMC. BMC Health Serv Res. 2012;12:P11.
50. Hollingsworth KG. Reducing acquisition time in clinical MRI by data undersampling and compressed sensing reconstruction. Phys Med Biol. 2015;60(21):R297–322.

51. Smith-Bindman R, Lipson J, Marcus R, Kim KP, Mahesh M, Gould R, et al. Radiation dose associated with common computed tomography examinations and the associated lifetime attributable risk of cancer. Arch Intern Med. 2009;169:2078–86.
52. Mah JK, Huang JC, Choo H. Practical applications of cone-beam computed tomography in orthodontics. J Am Dent Assoc. 1939;2010(141 Suppl 3):7S–13S.
53. Hodges RJ, Atchison KA, White SC. Impact of cone-beam computed tomography on orthodontic diagnosis and treatment planning. Am J Orthod Dentofacial Orthop. 2013;143:665–74.
54. Kapila SD, Nervina JM. CBCT in orthodontics: assessment of treatment outcomes and indications for its use. Dento Maxillo Facial Radiol. 2015;44:20140282.
55. Grauer D, Cevidanes LSH, Styner MA, Ackerman JL, Proffit WR. Pharyngeal airway volume and shape from cone-beam computed tomography: relationship to facial morphology. Am J Orthod Dentofacial Orthop. 2009;136:805–14.
56. Stokbro K, Aagaard E, Torkov P, Bell RB, Thygesen T. Virtual planning in orthognathic surgery. Int J Oral Maxillofac Surg. 2014;43:957–65.
57. Yang S, Liu DG, Gu Y. Comparison of linear measurements between CBCT orthogonally synthesized cephalograms and conventional cephalograms. Dentomaxillofac Radiol. 2014;43(7):20140024.
58. Kumar V, Ludlow JB, Mol A, Cevidanes L. Comparison of conventional and cone beam CT synthesized cephalograms. Dento Maxillo Facial Radiol. 2007;36:263–9.
59. De Grauwe A, Ayaz I, Shujaat S, Dimitrov S, Gbadegbegnon L, Vande Vannet B, et al. CBCT in orthodontics: a systematic review on justification of CBCT in a paediatric population prior to orthodontic treatment. Eur J Orthod. 2019;41:381–9.
60. Brooks SL. CBCT dosimetry: orthodontic considerations. Semin Orthod. 2009;15:14–8.
61. Abdelkarim A. Cone-beam computed tomography in orthodontics. Dent J. 2019;7:89.
62. Swennen GRJ, Mollemans W, Schutyser F. Three-dimensional treatment planning of orthognathic surgery in the era of virtual imaging. J Oral Maxillofac Surg. 2009;67:2080–92.
63. Broadbent BH, Golden WH. Bolton standards of Dentofacial developmental growth. Mosby; 1975.
64. Grayson BH, McCarthy JG, Bookstein F. Analysis of craniofacial asymmetry by multiplane cephalometry. Am J Orthod. 1983;84:217–24.
65. Swennen GRJ, Schutyser F. Three-dimensional cephalometry: spiral multi-slice vs cone-beam computed tomography. Am J Orthod Dentofacial Orthop. 2006;130:410–6.
66. Swennen GRJ, Schutyser F, Barth E-L, De Groeve P, De Mey A. A new method of 3-D cephalometry part I: the anatomic Cartesian 3-D reference system. J Craniofac Surg. 2006;17:314–25.
67. Farronato G, Garagiola U, Dominici A, Periti G, de Nardi S, Carletti V, et al. "Ten-point" 3D cephalometric analysis using low-dosage cone beam computed tomography. Prog Orthod. 2010;11:2–12.
68. Stamatakis HC, Steegman R, Dusseldorp J, Ren Y. Head positioning in a cone beam computed tomography unit and the effect on accuracy of the three-dimensional surface mode. Eur J Oral Sci. 2019;127:72–80.
69. Gurani SF, Di Carlo G, Cattaneo PM, Thorn JJ, Pinholt EM. Effect of head and tongue posture on the pharyngeal airway dimensions and morphology in three-dimensional imaging: a systematic review. J Oral Maxillofac Res. 2016;7:e1.
70. Zimmerman JN, Vora SR, Pliska BT. Reliability of upper airway assessment using CBCT. Eur J Orthod. 2019;41:101–8.
71. Hsung TC, Yeung WK, Choi WS, Luk WK, Cheng YY, Lam YH. Recording natural head position using cone beam computerized tomography. Sensors (Basel). 2021;21(24):8189.
72. Balachandran R, Kharbanda OP, Sennimalai K, Neelapu BC. Orientation of cone-beam computed tomography image: pursuit of perfect orientation plane in three dimensions—a retrospective cross-sectional study. Ann Natl Acad Med Sci India. 2019;55:202–9.
73. Cevidanes L, Oliveira AEF, Motta A, Phillips C, Burke B, Tyndall D. Head orientation in CBCT-generated cephalograms. Angle Orthod. 2009;79:971–7.
74. Zamora N, Llamas J, Cibrian R, Gandia Franco J, Paredes V. Cephalometric measurements from 3D reconstructed images compared with conventional 2D images. Angle Orthod. 2011;81:856–64.
75. Hassan B, Nijkamp P, Verheij H, Tairie J, Vink C, van der Stelt P, et al. Precision of identifying cephalometric landmarks with cone beam computed tomography in vivo. Eur J Orthod. 2013;35:38–44.
76. Fernandes TMF, Adamczyk J, Poleti ML, Henriques JFC, Friedland B, Garib DG. Comparison between 3D volumetric rendering and multiplanar slices on the reliability of linear measurements on CBCT images: an in vitro study. J Appl Oral Sci Rev FOB. 2015;23:56–63.
77. de Oliveira AEF, Cevidanes LHS, Phillips C, Motta A, Burke B, Tyndall D. Observer reliability of three-dimensional cephalometric landmark identification on cone-beam computerized tomography. Oral Surg Oral Med Oral Pathol Oral Radiol Endod. 2009;107:256–65.
78. Lam WY, Ngan HY, Wat PY, Luk HW, Pow EH, Goto TK. Novel geometric coordination registration in cone-beam computed tomogram. IEEE AIPR Workshop; 2014. pp. 1–6.
79. Al-Balkhi KM. Orthodontic treatment planning: do orthodontists treat to cephalometric norms? J Contemp Dent Pract. 2003;4:12–27.
80. Gribel BF, Gribel MN, Frazão DC, McNamara JA, Manzi FR. Accuracy and reliability of craniometric measurements on lateral cephalometry and

3D measurements on CBCT scans. Angle Orthod. 2011;81:26–35.
81. Teng C, Liu C, Yu Q, Liu S. Cone-beam computed tomography-based three-dimensional cephalometric analysis of mandible symmetry and the occlusal plane of adult patients with high-angle skeletal class III malocclusion and jaw deformity. Arch Oral Biol. 2021;127:105157.
82. Lagravère MO, Han J, Bogowicz P, Heo G. Cranial base growth in adolescence assessed through cone-beam computerized tomographies—pilot study. Int Orthod. 2015;13:302–19.
83. Maspero C, Farronato M, Bellincioni F, Cavagnetto D, Abate A. Assessing mandibular body changes in growing subjects: a comparison of CBCT and reconstructed lateral cephalogram measurements. Sci Rep. 2020;10:11722.
84. Gribel BF, Gribel MN, Manzi FR, Brooks SL, McNamara JA Jr. From 2D to 3D: an algorithm to derive normal values for 3-dimensional computerized assessment. Angle Orthod. 2011;81:3–10.
85. Bayome M, Park JH, Kook Y-A. New three-dimensional cephalometric analyses among adults with a skeletal class I pattern and normal occlusion. Korean J Orthod. 2013;43:62–73.
86. Lee S-H, Kil T-J, Park K-R, Kim BC, Kim J-G, Piao Z, et al. Three-dimensional architectural and structural analysis—a transition in concept and design from Delaire's cephalometric analysis. Int J Oral Maxillofac Surg. 2014;43:1154–60.
87. Liang C, Liu S, Liu Q, Zhang B, Li Z. Norms of McNamara's cephalometric analysis on lateral view of 3D CT imaging in adults from Northeast China. J Hard Tissue Biol. 2014;23:249–54.
88. Vahdettin L, Aksoy S, Öz U, Orhan K. Three-dimensional cephalometric norms of Turkish Cypriots using CBCTimages reconstructed from a volumetric rendering program in vivo. Turk J Med Sci. 2016;46(3):848–61.
89. Santos RMG, De Martino JM, Haiter Neto F, Passeri LA. Cone beam computed tomography-based cephalometric norms for Brazilian adults. Int J Oral Maxillofac Surg. 2018;47:64–71.
90. Ho C-T, Denadai R, Lai H-C, Lo L-J, Lin H-H. Computer-aided planning in orthognathic surgery: a comparative study with the establishment of Burstone analysis-derived 3D norms. J Clin Med. 2019;8:2106.
91. Wang RH, Ho C-T, Lin H-H, Lo L-J. Three-dimensional cephalometry for orthognathic planning: normative data and analyses. J Formos Med Assoc. 2020;119:191–203.
92. Dindaroğlu F, Yetkiner E. Cone beam computed tomography in orthodontics. Turk J Orthod. 2016;29:16–21.
93. Jaju PP, Jaju SP. Cone-beam computed tomography: time to move from ALARA to ALADA. Imaging Sci Dent. 2015;45:263–5.
94. van Bunningen RH, Dijkstra PU, Dieters A, van der Meer WJ, Kuijpers-Jagtman AM, Ren Y. Precision of orthodontic cephalometric measurements on ultra low dose-low dose CBCT reconstructed cephalograms. Clin Oral Investig. 2022;26:1543–50.
95. Berg B-I, Laville A, Courvoisier DS, Rouch P, Schouman T. Experiences with a new biplanar low-dose X-ray device for imaging the facial skeleton: a feasibility study. PLoS One. 2020;15:e0235032.
96. Sennimalai K, Selvaraj M, Kharbanda OP, Kandasamy D, Mohaideen K. MRI-based cephalometrics: a scoping review of current insights and future perspectives. Dentomaxillofac Radiol. 2023;52:20230024. https://doi.org/10.1259/dmfr.20230024. Epub ahead of print.
97. Heil A, Lazo Gonzalez E, Hilgenfeld T, Kickingereder P, Bendszus M, Heiland S, et al. Lateral cephalometric analysis for treatment planning in orthodontics based on MRI compared with radiographs: a feasibility study in children and adolescents. PLoS One. 2017;12:e0174524.
98. Abkai C, Hourfar J, Glockengießer J, Ulrici J, Hell E, Rasche V, et al. Ultra short time to Echo (UTE) MRI for cephalometric analysis–potential of an x-ray free fast cephalometric projection technique. PLoS One. 2021;16:e0257224.
99. Juerchott A, Saleem MA, Hilgenfeld T, Freudlsperger C, Zingler S, Lux CJ, et al. 3D cephalometric analysis using magnetic resonance imaging: validation of accuracy and reproducibility. Sci Rep. 2018;8:13029.
100. Juerchott A, Freudlsperger C, Zingler S, Saleem MA, Jende JME, Lux CJ, et al. In vivo reliability of 3D cephalometric landmark determination on magnetic resonance imaging: a feasibility study. Clin Oral Investig. 2020;24:1339–49.
101. Maspero C, Gaffuri F, Castro IO, Lanteri V, Ugolini A, Farronato M. Correlation between dental vestibular-palatal inclination and alveolar bone remodeling after orthodontic treatment: a CBCT analysis. Materials (Basel). 2019;12(24):4225.
102. Dobai A, Dembrovszky F, Vízkelety T, Barsi P, Juhász F, Dobó-Nagy C. MRI compatibility of orthodontic brackets and wires: systematic review article. BMC Oral Health. 2022;22:298.
103. Hung K, Yeung AWK, Tanaka R, Bornstein MM. Current applications, opportunities, and limitations of AI for 3D imaging in dental research and practice. Int J Environ Res Public Health. 2020;17:4424.
104. Hung KF, Ai QYH, Leung YY, Yeung AWK. Potential and impact of artificial intelligence algorithms in dento-maxillofacial radiology. Clin Oral Investig. 2022;26:5535–55.
105. Schwendicke F, Samek W, Krois J. Artificial intelligence in dentistry: chances and challenges. J Dent Res. 2020;99:769–74.
106. Kang SH, Jeon K, Kang S-H, Lee S-H. 3D cephalometric landmark detection by multiple stage deep reinforcement learning. Sci Rep. 2021;11:17509.
107. Al Turkestani N, Bianchi J, Deleat-Besson R, Le C, Tengfei L, Prieto JC, et al. Clinical decision support systems in orthodontics: a narrative review of

data science approaches. Orthod Craniofac Res. 2021;24:26–36.

108. Shahidi S, Bahrampour E, Soltanimehr E, Zamani A, Oshagh M, Moattari M, et al. The accuracy of a designed software for automated localization of craniofacial landmarks on CBCT images. BMC Med Imaging. 2014;14:32.
109. Gupta A, Kharbanda OP, Sardana V, Balachandran R, Sardana HK. A knowledge-based algorithm for automatic detection of cephalometric landmarks on CBCT images. Int J Comput Assist Radiol Surg. 2015;10:1737–52.
110. Neelapu BC, Kharbanda OP, Sardana V, Gupta A, Vasamsetti S, Balachandran R, et al. Automatic localization of three-dimensional cephalometric landmarks on CBCT images by extracting symmetry features of the skull. Dentomaxillofacial Radiol. 2018;47:20170054.
111. Zhang J, Liu M, Wang L, Chen S, Yuan P, Li J, et al. Joint Craniomaxillofacial bone segmentation and landmark digitization by context-guided fully convolutional networks. Med Image Comput Comput-Assist Interv MICCAI Int Conf Med Image Comput Comput-Assist Interv. 2017;10434:720–8.
112. Lee SM, Kim HP, Jeon K, Lee S-H, Seo JK. Automatic 3D cephalometric annotation system using shadowed 2D image-based machine learning. Phys Med Biol. 2019;64:055002.
113. Yun HS, Hyun CM, Baek SH, Lee S-H, Seo JK. A semi-supervised learning approach for automated 3D cephalometric landmark identification using computed tomography. PLoS One. 2022;17:e0275114.
114. Ghesu FC, Georgescu B, Mansi T, Neumann D, Hornegger J, Comaniciu D. An artificial agent for anatomical landmark detection in medical images. In: Ourselin S, Joskowicz L, Sabuncu MR, Unal G, Wells W, editors. Medical image computing and computer-assisted intervention—MICCAI 2016. Cham: Springer International Publishing; 2016. p. 229–37.
115. Ghesu FC, Georgescu B, Grbic S, Maier A, Hornegger J, Comaniciu D. Towards intelligent robust detection of anatomical structures in incomplete volumetric data. Med Image Anal. 2018;48:203–13.
116. Alansary A, Oktay O, Li Y, Folgoc LL, Hou B, Vaillant G, et al. Evaluating reinforcement learning agents for anatomical landmark detection. Med Image Anal. 2019;53:156–64.
117. Norori N, Hu Q, Aellen FM, Faraci FD, Tzovara A. Addressing bias in big data and AI for health care: a call for open science. Patterns. 2021;2:100347.

Three-Dimensional Virtual Planning in Orthodontics

12

Vinay Kumar, Sanjeev Verma, Raj Kumar Verma, and Satinder Pal Singh

12.1 Introduction

The craniofacial morphology and its assessment are critical in the various disciplines of dentistry, viz., cranio-maxillo-facial surgery, orthodontics, prosthodontics and implantology, conservative and endodontics, and forensics. Its recognition is necessary for any preoperative, postoperative, and facial balance and harmony. With the advent of three-dimensional technology, it is now possible to create or morph a virtual digital clone of the patient using 3D facial scan, intraoral scan made either directly (intraoral scanners) or indirectly (tabletop or desktop scanners), and cone-beam computed tomography (CBCT) [1]. The literature is enriched with the multifaceted application of "the state-of-art" digital technologies in the orthodontic discipline [2].

To assess the applications or utilities of 3D virtual planning in dentistry as general and orthodontics as particular, we conducted bibliometric analyses using the keywords "3D virtual planning" AND "Dentistry" and "3D virtual planning" AND "Orthodontics" in all field section, and a total of 143 articles were found in the PUBMED database https://pubmed.ncbi.nlm.nih.gov/?term=%283D+virtual+planning%29+AND+%28orthodontics%29&size=20. The bibliometric analysis of these 143 articles revealed that almost every domain, viz., cephalometry, orthognathic surgery, CBCT, computer-assisted appliance fabrication, CAD-CAM, splint fabrication, indirect bracket bonding, model analysis, etc., has shown co-occurrence network for 3D virtual planning and orthodontics (Fig. 12.1). The purpose of this chapter is to explore the multifacted clinical applications of digital technologies in orthodontics, beginning with the creation of a "virtual clone" of patient to the diagnosis, planning appropriate treatment and its execution, appraisal, and assessing the prognosis.

V. Kumar (✉) · S. Verma · R. K. Verma · S. P. Singh
Unit of Orthodontics, Oral Health Sciences Centre, Postgraduate Institute of Medical Education and Research, Chandigarh, India

S. S. Rana et al. (eds.), *Applications of Three-dimensional Imaging for Craniofacial Region*,
https://doi.org/10.1007/978-981-97-4608-8_12

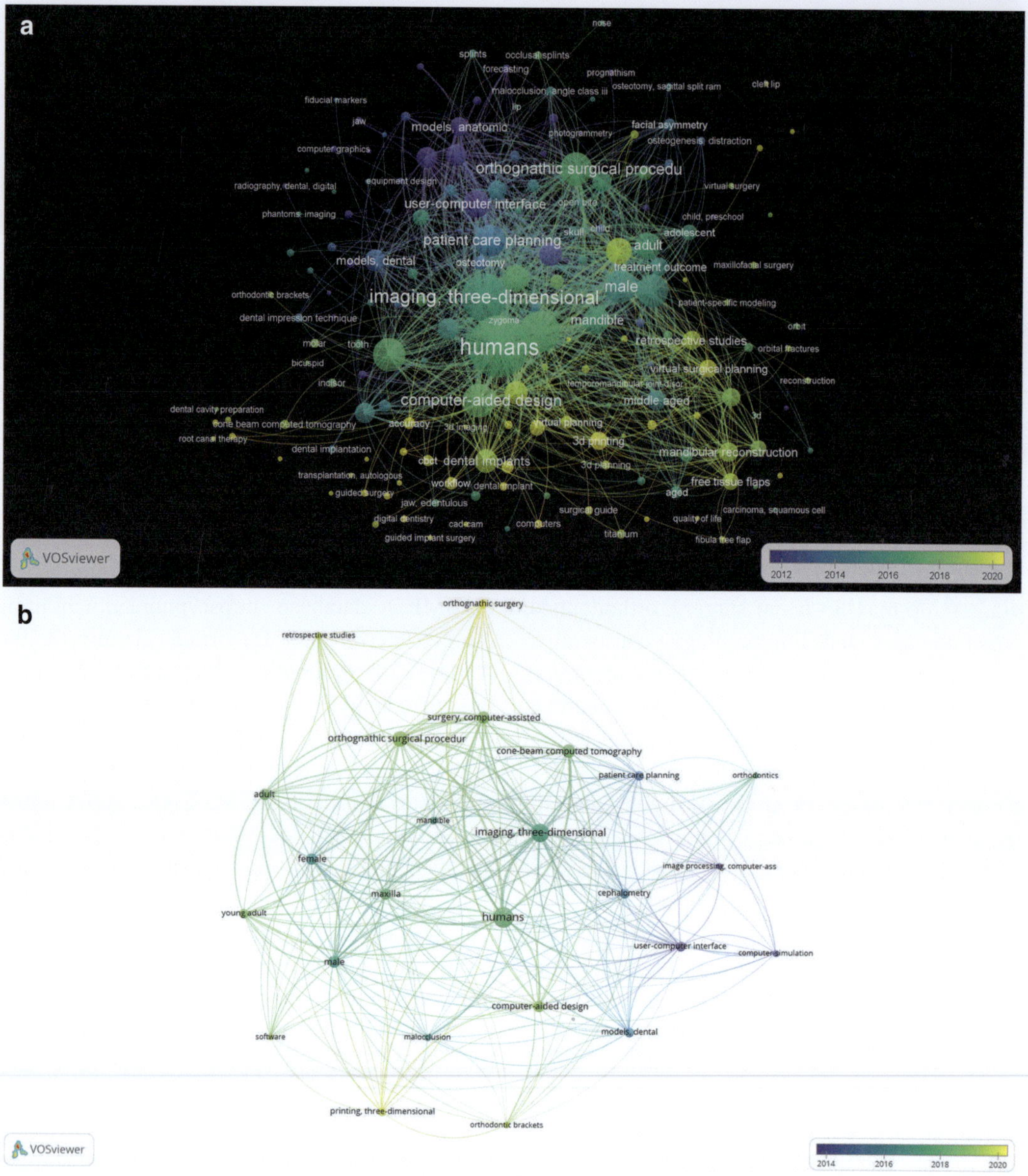

Fig. 12.1 (**a**) VOS viewer visualization of co-occurrence network of the 3D virtual planning in Dentistry. (**b**) VOSviewer visualization of co-occurrence network of the 3D virtual planning in orthodontics

12.2 The Analogy Between Conventional and Digital Technique

With the advent of digital technology, several processes, materials, and imaging in conventional orthodontics have been replaced as shown in Table 12.1.

12.2.1 Various Equipment Used in Digital Technique

1. Intraoral scanner: iTero by Align Technology, Trios series by 3Shape, and CS3700 by Carestream Dentals.
2. Tabletop or desktop scanner: Maestro3D (MDS 500 dental scanner).

Table 12.1 Analogy between conventional and digital technique

Conventional technique	Digital/3D technique
Impression making	Intraoral scanning
Extraoral/intraoral photographs	Facial/intraoral scans
Plaster of Paris	Standard tessellation language (STL), 3D printing
2D radiography (IOPA, occlusal view, dental panoramic tomography, PA, and lateral cephalograms)	Cone-beam computed tomography

3. 3D facial scanner: Fixed-type (OBI scanner); Moveable-type (Artec Evan scan).
4. Cone-beam computed tomographic scan: NewTom, Carestream, Planmeca, etc.
5. Video camera (4D imaging and video stereophotogrammetry).
6. MRI and surface scanning

12.2.1.1 Advantages

The intraoral scans are clinically acceptable for diagnosis and treatment planning in dentistry as well as in orthodontics and can be used in place of plaster models [3].

12.2.1.2 Limitations

The digital technic requires more time than the plaster models for analysis. Moreover, intraoral conditions such as saliva, tongue, and limited oral space can also contribute to scanning inaccuracies [3]. Clinicians should keep in mind that scanning distortion might occur in the posterior areas of the mandible. In the clinical setting, careful scanning procedures and additional scans of the mandibular posterior areas might improve scanning accuracy.

12.3 Application of 3D Technology

12.3.1 Dental Measurements and Surface Analysis

With conventional methods, the mesiodistal width or labiolingual dimension of the teeth is measured on a study model obtained from plaster of Paris using alginate impressions and is subjected to different analyses for tooth size arch length, arch perimeter, Bolton's analysis, overjet, and overbite determination. However, digital models obtained from the direct intraoral scan or CBCT or desktop scan (indirect scanning of study models) are clinically acceptable. They can be used for performing dental measurements and model analysis for diagnosing and planning treatment (Fig. 12.2). The dental models obtained from intraoral scans and plaster of Paris were analyzed for linear tooth measurements for height and mesiodistal width obtained from a digital caliper and 3D software (reverse engineering). The surface analysis of the two models was done by the "best-fit method" as shown in Fig. 12.3. The authors found no significant difference between the intraoral scan and plaster models [4, 5]. Similarly, digital models obtained from intraoral scanners and cone-beam computed tomography scans of alginate impressions for tooth-width measurements and the Bolton analysis also showed that they are reliable, valid, and reproducible for dental measurements for diagnostic procedures [6]. The assessment of the degree of crowding in the maxillary or mandibular arch has also been accurately measured on 3D software (OrthoCad) by Leifert et al. (2009) and concluded that this software is accurate, clinically acceptable, and reproducible as compared to conventional study model analysis using a vernier calliper [7].

12.3.2 Digital Indirect Bonding (Virtual Bonding)

Indirect bonding is there in the field of orthodontics for a long time. The conventional process goes through multiple steps, which involve the temporary adhesion of brackets to the plaster cast and making of the semi-rigid transfer tray from thermoplastic material. Brackets are then transferred to the patient's mouth and bonded with a bonding agent with bracket siting guided by that thermoplastic bracket transfer tray. There is recent software that can facilitate virtual bracket placement (with slot size, tip, and torque specifi-

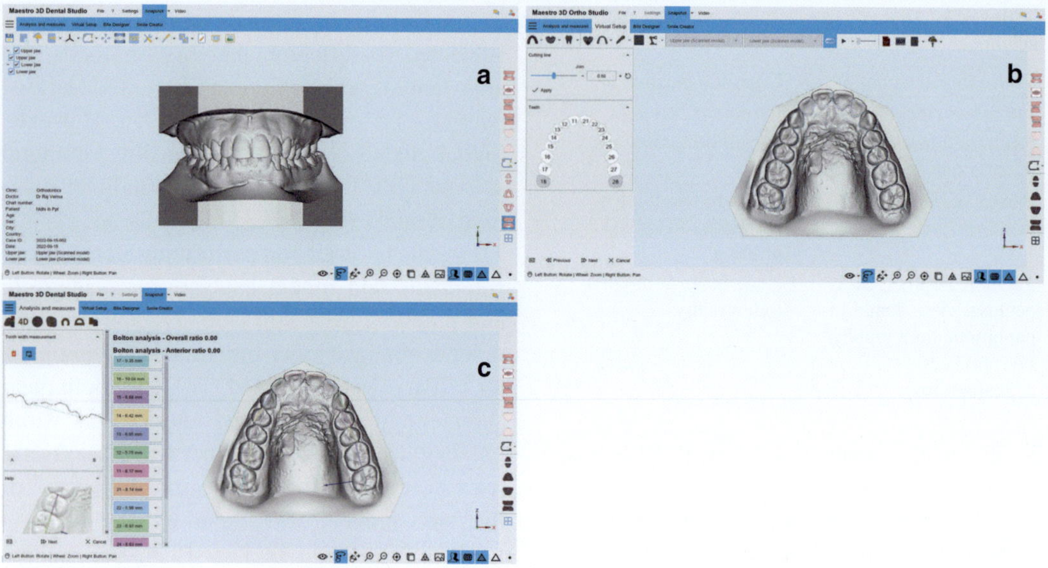

Fig. 12.2 Model analyses. (a) STL file; (b) Teeth segmentation; (c) Measurement for model analyses

Fig. 12.3 Surface superimposition

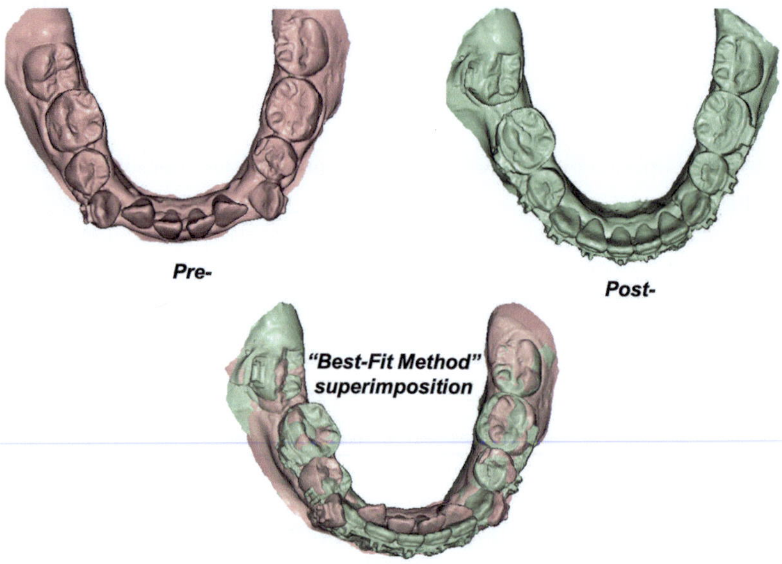

cation) on virtual models. Further, we can design the bracket transfer tray whose SLT file can be printed from compatible material. This 3D-printed tray can be used to transfer brackets in patients' mouths, and it will guide the final bracket placement.

The stepwise procedure of digital indirect bonding (Fig. 12.4) is described as follows:

Step 1. STL files of the 3D digital models are uploaded to the software.

Step 2. The individual tooth is isolated and marked in the digital model.

Step 3. The clinical crown of individual teeth is isolated and segmentations of these teeth are done.

Step 4. The software generates the virtual roots. Roots can also be imported from CBCT-generated STL files of individual patients. The latter is an accurate method as roots developed by the software are arbitrary.

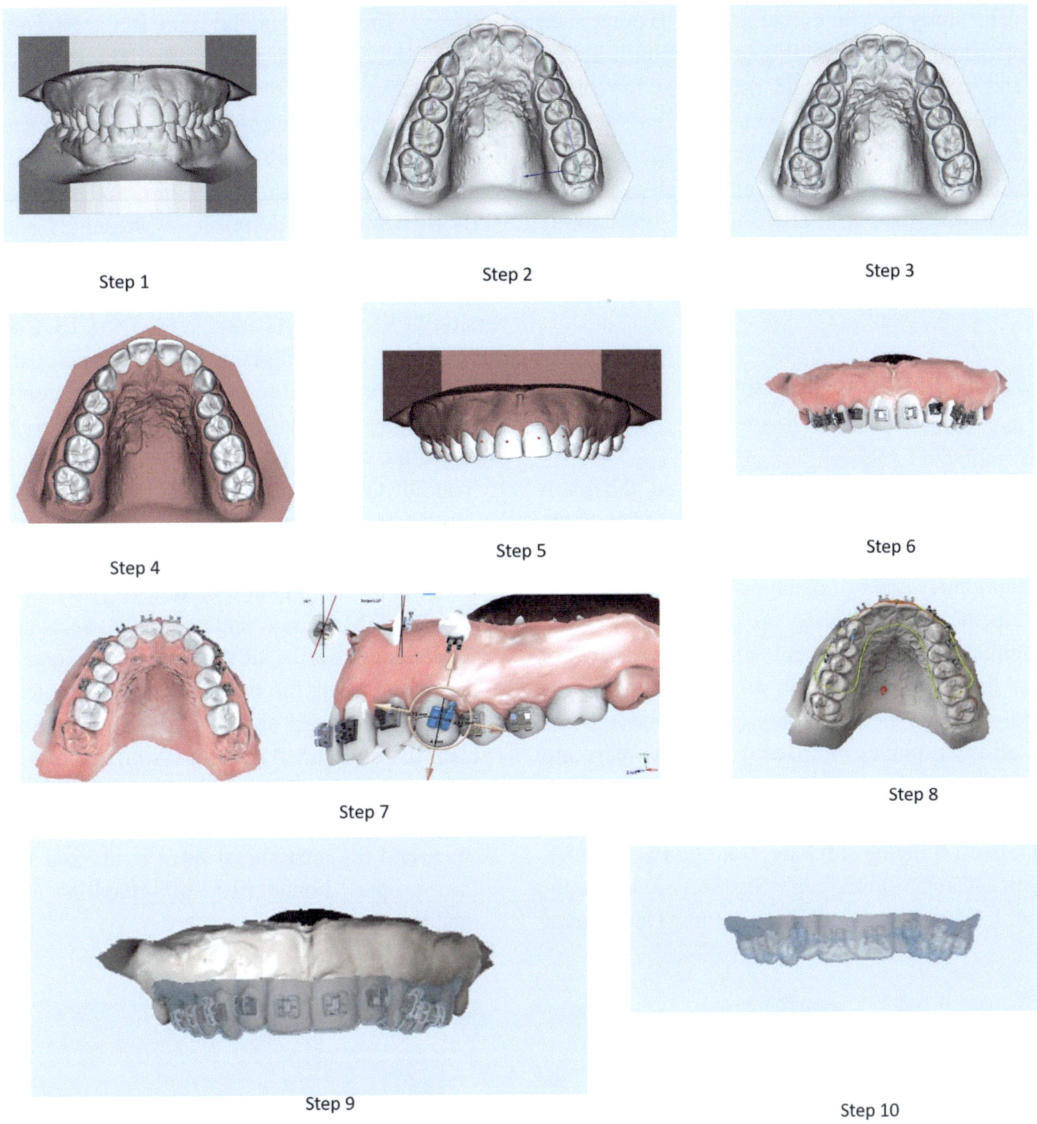

Fig. 12.4 Step-by-step procedure of virtual indirect bonding and tray fabrication

Step 5. The individual center of the clinical crown is marked and adjusted according to the individual requirements of the patients.

Step 6. Virtual brackets are placed on the center of the clinical crown. This can be done for individual teeth or the whole arch as per convenience.

Step 7. Individual brackets can be adjusted depending on tooth rotation, occlusal-gingival height, and interferences from opposite teeth/brackets.

Step 8. Demarcation of the area was done for making the hollow bracket transfer tray. It can be kept with full or partial coverage of the brackets.

Step 9. The brackets transfer tray/shell can be isolated and exported in STL format for 3D printing.

Step 10. Brackets with adhesive can be placed in a transfer tray inside the housing of the individual brackets and transferred to the patient's mouth. The transfer tray can be removed after sufficient curing of the adhesive.

The study by Oliveira et al. (2019) confirmed that virtual indirect bonding of orthodontic accessories is as accurate and precise as the direct bonding technic [8]; however, there is also a profound role of clinician's personnel experience [9] in terms of the "learning curve" achieved with experience, that is, the bonding of orthodontic attachments virtually to the same level of correctness, when compared to the direct procedures.

12.3.3 Orthognathic Surgical Planning

Facial esthetics has been considered the main driving force for approximately 70% of patients with various dentofacial deformities to seek orthodontics and orthognathic surgery treatment. From the profile tracing on photographs to the computer-based treatment simulation, software has helped maxillofacial surgeons to optimize and visualize the osteotomy cut and movements in all three planes of space. Currently, there are so many surgical planning software available in the market, viz., Dolphin imaging software (Dolphin Imaging software, Canoga Park, USA), Quick Ceph (Quick ceph Systems, San Diego, CA, USA), Dentofacial Planner Plus (Dentofacial Software, Toronto, Canada), and IPS (IPS case Designer KLS Martin group) [10]. The step-by-step digital workflow of the orthognathic surgical planning for maxillary superior repositioning and mandibular setback in a 19-year-old patient with an anterior open bite of the 3 mm and skeletal Class III dentofacial deformity is presented and described in Figs. 12.5 and 12.6, using Dolphin imaging software (Dolphin Imaging software version 11.95, Canoga Park, USA). The CBCT of full FOV and intraoral scans of the dental models have been considered to be the most commonly used imaging records for contemplating virtual orthognathic surgery [1].

1. The DICOM file of the CBCT scan and STL file of the maxillary and mandibular dental models are acquired and transported to the Dolphin 3D surgery software.
2. The DICOM file is orientated on the software to standardize it in all three planes of space; then by clicking the next button, the segmentation of the hard and soft tissue is done to clear the underlined structure from noise.
3. Using the build X-ray tool, the OPG is constructed from the sagittal view of the CBCT scan, and the anatomical limit is marked for the proper boundaries of maxilla and mandible.

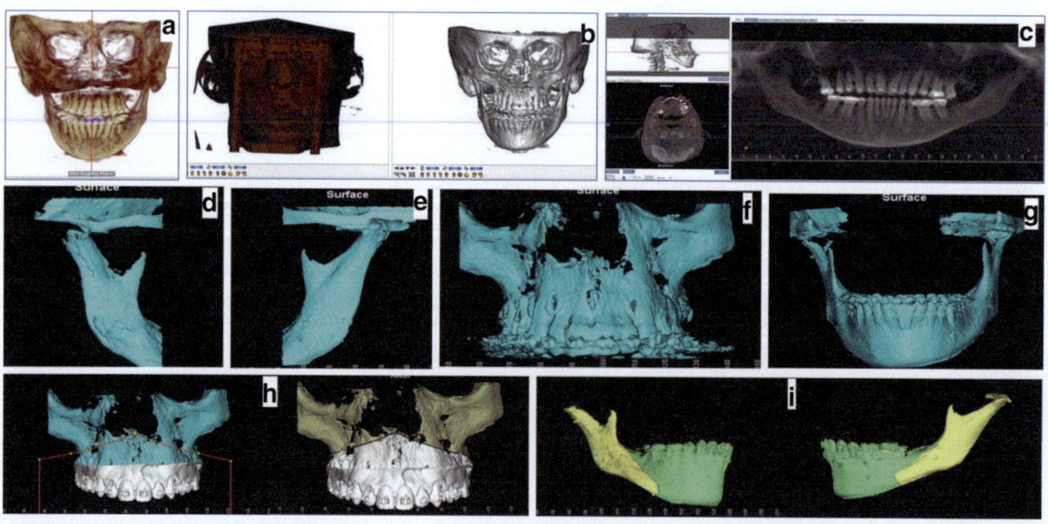

Fig. 12.5 Workflow for orthognathic surgery; (**a**) Orientation of DICOM file (CBCT); (**b**) Segmentation of soft and hard tissue; (**c**) X-ray build-up; (**d–g**) Segmentation and Clean-up of maxillary and mandibular section using Crop Tool; (**h** and **i**) Defining osteotomy line for maxilla and mandible

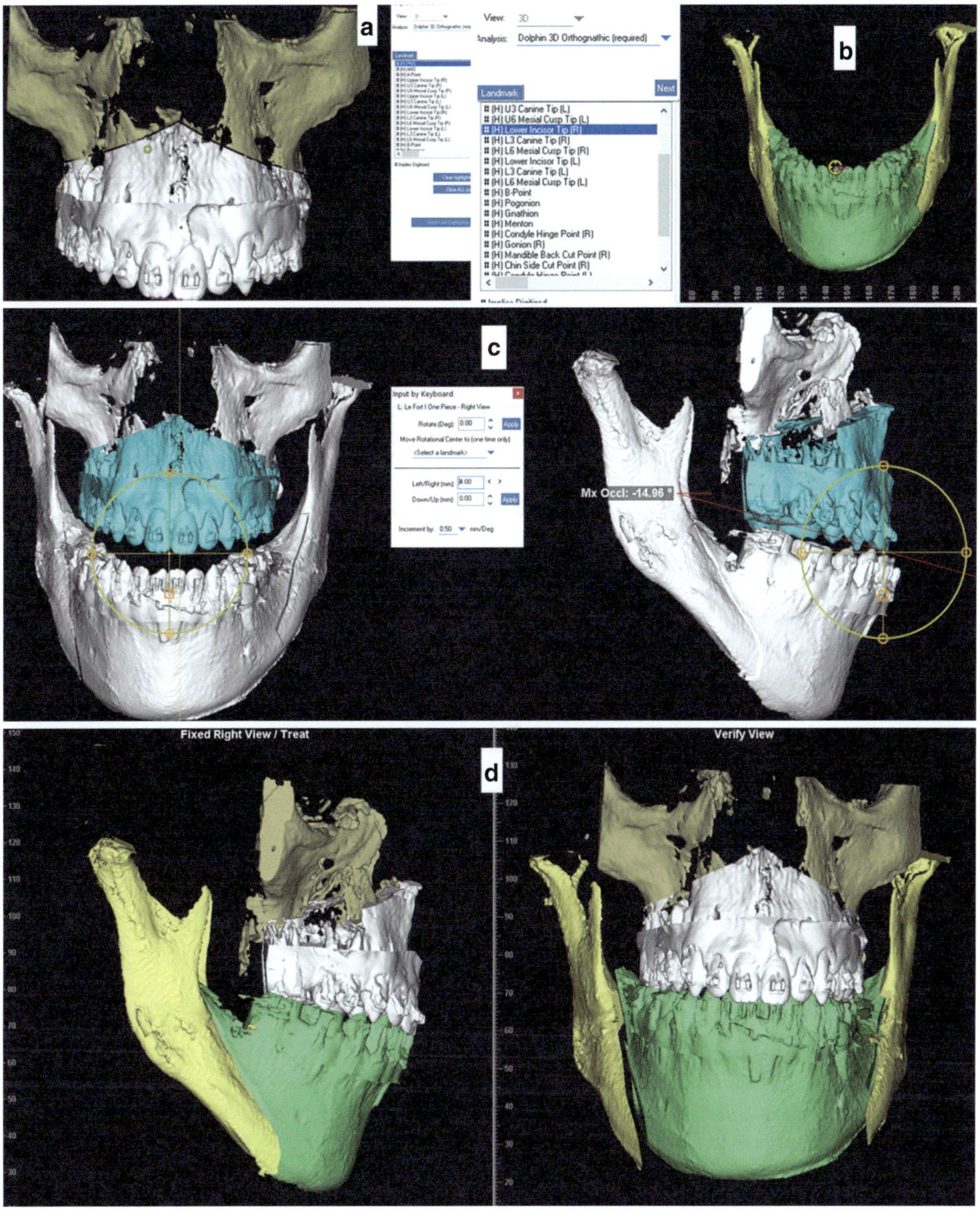

Fig. 12.6 Workflow for orthognathic surgery (cont.); (**a** and **b**) localization of various landmarks in maxilla and mandible; (**c** and d) maxillary and mandibular surgery (treatment planning)

4. The cropping tool is used to remove the extra structures from the isolated anatomic boundary of the maxilla, mandibular right and left proximal segments, and mandible as a whole (mandible with right and left proximal segments). This process is called as 'segmentation and clean-up' of the maxilla and mandible.
5. The STL files of the maxillary and mandibular dental models can be overlayed to the DICOM file of the CBCT using edit models and can be verified for an accurate position in the DICOM file. They shall help in the accurate fabrication of surgical splints required for orthognathic surgery.
6. The osteotomy cut is defined in the maxilla and mandible at the desired level. Here we have chosen a Lefort-1 osteotomy cut for the maxilla and bilateral sagittal split in the mandible.
7. The landmarks are identified and located in the maxillary and mandibular regions.
8. With the help of a treatment planning tool, the surgical movements of maxillary and mandibular segments are planned as required for the individual case. In this illustrated case, the maxillary segment was cut at Leforte-1 (one piece) level, with advancement by 4 mm and superior positioning by 3 mm. The mandible was osteotomized at BSSO level, setback by 4 mm and 6 mm superior positioning to achieve the occlusion.
9. The Splint tool allows you in selecting the width and thickness of the wafer based on treatment plans and helps in making an intermediate and or final- splint to position the maxilla or mandible based on the preferred order of your operation. In the preview section, the splint is verified for details and saved in the STL format for printing (Fig. 12.7)

A systematic review reported by Alkhayer et al. (2020) has claimed that a nonsignificant mean change of less than 2 mm in the upper and lower jaw is anticipated for the accuracy between digital and conventional orthognathic workflow [11]. The accuracy values for pitch, yaw, and roll were < 2.75, < 1.7, and < 1.1 degrees for the upper jaw, respectively, and < 2.75, < 1.8, and < 1.1 degree for the lower jaw. Furthermore, calculation of the linear and angular differences between the virtual plan and postoperative outcomes was the most frequently used method used for accuracy assessment (10 out of 12 studies), and a difference of less than 2 mm/° was considered acceptable and accurate [11].

Data retrieved from 22 patients [12] consecutively treated for computer-assisted bimaxillary orthognathic surgery with maxillary segmentation have shown the error rate (total) for maxillary repositioning as 0.62 mm when the cone-beam computed tomography images after surgery and the planned 3D skull before surgery were superimposed. When comparing this technique with classical planning, virtual planning appears to be more accurate, especially in terms of achieving frontal symmetry.

The limitation of the virtual planning approach is that there is variation in the level of precision and accuracy for different anatomical units of the maxilla and mandible. A study by Zinser et al. (2012) [13], who treated eight skeletal Class III patients with a "patented three-surgical splint" protocol, found that for the position of maxilla and condyle, a clinically acceptable level of precision was achieved. However, for mandible and soft tissue, the level of precision was marginal to low, respectively [13].

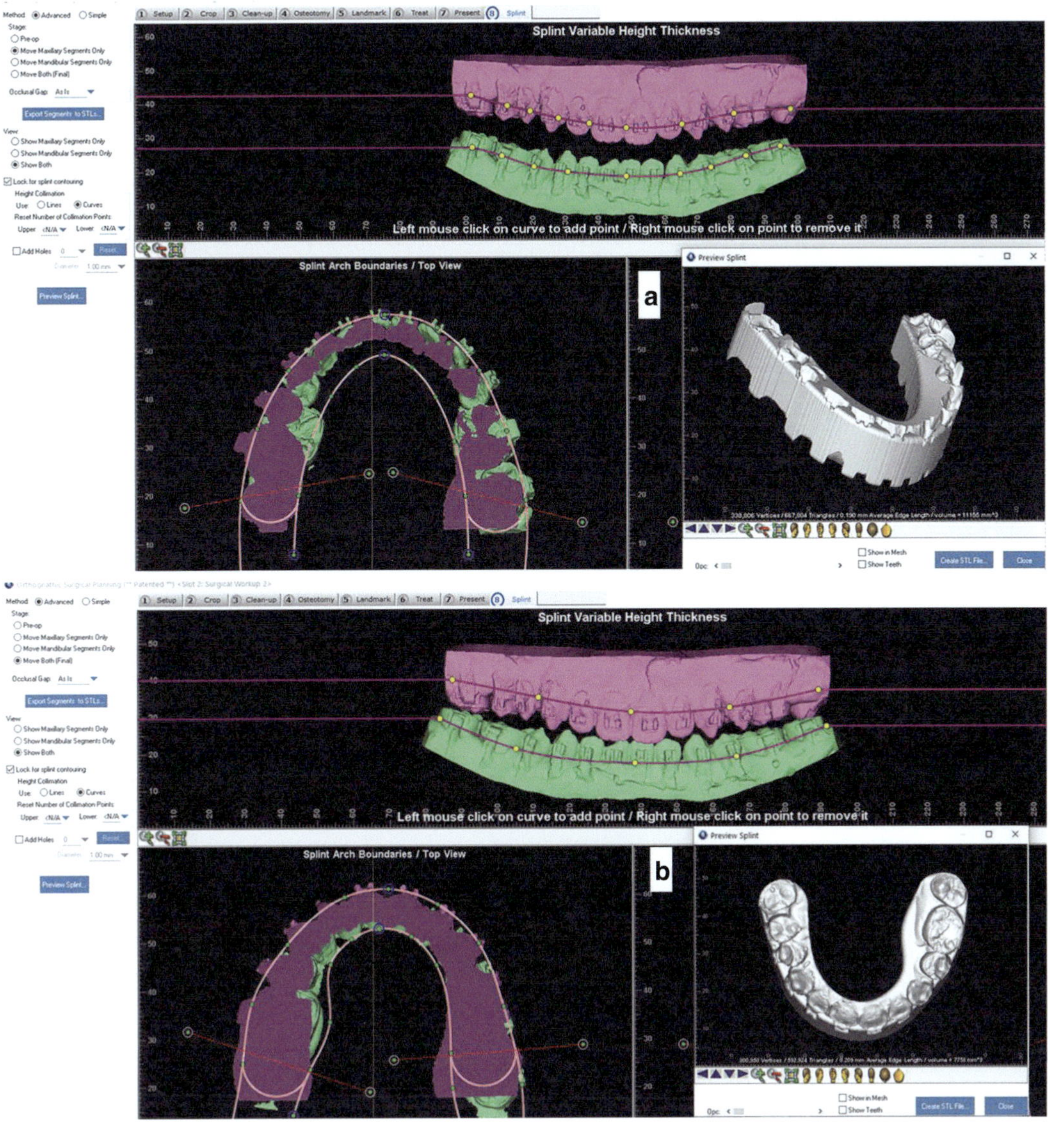

Fig. 12.7 Splint fabrication; (**a**) Splint designing with STL file of the splint for Maxillary Surgery (Intermediate-splint); (**b**) Splint designing with STL file of the splint for mandibular surgery (Final Splint)

12.3.4 Orthodontic Virtual Setup

To determine the final occlusal scheme, optimization of the discrepancies of tooth size and arch length, and the need for asymmetrical extraction in some cases, Kesling HD proposed the conventional diagnostic setup [14, 15]. It serves as a clinical aid in diagnosis and treatment planning with the aforementioned advantages. The conventional method [14] of diagnostic setup has been modified [16, 17], to ease the step-by-step procedure; however, with the advent of the digital era, the virtual setup has become too easy to perform and a more sophisticated method than conventional one. Maestro 3D dental studio version 6 and OrthoAnalyzer (3Shape, Copenhagen, Denmark) are the most commonly used software to perform a virtual orthodontic setup on the pretreatment dental model. Creating a virtual setup, starts with the determination of the arch form and

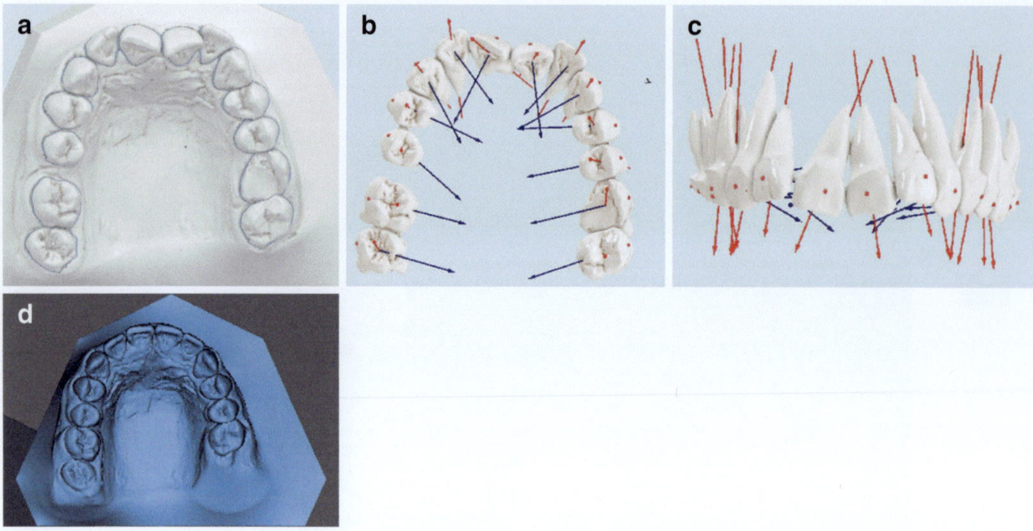

Fig. 12.8 Virtual setup: A. semiautomatic segmentation of the STL file of maxillary arch; (**b** and **c**) axial inclination and arch form of teeth; and (**d**) teeth setup done (virtual). (**a**) Semiautomatic determination of the border of each tooth using software for segmentation of each tooth in the respective arches. (**b** and **c**) Confirming the arch form and tooth axis in the occlusal and sagittal plane. (**d**) Finally, a virtual setup is created by displacing each tooth to the desired position to create a harmonious arch or maxilla-mandibular relationship

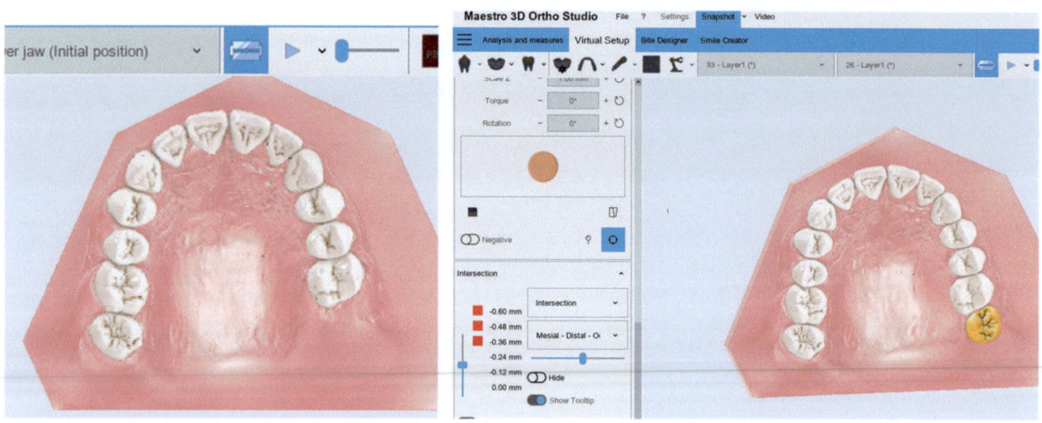

Fig. 12.9 Virtual setup with pontic for #27 tooth

tooth axis. Each of the individual teeth is segmented semiautomatically using the software. An overview of the virtual setup for the maxilla is shown in Fig. 12.8.

The virtual "pontic tool" application in the software also addresses the replacement of any missing teeth and residual spaces after the completion of orthodontic therapy (Fig. 12.9).

The spatial position of roots achieved using a virtual setup of the crown only has shown errors when compared with those achieved in the actual treatment. Therefore, the study conducted by Park M et al. have recommended performing the virtual setup using crowns and roots for accurate and precise treatment simulation, especially in planning extraction treatment [18].

In the question of whether digital treatment simulations have any impact on the orthodontic treatment-planning decisions or practitioners' confidence in their selected plans, the literature suggested that digital setup resulted in a change in the treatment plans in about 24% of the cases

[19]. The results from 22 orthodontists and 7 orthodontic residents who examined the records of 6 patients with different case types found that there was a significant change in the treatment plan for 9.2 percent of the cases. This includes some modifications, viz., change in the pattern of extraction of teeth, proposing space closure than creation of space and its rehabilitation with implants, partial change in the treatment plan (14.4% of the cases) with adding interproximal reduction or inclusion of temporary anchorage devices [19]. There was a marked improvement in the confidence level of the practitioner and reported that the most helpful features of digital setups were the ability to superimpose the setup with the original model, determine the amount of tooth movement needed, check the final incisal relationship, and establish the amount of interproximal reduction required [19].

12.3.5 Splint-Less Orthognathic Surgery

The literature has compared the accuracy of printed splints with conventional acrylic splints and satisfied the inclusion criteria. Cheng-Ting Ho et al. [20] in their study evaluated the fit of 30 printed splints clinically all of which were deemed fit, while 2 conventional splints were deemed unfit. The average difference between the conventional and the STL splints in the air-space calculated between the splints and the teeth surface was 0.24 ± 0.23 mm as measured by Gateno et al. [21] The splints generated by PolyJet technology were accurate enough for clinical use with a root mean square for the reproducibility and comparison tests of 0.15 mm and 0.19 mm, respectively, as reported by Shaheen et al. [22] None of the variables measured on SLA-printed splints and conventional acrylic splints showed statistical significance in the study by Song and Baek [23]. They stated that only the vertical parameters showed clinical significance, and thus the accuracy of SLA-printed splints needed to be approved. However, with the use of patient-specific implant (PSI), several error-prone and time-consuming clinical steps, viz., impression making, plaster study models and face bow transfer, model surgery, and fabrication of acrylic splint, have been eliminated. The authors [24] have reported the use of PSI for the management of an 18-year-old female with micro gnathic maxilla with hypodontia. The preoperative CBCT scan was used to fabricate a PSI, and the operation was done without the need for a surgical splint to facilitate maxillomandibular osteotomies and plan the occlusion. The authors have claimed this method is rapid and reliable for the repositioning of the maxilla [24].

12.3.6 Orthodontic Appliance Designing and Fabrication

Orthodontic treatment in adolescent and adult using clear aligner therapy (invisible braces) has been only possible with digital technology. The segmented tooth movement permitted with these appliances has certainly reduced the treatment time as compared to conventional labial braces; however, a recent systematic review has concluded that these braces are not so effective in producing proper occlusal contact, control of teeth torque, and retention [25, 26].

When the orthodontic treatment is completed and the patient is ready to remove the upper and lower fixed appliances, the maxillary and mandibular archwires and molar tubes are removed and an intraoral scan is performed. The brackets are virtually removed using Mesh-mixer (Autodesk Inc., USA) software [27]. An STL file of the virtual models without brackets is generated and exported to a 3D printer. The printed models allow the manufacturing of thermoformed, lingual-bonded, or Hawley-type retainer which can be placed with high precision immediately at the debonding appointment. It reduces the number of visits to deliver the retainer appliances and has the advantage of re-fabrication of the retainer appliance in case of any loss or damage [27]. It can also correct the teeth's positions virtually if any relapse is evident. A new thermoformed appliance can be fabricated for realignment [27].

12.3.7 Guides for Temporary Anchorage Devices (TAD)

The placement of TAD in the different anatomic locations of the maxilla and mandible has become an easy task with the least or minimal complications using 3D virtual planning. The fabrication of the insertion guides to facilitate the insertion of TADs using 3D-printing technology is so accurate that it is considered to be a superior method of implant insertion. In the study by Bae et al. [28], the accuracy of the placement of orthodontic mini-screws was improved with mesiodistal deviations of 0.29 mm (range, 0.03–0.73 mm) coronally and 0.21 mm (range, 0.03–0.97 mm) apically. This suggests that root contact was rare and the mini-screws could be stably placed. The lesser deviation may be due to the limited coverage of the surgical guide and control of artifacts that was possible in this study which was on cadavers. However, Liu et al. [29] reported that the angular deviation was 1.2° ± 0.43° and the mesiodistal deviation was 0.42 ± 0.13 mm at the apical area with surgical guides; Morea et al. [30] reported that the angular deviation was 1.76° and the 3D linear distance deviations were 0.86 mm (coronal) and 0.87 mm (apex) using surgical guides. All the above studies have evaluated the mini-screw position on CBCT or CT scans. The mini-screws that appeared to be invading the root on 2D images were found to be placed between the roots, without damage to the roots, on the 3D images. CBCT evaluation also gave a better idea of the interradicular space and adjacent structures like the maxillary sinus, mandibular canal, which can be adequately protected during mini-screw insertion.

12.3.8 Miscellaneous Application of 3D Virtual Technology

1. The manufacturing of palatal plates for infants with trisomy 21 using intraoral scanning [31].
2. To strengthen the practitioner's learning from a treated case by prompt diagnosis, executing proper treatment plan, computer-aided manufacturing, and therapeutic follow-up [32].
3. 3D-printed Band and Loop space maintainer [33].
4. Vacuum-formed space maintainers for deciduous second molar during the mixed dentition [34].
5. Visualization of the alveolar cleft and planning of the patient-specific graft [35, 36].
6. Nasoalveolar bone graft in patients with unilateral cleft lip and palate [37].
7. Presurgical nasoalveolar molding [38, 39].

12.4 Summary

Although virtual technology is still in the stage of infancy, it has successfully overcome the inherent problem of data loss as a part of reducing the 3D structures to a two-dimensional view. The three-dimensional virtual planning in orthodontics seems to have the advantages of being reproducible and an accurate modality in the management of challenging or complex malocclusions and dentofacial deformities. Its application in varied domains has shown the outcome at par with conventional technologies. However, more and more clinical trials are required to transform the conventional technic into a digital or virtual paradigm.

References

1. Conejo J, Dayo AF, Syed AZ, Mupparapu M. The digital clone: intraoral scanning, face scans and cone beam computed tomography integration for diagnosis and treatment planning. Dent Clin N Am. 2021;65(3):529–53.
2. Francisco I, Ribeiro MP, Marques F, Travassos R, Nunes C, Pereira F, Caramelo F, Paula AB, Vale F. Application of three-dimensional digital Technology in Orthodontics: the state of the art. Biomimetics (Basel). 2022;7(1):23.
3. Aragón ML, Pontes LF, Bichara LM, Flores-Mir C, Normando D. Validity and reliability of intraoral scanners compared to conventional gypsum models measurements: a systematic review. Eur J Orthod. 2016;38(4):429–34.
4. Verma RK, Singh SP, Verma S, Kumar V, Bhupali NR, Arora S. Comparison of reliability, validity, and accuracy of linear measurements made on pre- and posttreatment digital study models with conventional plaster study models. J Orthod Sci. 2019;8:18.

5. Zhang F, Suh KJ, Lee KM. Validity of intraoral scans compared with plaster models: an in-vivo comparison of dental measurements and 3D surface analysis. PLoS One. 2016;11(6):e0157713.
6. Wiranto MG, Engelbrecht WP, Tutein Nolthenius HE, van der Meer WJ, Ren Y. Validity, reliability, and reproducibility of linear measurements on digital models obtained from intraoral and cone-beam computed tomography scans of alginate impressions. Am J Orthod Dentofacial Orthop. 2013;143(1):140–7.
7. Leifert MF, Leifert MM, Efstratiadis SS, Cangialosi TJ. Comparison of space analysis evaluations with digital models and plaster dental casts. Am J Orthod Dentofacial Orthop. 2009;136(1):16.e1–4; discussion 16.
8. Oliveira NS, Gribel BF, Neves LS, Lages EMB, Macari S, Pretti H. Comparison of the accuracy of virtual and direct bonding of orthodontic accessories. Dental Press J Orthod. 2019;24(4):46–53.
9. De Oliveira NS, Rossouw E, Lages EMB, Macari S, Pretti H. Influence of clinical experience on accuracy of virtual orthodontic attachment bonding in comparison with the direct procedure. Angle Orthod. 2019;89(5):734–41.
10. Smith JD, Thomas PM, Proffit WR. A comparison of current prediction imaging programs. Am J Orthod Dentofacial Orthop. 2004;125(5):527–36.
11. Alkhayer A, Piffkó J, Lippold C, Segatto E. Accuracy of virtual planning in orthognathic surgery: a systematic review. Head Face Med. 2020;16(1):34.
12. Rios O, Lerhe B, Chamorey E, Savoldelli C. Accuracy of segmented Le fort I osteotomy with virtual planning in Orthognathic surgery using patient-specific implants: a case series. J Clin Med. 2022;11(19):5495.
13. Zinser MJ, Mischkowski RA, Sailer HF, Zöller JE. Computer-assisted orthognathic surgery: feasibility study using multiple CAD/CAM surgical splints. Oral Surg. Oral med. Oral Pathol. Oral Radiol. 2012;113:673–87.
14. Kesling HD. The philosophy of the tooth positioning appliance. Am J Orthod Oral Surg. 1945;31(6):297–304.
15. Kesling HD. The diagnostic setup with consideration of the third dimension. Am J Orthod. 1956;42(10):740–8.
16. Kannan S, Singh AK, Gupta G. An edge over diagnostic setup. APOS Trends Orthod. 2017;7:294–5.
17. Macchi A, Carrafiello G, Cacciafesta V, Norcini A. Three-dimensional digital modeling and setup. Am J Orthod Dentofacial Orthop. 2006;129(5):605–10.
18. Park M, Allareddy V, Atsawasuwan P, Lee MK, Lee KC. Consideration of root position in virtual tooth setup for extraction treatment: a comparative study of simulated and actual treatment results. Korean J Orthod. 2023;53(1):26–34.
19. Hou D, Capote R, Bayirli B, Chan DCN, Huang G. The effect of digital diagnostic setups on orthodontic treatment planning. Am J Orthod Dentofacial Orthop. 2020;157(4):542–9.
20. Ho C-T, Lin H-H, Lo L-J. Intraoral scanning and setting up the digital final occlusion in three-dimensional planning of Orthognathic surgery: its comparison with the dental model approach. Plast Reconstr Surg. 2019;143(5):1027e–36e.
21. Gateno J, Xia J, Teichgraeber JF, Rosen A, Hultgren B, Vadnais T. The precision of computer-generated surgical splints. J Oral Maxillofac Surg. 2003;61(7):814–7.
22. Shaheen E, Coopman R, Jacobs R, Politis C. Optimized 3D virtually planned intermediate splints for bimaxillary orthognathic surgery: a clinical validation study in 20 patients. J Craniofac Surg. 2018;46(9):1441–7.
23. Song K-G, Baek S-H. Comparison of the accuracy of the three-dimensional virtual method and the conventional manual method for model surgery and intermediate wafer fabrication. Oral Surg Oral Med Oral Pathol Oral Radiol Endodontology. 2009;107(1):13–21.
24. Gander T, Bredell M, Eliades T, Rücker M, Essig H. Splintless orthognathic surgery: a novel technique using patient-specific implants (PSI). J Craniomaxillofac Surg. 2015;43(3):319–22.
25. Ke Y, Zhu Y, Zhu M. A comparison of treatment effectiveness between clear aligner and fixed appliance therapies. BMC Oral Health. 2019;19(1):24.
26. Kassam SK, Stoops FR. Are clear aligners as effective as conventional fixed appliances? Evid Based Dent. 2020;21(1):30–1.
27. Groth C, Kravitz ND, Shirck JM. Incorporating three-dimensional printing in orthodontics. J Clin Orthod. 2018;52(1):28–33.
28. Bae M-J, Kim J-Y, Park J-T, Cha J-Y, Kim H-J, Yu H-S, et al. Accuracy of miniscrew surgical guides assessed from cone-beam computed tomography and digital models. Am J Orthod Dentofacial Orthop. 2013;143(6):893–901.
29. Liu H, Liu D, Wang G, Wang C, Zhao Z. Accuracy of surgical positioning of orthodontic miniscrews with a computer-aided design and manufacturing template. Am J Orthod Dentofacial Orthop. 2010;137(6):728.e1–728.e10.
30. Morea C, Hayek JE, Oleskovicz C, Dominguez GC, Chilvarquer I. Precise insertion of orthodontic miniscrews with a stereolithographic surgical guide based on cone beam computed tomography data: a pilot study. Int J Oral Maxillofac Implants. 2011;26(4):860–5.
31. Xepapadeas AB, Weise C, Frank K, Spintzyk S, Poets CF, Wiechers C, Arand J, Koos B. Technical note on introducing a digital workflow for newborns with craniofacial anomalies based on intraoral scans - part I: 3D printed and milled palatal stimulation plate for trisomy 21. BMC Oral Health. 2020;20(1):20.
32. Makaremi M, de Brondeau F, Lacaule C, N'Kaoua B. Le workflow numérique au service de l'apprentissage clinique du praticien [the digital workflow at the service of the practitioner's clinical learning]. Orthod Fr. 2020;91(1–2):93–9.

33. Khanna S, Rao D, Panwar S, Pawar BA, Ameen S. 3D printed band and loop space maintainer: a digital game changer in preventive orthodontics. J Clin Pediatr Dent. 2021;45(3):147–51.
34. Barros SE, Siqueira SP, Janson G, Chiqueto K. Short-term efficacy of vacuum-formed maintainer for deciduous second molar space maintenance in the mixed dentition: a single-Centre, randomized controlled clinical trial. Orthod Craniofac Res. 2021;24(4):502–10.
35. Kesztyűs A, Würsching T, Nemes B, Pálvölgyi L, Nagy K. Evaluation of 3D visualization, planning and printing techniques in alveolar cleft repair, and their effect on patients' burden. J Stomatol Oral Maxillofac Surg. 2022;123(4):484–9.
36. Zhou WN, Xu YB, Jiang HB, Wan L, Du YF. Accurate evaluation of cone-beam computed tomography to volumetrically assess bone grafting in alveolar cleft patients. J Craniofac Surg. 2015;26(6):e535–9.
37. Pálházi P, Nemes B, Swennen G, Nagy K. Three-dimensional simulation of the nasoalveolar cleft defect. Cleft Palate Craniofac J. 2014;51(5):593–6.
38. Zheng J, He H, Kuang W, Yuan W. Presurgical nasoalveolar molding with 3D printing for a patient with unilateral cleft lip, alveolus, and palate. Am J Orthod Dentofacial Orthop. 2019;156(3):412–9.
39. Dalessandri D, Tonni I, Laffranchi L, Migliorati M, Isola G, Bonetti S, Visconti L, Paganelli C. Evaluation of a digital protocol for pre-surgical orthopedic treatment of cleft lip and palate in newborn patients: a pilot study. Dent J (Basel). 2019;7(4):111.

13 Three-Dimensional Superimposition of Craniofacial Structures

Sakshi Katyal, Sharvari Vichare, Shailendra Singh Rana, Payal Maken, and Abhishek Gupta

13.1 Introduction

Medical, Dental and other allied fields have made extensive use of superimpositions of serial craniofacial scans to depict treatment changes with time. Superimposition is also a valuable tool to better evaluate how dental and craniofacial morphology is affected by treatment or growth. Traditionally, the superimposition of 2D cephalograms has been used widely to evaluate the growth and treatment effects on jaws, associated soft tissue, and dentition. With the digitization of dentistry and invent of CBCT and scanners, 3D cephalometry has started to occupy space but yet has not gained its full potential. This is due to the inherent errors of landmarking and the difficulty in the quantification of change.

S. Katyal
Department of Dentistry, All India Institute of Medical Sciences, Bibinagar, Hyderabad, India

S. Vichare · S. S. Rana (✉)
Department of Dentistry, All India Institute of Medical Sciences, Bathinda, Punjab, India

P. Maken
School of Computer science and Engineering, Shri Mata Vaishno Devi University, Katra, India

A. Gupta
Biomedical Applications division, CSIR-Central Scientific Instruments Organisation, Chandigarh, India

The fields of Maxillofacial Surgery [1], Dentistry, Orthodontics, Implantology [2], and numerous other medical disciplines have made extensive use of 3D imaging methods in the recent years [3]. The 3D models of same or different patients are superimposed [4].

In dentofacial orthopedics, superimpositions were carried out on two-dimensional pictures, or radiographs traditionally. Stable anatomical traits from the same patient at various times could be utilized to assess changes brought on by growth or treatment [4]. Since the morphology of most cranial structures varies significantly over time, it may be more challenging to identify stable superimposition reference locations for growing people. Instances where the first set of reference regions is not perfectly matched, errors in reference sets might impact the superimposition results on the outcome sets. Since the anterior cranial base's development is almost complete by the time a child reaches the age of 7, it continues to serve as the gold standard reference region, much like 2D registration [5, 6].

3D cone-beam computed tomography (CBCT) images can be superimposed through the process of manual registration, where corresponding landmarks are identified and matched, or by employing the best-fit technique, which involves aligning stable anatomical regions to achieve the desired outcome. Three

S. S. Rana et al. (eds.), *Applications of Three-dimensional Imaging for Craniofacial Region*, https://doi.org/10.1007/978-981-97-4608-8_13

Table 13.1 Three primary methods for 3D cephalometric superimposition

S. No.	Superimposition method	Description	Methodology	Examples
1	Landmark-based superimposition [7]	This method identifies specific landmarks on anatomical structure and then aligns based on those landmark points	Transformation algorithms match corresponding landmarks	Skeletal comparison, facial recognition
2	Surface-based superimposition [8]	It aligns the surfaces or the contours of the anatomical structure together	Register the surface geometry based on features like texture or curvature	3D model alignment in computer graphics and medical imaging for various organ surface alignments
3	Voxel-based superimposition [9]	It aligns the 3D images together based on the voxel intensity of the images	Comparing the voxel intensity based on similarity metrics such as some squared differences, mutual information, etc.	CT/CBCT or MRI alignment in medical imaging

primary methods of 3D cephalometric superimposition are as follows: [4].

1. Landmark-based superimposition.
2. Surface-based superimposition.
3. Voxel-Based Superimposition.

Table 13.1 shows the comparative table of the primary 3D cephalometric superimposition methods. The superimposition of 3D data sets obtained from cone-beam CT (CBCT) images or conventional computed tomography (CT) has been documented using a variety of methods [10]. Some examples of this kind of superimposition include those based on landmarks, surfaces, or voxels, and they are employed for form-stable anatomical structures [11].

13.2 History of Craniofacial Superimposition

The first documented superimposition that was recorded involved the comparison of pre-death images against cranial remnants which was utilized as substantiating proof to be submitted in a court of law. Subsequently, it gained significant importance in forensic situations worldwide. Methodology in craniofacial superimposition has evolved with technological advances. Computer-aided superimposition, through the orientation of three-dimensional face models onto CBCT cranial structures, represents a novel advancement in this field. For 2D craniofacial radiographs, the gold standard superimposition approach is the "structural method" that was devised by Björk [12] and Björk and Skieller [13].

13.3 Landmark-Based Superimposition

Landmark-based 3D superimposition is a method that involves the orientation of one DICOM onto another, such that the respective landmarks coincide as closely in a certain manner with the positions of the corresponding landmarks on the second.

It involves identifying landmarks on an isosurface visualized from CT-generated craniofacial data in a 3D environment [14]. Points are initially marked on the surface of 3D reconstructed cone-beam computed tomography (CBCT) and subsequently adjusted on multiplanar reformation (MPR) images.

Shape differences are established through the change in the location of corresponding landmarks. Variations in form are ascertained through the inspection of these changes between two data sets. It relies on stable reference points for the orientation of consecutive DICOM data followed by an evaluation of treatment outcomes around the area of interest. If the accuracy of landmark detection and the precision of 3D surface models are high, then the use of landmark-based superimposition methodologies will be effective [15]. Following are some of the landmark-based registration approaches:

13.3.1 Thin-Plate Spline

The registration results can also have many-to-one correspondence [17]. Spline transformations can represent the variations in 3D surface shape very well. Thin-plate spline (TPS) transformation is a widely used method for 3D registration based on landmarks as follows:

1. Compute the transformation matrix using the correspondences between landmarks of 3D surfaces as Eq. 13.3.

$$T(x,y,z) = \left[1 x y z f(x,y,z)\right] \begin{bmatrix} c1 \\ c2 \\ c3 \\ c4 \\ c5 \end{bmatrix} \quad (13.3)$$

   where T (x, y, z) are the transformed coordinates of the points, f (x, y,z) is the function for deformation which maps the original coordinates to the transformed coordinates, and c1, c2, c3, c4, and c5 are the coefficients of the thin-plate spline transformation.
2. Apply the Transformation to the Surface to Deform its Shape to Match the Shape with Other while Minimizing the Bending Energy as Eq. 13.4

$$E = , \quad D^2 f^2 dA \quad (13.4)$$

where $D^2 f$ is the Hessian matrix of f.

13.3.1.1 The Reference System

The reference system allows the superimposition of serial 3D surface representations using stable anatomical areas [18]. For overall superimposition (full FOV scans), the landmarks of the anterior cranial base can be employed as a point of reference, as it is widely acknowledged that this region has completed a majority of its growth before the adolescent growth spurt. Thus, it serves as a remarkably stable reference structure to compare changes in the face, or specifically the maxilla and mandible.

Some of the landmarks that have been used to define the 3D reference plane are the right and left auditory external meatus (AEML and AEMR), the dorsum foramen magnum (DFM) (Fig. 13.1), left and right foramen ovale (RFO and LFO), and the midpoint of the right and left foramen spinosum (ELSA) as a stable reference system for superimposition [19]. Another reference plane involving nasion (Na), sella turcica (S), and basion (Ba) can be identified on the cranial base for orientation in the sagittal dimension.

For medium FOV scans, nasion, infraorbital foramen R/L (IOF), zygomatic frontal sutures (ZF) (Fig. 13.1), and incisive foramen can be used to evaluate the changes posttreatment [20].

The 3D automated referencing system enables the creation of a three-dimensional cephalometric reference system in the form of an anatomical Cartesian coordinate system. It incorporates a 3D reference plane, with a horizontal (x) orientation, that is calculated as a plane positioned six degrees below the anterior cranial base (S-N) plane. This reference plane

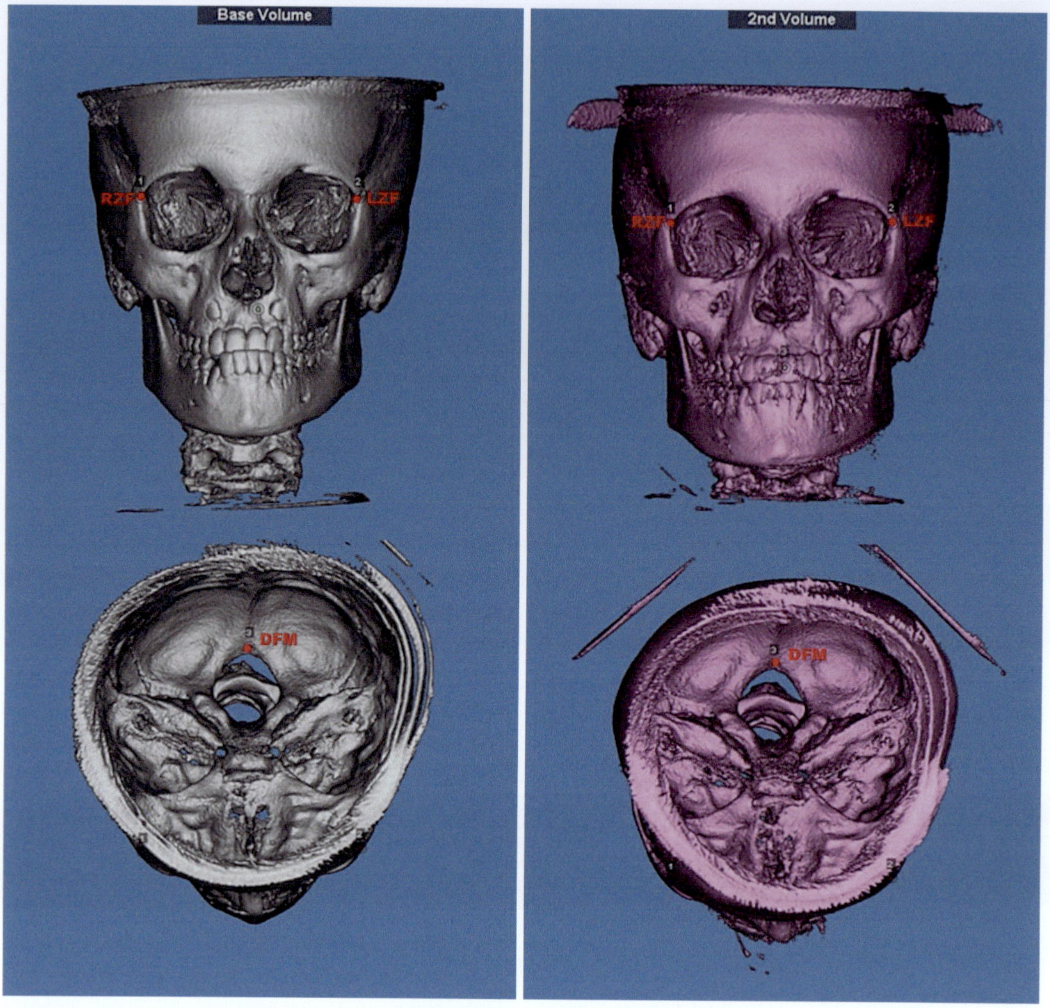

Fig. 13.1 Three-point reference plane comprising of Dorsal Foramen Magnum [DFR], Right and Left Zygomatic Frontal Suture [RZF, LZF] for landmark-based superimposition of pretreatment and posttreatment volumetric images

has its origin in sella and is perpendicular to the virtual lateral cephalogram.

The horizontal (x) 3D cephalometric reference plane and the vertical (y) plane, which both originate in sella, are perpendicular to one another. Furthermore, a third plane with its origin in sella that is perpendicular to both vertical (y) and horizontal (x) 3D cephalometric reference planes is calculated as the median (z) plane [18].

Figure 13.2 depicts the landmark-based superimposition of pretreatment and posttreatment CBCT by side-to-side method, where the same landmarks are identified on the reference plane of each DICOM data, and changes in the area of interest can be qualitatively seen in all planes.

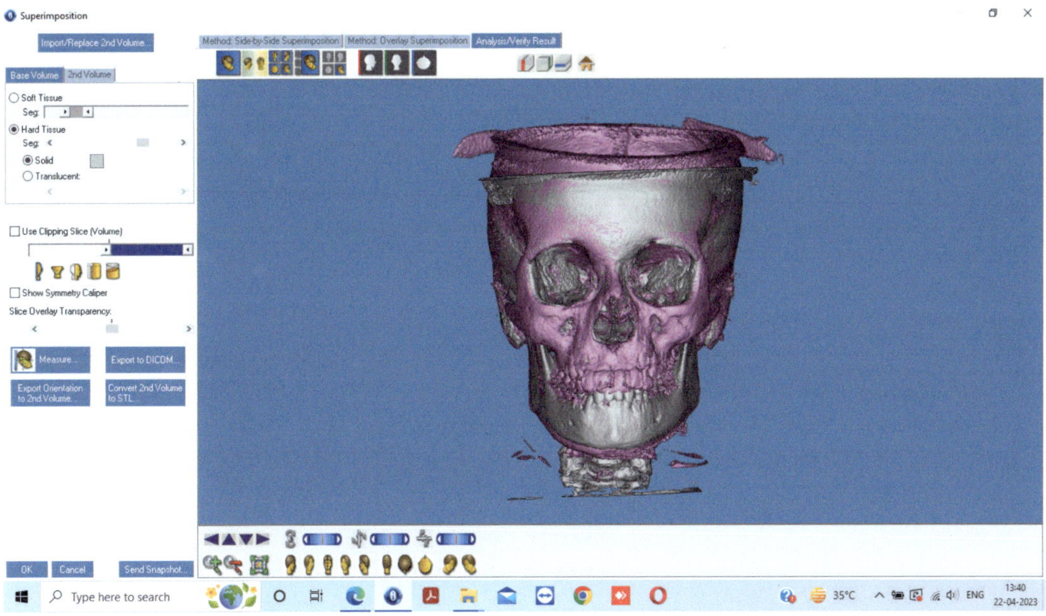

Fig. 13.2 Landmark-based superimposition of pretreatment (gray) and posttreatment volumetric models (purple) depicts maxillary saggital advancement in a Skeletal Class III case treated with facemask

13.3.1.2 Errors in Landmark Reproducibility

Studies report large errors in the localization of landmarks in the x-coordinate for orbitale [OrR (error = 0.89 mm), OrL (0.68 mm)] and porion [PoR (0.61 mm)], whereas Na, S, Ba, Co, and ANS showed good reproducibility as reference landmarks [20].

Landmark-based 3D superimposition may pose challenges due to the following reasons: [21, 22].

- Manual placement of landmarks requires a well-trained personnel and can be time-consuming.
- Prescise identification of landmarks may be hampered due to the summation of positioning errors in all three planes.
- The accuracy of landmark identification can be affected by the quality of the imaging data, such as noise, artifacts, and resolution.
- 3D superimposition techniques have limitations depending on image quality, reference areas, landmark consistency, and software/hardware performance.
- Majorly, the choice of landmarks can affect the accuracy of the superimposition process.

13.4 Surface-Based Superimposition (SBR)

Surface-based superimposition was proposed by Hajeer et al., [23] as a method of 3D superimposition to study facial symmetry in orthognathic surgery. This is based on the principle of triangular representations of corresponding 3D geometries and involves evaluation of surface structures to assess treatment results or proposed change. An additional step is necessary to transform DICOM files into Standard Tessellation Language (STL) files, followed by image segmentation.

The method employed is the iterative closest point (ICP) technique, which carries out superimposition by aligning the corresponding closest points on the identical three-dimensional (3D) surface, as opposed to utilizing landmarks for registration. The stable anatomic surfaces are registered as reference regions while overlaying images from subsequent time points, and the ICP algorithm then automatically superimposes two or more DICOM data sets. This method is also called as "best-fit method" because of the iterative process used in the ICP algorithm to minimize the distance between the surfaces approximated [24].

13.4.1 Iterative Closest Point (ICP)

ICP aligns or registers iteratively the two 3D surfaces by aligning the sets of landmark points by minimizing the corresponding distance between points [16]. The method flow is as follows:

1. Initialize identity matrix T (called transformation matrix).
2. Iterate until convergence following:
   (a) Find correspondence between landmark points in source 3D surface A and target 3D surface B using distance metrics like Euclidean distance as Eq. 13.1.

$$d(pi,qj)=\sqrt{(pix-qjx)^2+(piy-qjy)^2+(piz-qjz)^2} \quad (13.1)$$

   where pi (x, y, z) are points of surface A and qj (x, y, z) are points of surface B.
   (b) Compute the transformation matrix which minimizes the distance between the calculated corresponding 3D_3D points. Update the T using a least square method or any other optimization technique.
   (c) Update the transformation matrix T, i.e., T = ΔT ·T as Eq. 13.2.

$$\Delta T=\left(\sum_{N}^{i} qi\,p_i^T\right)\left(\sum_{N}^{i} qi\,p_i^T\right)^{-1} \quad (13.2)$$

   N is the total number of points in surface A or B.
3. Repeat until convergence.

The workflow of the surface superimposition technique (where T0 denotes the pretreatment phase and T1 refers to the posttreatment phase) is shown as follows in a stepwise manner and also in Fig. 13.3:

1. Step 1—The process of converting DICOM files to STL format is undertaken.
2. Step 2—In the first stage of registration, the two models are initially superimposed manually. The 3D cephalograms are oriented and grossly registered using the true horizontal or FH-plane. This shortens the time needed for the subsequent automatic superimposition.

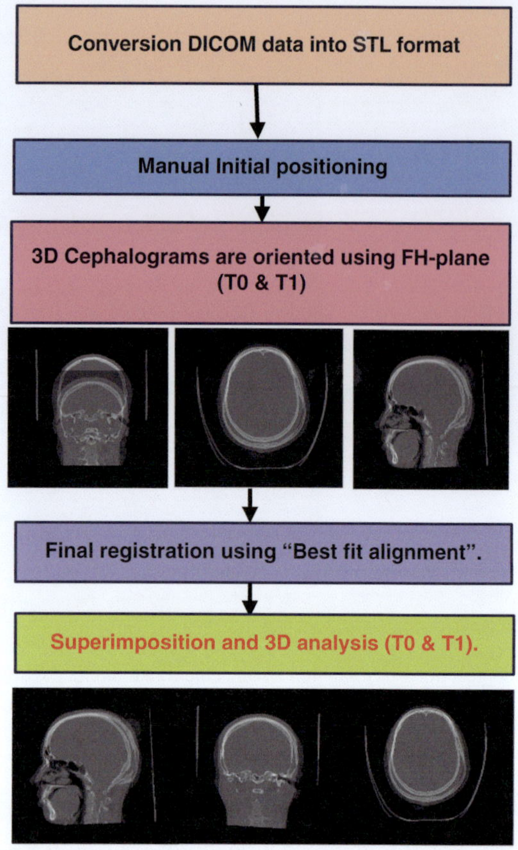

Fig. 13.3 Workflow of the surface superimposition technique

3. Step 3—Final registration is performed using the "Best fit alignment" of 3D reference surfaces using an iterative closest point (ICP) algorithm.
4. Step 4—Superimposition and 3-D analysis encompass the process of visualizing the color-coded distances between corresponding regions of T0 and T1 on the overlaid models. This technique facilitates the quantification of the outcome, which can be assessed comprehensively and in all three spatial dimensions.

The surface-based registration method is further divided into three phases, shown in Fig. 13.4: "choice of transformation; surface representation and similarity criterion; and matching & global optimization" [25].

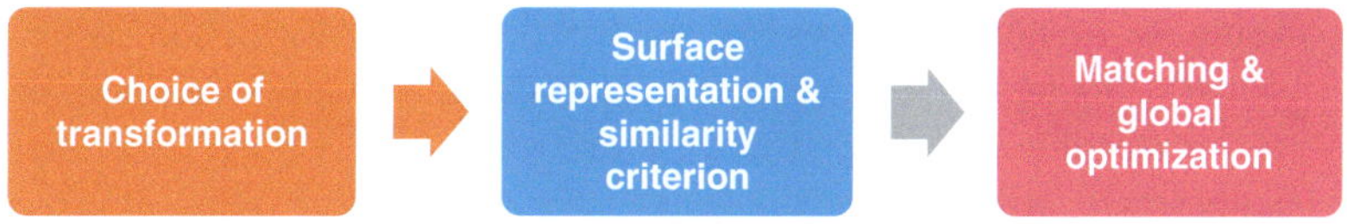

Fig. 13.4 Surface-based registration (SBR) framework

13.4.2 Choice of Transformation

To map the points of two surfaces A onto B, this phase involves making assumptions about the nature of the relationship T between the two images. The issue addresses the applicability of rigid-body principles and, if not, what nature and kind of relationship best transforms one modality to another. Here, T stands for the change in anatomy between two or more modalities of the same kind.

1. *Rigid-body transformation*: If the necessary precision of the transformation outweighs the anatomical deformations, rigid-body transformation is offered. A rigid-body transformation can be expressed generally as a combination of rotation and a translation as follows in Eq. 13.5.

$$Tp = R.x + T \tag{13.5}$$

   where R is a rotation around the origin first of surface A to B and T is translation around the origin second of surface A.

   Thus, the rigid-body registration provides the least values of R and t, giving the points of A and B their 3D-to-3D correspondences. This approach works with any collection of point pairs, not simply surface registration.
2. *Non-rigid transformations*: Any major deformations between surfaces that are not due to noise or distortions but are instead generated by other variables are considered to be non-rigid transformations. Whether they are described using local or global fitting also affects the use of non-rigid transformation. The generalizations of rigid-body transformations fall within the domain of non-rigid transformations. Using global polynomials, a generic formula is a function that maps surface A to surface B. One possible alternative to the global polynomial function is to use splines or piecewise polynomials [25].

13.4.3 Surface Representation and Similarity Criterion

The subsequent phase of SBR consists of computing the surface representation and determining the similarity criteria for the two surfaces. The surface representation should be stable for the examined two modalities. The similarity criteria should link a homologous point. The four approaches utilized for surface representation are feature-based, point-based, model-based, and global-based similarity [25]. The similarity criteria definition is connected to the choice of matching component. The criteria for matching component selection rely on whether the anatomy is smooth, cranial, or angular (application-specific) and also on transformation that is rigid or nonrigid.

1. *Feature-based methods* express the surface shape as a set of features. The features that describe the surface shape are, first, point features (sparse) such as local peaks, saddle points, or pits and, second, regions such as consistent curvature signs and curves such as ridges or boundaries [26].
2. *Point-based methods* perform the registration based on dense point sets with correspondence points, where these points can be a subset of the available surface points. It is also called free-form matching [27]. These methods work by two-point sets being relatively close to each other. To register the method, a global function connecting surfaces A and B, such as SSD (Sum of squared distances between nearest points), must be minimized. Minimizing a global function, such as SSD

(Sum of squared distances between closest points), linking surfaces A and B is necessary to register the technique. The differences in the result lie in the choice of distance measure and the likelihood of finding a match. Eq. 13.6 is a commonly used metric to calculate the distance between point an in set A and point b in set B.

$$\text{distance} = \sqrt{(x_2\ \ x_1)^2 + (y_2\ \ y_1)^2} \quad (13.6)$$

where a (x1, y1) and b (x2, y2) are the points of surface A and B, respectively.

3. *Model-based approaches*: A deformable surface model uses raw image data and an expression based on physical principles or surface evolution to predict the surface's shape and/or dynamic behavior. This model can be expressed as surface identification (segmentation) in a single volume or as surface tracking over a sequence of volumes. Aside from a few notable cases, these methods typically calculate surface and curve motion without explicit matching.
4. *Global shape-based methods*: These methods provide surface registration based on global surface geometry and do not largely rely on prior estimates of the transformation because it also does not rely on local shape information. Consequently, these methods might address featureless regions of the surfaces [28, 29].

13.4.4 Matching and Global Optimization

The final phase is to search for matching or corresponding feature point pairs based on surface representation and optimal transformation as defined in the first two phases. This could be performed by doing comparisons of finite candidates or iteratively minimization of an objective function. The computation depends on the assumptions made in earlier stages. Some of the methods could be discrete feature matching and transformation using pose clustering matches, sequential hypothesis and testing, and geometric hashing. Other methods involve closest point finding with global optimization and model-based motion estimation using finite element modeling [25].

The surface-based registration method is considered more precise than the landmark-based method due to the larger surface area available for registration [30]. Although it is a reliable method for assessing changes in craniofacial structures, variations in image quality can introduce potential errors. Potential errors related to variations in image quality, image resolution, noise, imaging artifacts such as motion artifacts or metal artifacts, and quality of surface segmentation can affect the accuracy of surface-based superimposition [4, 31]. These factors should be taken into consideration when using surface-based superimposition for dental imaging. Surface-based registration has the potential to be a viable substitute for the prevalent voxel-based methods in medical imaging. Similar to Digital Imaging and Communications in Medicine (DICOM) for voxel data, the open-source STL format is readily available via most commercial and freeware software packages. Rapid prototyping and computer-aided manufacturing have made extensive use of such surface models in industry, especially in the engineering and architectural fields.

13.5 Voxel-Based Superimposition

The technique of voxel-based superimposition for dentofacial applications was introduced by Cevidanes et al. in 2005 [32]. It is the most commonly described, only fully automated technique. It allows for image analysis to be conducted in a manner that is not dependent on operator-related factors [33].

Voxel-based methods employ the best-fit strategy to superimpose voxel grayscale values from multiple data sets. This method is based on

Mutual Information Maximization (MIM) algorithm [34], wherein it compares and matches reference areas based on their grayscale values, of CT scan or CBCT images, thus avoiding segmentation errors [30].

The initial step involves the selection of the volume of interest, also known as the registration area, as depicted in Fig. 13.5. Following this, a rough alignment of the 3D models is achieved. Anterior cranial fossa for large field-of-view scans (FOV) and zygomatic arches for smaller FOV scans are commonly used as registration areas [35]. Consequently, based on the gray values of the corresponding voxels, the software calculates the necessary translation and rotation to achieve geometric alignment between the two DICOM images. Subsequently, this alignment is applied to the constructed 3D models, as shown in Fig. 13.6.

Some methods for voxel-based registration are mutual information (MI)-based registration, demon's registration, and fluid registration.

13.5.1 Mutual Information-Based Registration [36]

This method was proposed by Viola and Wells (MIT) in 1994. The registration technique was based on the assumption that surfaces having similar grayscale values in one surface or image could correspond to the regions in another image that consist of similar grayscale values (but not the same). The joint histogram of the two surfaces would show the clusters of gray tomes of matching structures. The steps of performing 3D registration using MI are as follows:

1. Compute the mutual information (MI) between the intensity values of the voxels of the two 3D surfaces as Eq. 13.7

   $$MI(A,B) = H(A) + H(B) - H(A,B) \quad (13.7)$$

   where H (A) and H (B) are the entropies of surfaces A and B and H (A, B) is the joint entropy of A and B.

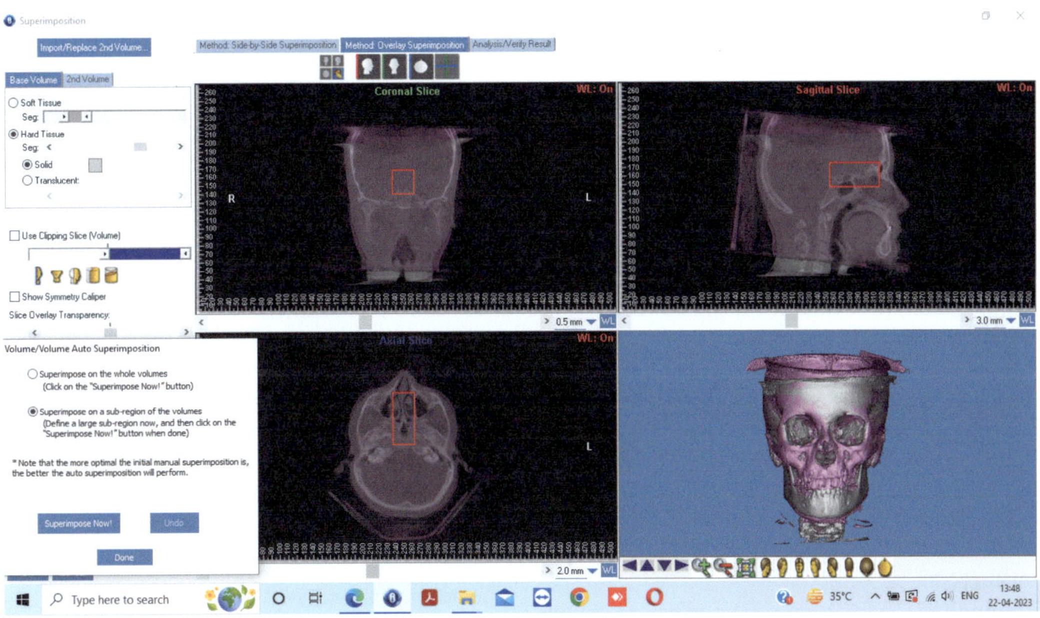

Fig. 13.5 Voxel-based superimposition; the registration area (anterior cranial base) is demarcated, and depending on the gray value and voxel by voxel, the two subsequent volume data sets are oriented

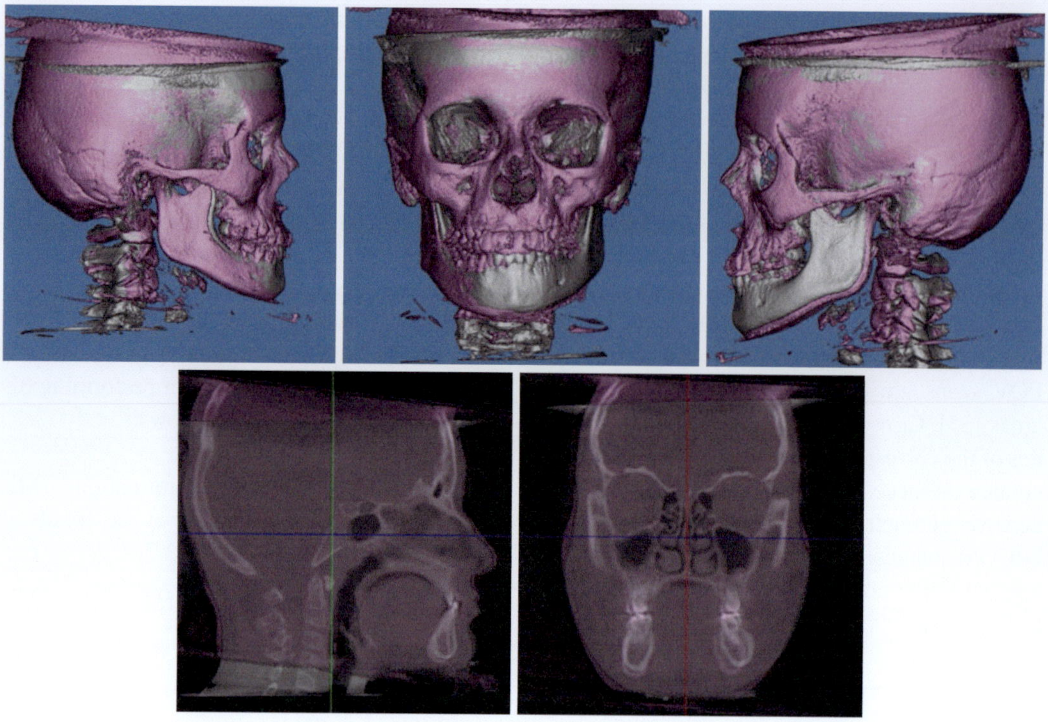

Fig. 13.6 Outcomes of voxel-based superimposition for two subsequent volume datasets, after automated orientation to the anterior cranial base

2. Maximize the mutual information by optimizing the transformation between two surfaces (translation, rotation, and scaling).
3. Repeat steps until convergence.

13.5.2 Demons Registration [37]

Demons algorithm is used for the registration of images for deformation by iteratively solving gradient descent constraint and having a voxel correspondence between the reference and the second 3D surface. The process is as follows:

1. Compute the gradient descent constraint of the intensity values of voxels on both surfaces.
2. Iteratively deform one 3D surface to match the other by applying the displacement field as in Eq. 13. 8

$$\Delta u = \nabla '' \left(\frac{\nabla I(x+u) - \nabla J(x)}{\nabla I(x+u) - \nabla J(x)^2 + \alpha} \right) \quad (13.8)$$

where u is the displacement field, J and I are the intensities of the fixed and moving images, and α is the regularization parameter.
3. Repeat until convergence.

13.5.3 Fluid Registration [38]

This method models the deformation between two 3D surfaces as a fluid flow problem where the intensities are treated as fluid densities. The target is to calculate a velocity field of the image which describes the movement of points in one surface A to align it with the corresponding points in other surface B. The velocity field is applied to deform the 3D image to match another. The process is followed by minimizing a similarity metric such as SSD or MI between intensities of two surfaces. The Navier-Stokes Equation can be used for fluid flow as Eq.13.9:

$$\rho \left(\frac{dv}{dt} + (v '' \nabla) V \right) = -\nabla p + \mu \nabla^2 V + f \quad (13.9)$$

where v is the velocity field, ρ is the fluid density, p is the pressure, μ is the viscosity, and f is the external force.

Voxel-based superimposition has several applications in orthodontics and craniofacial surgery. Here are some of the applications of voxel-based superimposition in these fields:

1. Voxel-based superimposition can be used to assess changes in facial soft tissue over time [22].
2. It is a reliable and reproducible method for assessment of craniofacial skeletal structures [39].
3. For evaluation of stable reference areas: Voxel-based superimposition can be used to evaluate the reliability and reproducibility of different anterior cranial base reference areas for craniofacial CBCTs [40, 41]. The anterior cranial base is commonly used as a reference area for voxel-based superimposition in orthognathic surgical planning.
4. This method permits the assessment of changes in the size of pathological hard tissues or their progression with high efficiency and reproducibility [42].

13.6 Quantification of Three-Dimensional Change

One may use either two-dimensional (2D) slices or three-dimensional (3D) models to measure linear distances and angles between particular reference sites. Three-dimensional linear measurements in every plane of space transform into Euclidean distances between landmarks that are overlaid at two separate periods. This quantification is derived using numerous approaches and is based on hundreds of points in triangular meshes of surface models [39].

1. Color-coded maps: By utilizing semitransparent overlays, the visual representation of color-coded maps can assist clinicians and researchers in comprehending the intricate changes occurring across the entire surface. Moreover, localized measurements within these maps can be obtained at a single point or within a defined radius surrounding a landmark. The measurement of 3D linear distances between the nearest vertices of triangular meshes on two surfaces constitutes the basis for closest point analysis, and these changes are presented by coding with different colors.
2. Shape correspondence: The process of calculating point-based surface models, in which every model has an equal number of homologous vertices and triangular meshes. After that, appropriate surface vectors and distances may be calculated and visually presented. One may take localized measurements at a single point or any specified radius around a landmark on maps by utilizing the closest point feature.
3. Quantification of directional changes in each plane of the 3D space: Measuring the elements in every plane of the space is feasible using automated or observer-defined landmarks. There are three techniques to estimate the distances between landmarks: vertical (z-axis), anteroposterior (y-axis), and transversal (x-axis).
4. 3D angular measurements: The quantification of pitch, roll, and yaw of a model can be achieved by employing 3D angular measurements between lines or planes that are defined within a common 3D coordinate system. The indication of rotations in different directions, such as clockwise or counterclockwise rotation, can be conveyed through positive and negative values. For instance, the assessment of mandibular rotations can be carried out in the following manner: pitch can be measured by examining the angle obtained in the sagittal view, roll can be measured in the coronal view, and yaw can be measured in the axial view amidst two time frames.

13.7 Comparative Accuracy of Superimposition Methods

Cevidanes et al. investigated the intra-observer reliability for quantifying treatment outcomes using color-coded distance maps. CBCT images were registered on the anterior cranial base. The

Table 13.2 Different 3D superimposition methods with their applications, advantages, and disadvantages [44]

S.No.	Methods	Applications	Advantages	Disadvantages
1.	Registration-based or point-based.—Arbitrary selected points are registered [44]	Assessing the growth of patient's craniofacial structures and before and after orthodontic treatment results	1. It helps in evaluating the growth of patients or the orthodontic treatment process with the help of the fusion of two 3D images 2. Observing bilateral structures in real size	1. Extensive and time-consuming 2. Measurement outcomes differentiate depending on the plane definition, slice thickness, and number of sections selected
2.	Mathematical algorithms and information theory based [44]: Software assisted Voxel based Landmark based	Observing and analyzing the hard and soft tissue changes between two scans relative to registered landmarks	1. Provide a more realistic way to evaluate the changes 2. Human error is eliminated 3. Create accurate surface models and accurate measurements with multi-planar reconstruction and color-coded images 4. Create an unbiased scientific setup for the superimposition process	1. Slightly inferior to the threshold-based method 2. Since the software is used, clinical measurements may be impacted by the segmentation process 3. There might be some landmark identification and registration errors

inter-examiner variability was found to be small (measurement error $\leq$ 0.5 mm). This precision was attributed to the automation of voxel-based superimposition and independence on the surface characteristics of models [39].

In another study, Ghoneima et al. discovered that the landmark-based method was similarly dependable but less accurate than the surface-based and voxel-based superimposition methods [20], which both employed the anterior cranial base as a reference structure to detect changes in landmark positions during superimposition [43].

13.7.1 Various 3D Superimpositions Methods

Two common methods for 3D superimpositions are the structural method and the best-fit method. Among these, mathematical algorithms or registration are the common methods. A registration-based technique selects landmarks that will coincide after superimposition and uses them for volumetric image registration. The operator may then manually manipulate the superimposed for further fine-tuning after initial superimposition. An initial 3D scan is taken into account for a referenced volume of interest (VOI) using a mathematical approach. The program immediately applies the second scan's best-fit algorithm over the first VOI. The software-based approach does not need operator knowledge. The landmarks were used by an operator to do the first alignment of the two anatomic components, much as in most software applications. Next, the changes are measured by the software in concern with the registered points. After that, the final image is placed, revealing the outcomes of the growth or therapy. Table 13.2 shows various 3D superimposition methods with their applications, advantages, and disadvantages.

13.8 The Virtual Face

The process of overlaying a three-dimensional image of a face on a cone-beam computed tomography (CBCT) scan is founded upon the principle of surface-based registration, yielding a highly precise depiction of a patient's facial structure.

The utilization of 3D photographic techniques, such as 3D-MD, enables the acquisition of surface data, resulting in a more intricate and textured depiction of facial surface structures, including the hairline, eyebrows, and eyelashes allowing the demarcation of the soft tissue landmarks [45]. However, it is important to note that due to the absence of stable references in 3D photogrammetry, 3D photography, and laser scanning, accurately quantifying soft tissue changes through these methods is challenging [11]. To address this issue, a stable reference for image superimposition is necessary to establish a standardized record of the relationship between facial soft tissues and the underlying skeletal and dental structures. Currently, CBCT technology provides the means to utilize stable reference structures. Consequently, the untextured soft tissue surface of CBCT scans and the wavefront object files of stereophotographic images are exported as a stereolithography file (*.stl) to facilitate the superimposition of soft tissue images onto the CBCT model.

Using this method, Cevidanes et al. (2010) have demonstrated 3D soft tissue changes with voxel-based registration at the cranial base. Gerig et al. suggested the measurement of soft tissue changes with color maps serving as a visual tool to assess and quantify these changes [46]. These color maps depict the inward displacement (blue) or outward displacement (red) of superimposed structures.

13.9 Airway Superimposition

Semiautomated segmentation of the upper airways and facial skeleton is possible using mean thresholds of −1000 to −299.39 Hounsfield for airways and + 620 to +1000 Hounsfield for hard tissue [47].

A 3D model of the airway is aligned using defined landmarks to create a new coordinate system, allowing for a point-based analysis that volumetrically compares the airway model at two different time points. This analysis measures the distances between triangular nodes on the target object and the closest triangular nodes on the reference object, providing mean, minimum, and maximum values that are visualized through a color map.

13.10 Multimodal Image Registration

Multimodal image registration (MMIR) includes the merging of various imaging modalities such as CT, positron emission tomography (PET), and MRI for viewing and displaying both osseous and soft tissues into a single image [25]. With the advent of CBCT in dental imaging, the drawbacks of 2D image superimposition have been overcome, and it is now possible to superimpose CBCTs using a skull base to analyze the changes in the craniofacial bones [4].

Variations in voxel size, pixel intensity, identification of anatomical structures, picture orientation, and range of vision make it challenging to register multimodality images between MRI and CBCT. Nevertheless, the technique was first used in 1998 when lateral cephalometric radiographs were combined with sagittal MRI slices [48]. However, as it offers a complimentary view of both hard and soft tissues in a single imaging frame, the registration of 3D data from MRI and CBCT is preferred.

Multimodal image registration is commonly used for visualization of tumors in the head and neck region [49, 50]; it is extremely beneficial in TMJ imaging to comprehend the complex osseous, cartilaginous, and soft tissue components. However, unlike the conventional single-step superimposition process, multimodal image registration is a two-step process as follows:

1. Registration – involves alignment of target images
2. Fusion – involves the fused display of the target images.

Various terms have been used interchangeably to refer to this process, such as superimposition, matching, merging, integration, and correlation; however, it is an important arena for exploration within the scope of this topic.

Both extrinsic and intrinsic models of the registration process were identified by Van den Elsen et al. and Maintz et al. [51, 52]. The intrinsic model is dependent on segmented bodies, anatomical landmarks, and voxel values. The fiducial markers used in the extrinsic model are either noninvasively adhered to the skin's surface or invasively positioned/screwed into the tissues. For many years, the gold standard method to assess the correctness of the registration process was screw-mounted fiducial markers. However, the invasiveness of this method limits its application to in vitro studies and surgical procedures. Anatomical landmarks are frequently obvious and simple to find in the human skull when using intrinsic registration models; however, registering vast tissues in complex locations necessitates the discovery of several anatomical landmarks [53]. To identify the landmarks, user input is also necessary, which raises the possibility of operator bias, particularly with less-experienced operators. Monomodal image registration is thought to be a lot simpler method than multimodality picture registration because of the high degree of similarity between images of the same modality. Finding matched anatomical landmarks in multimodality image registration, such as MRI and CBCT/CT, is difficult.

Another intrinsic method is to align the primary orientation and center of gravity of two images by using the voxel values (gray values) of the image. The "maximization of mutual information" strategy, which makes use of the entire image's gray values in a relative entropy histogram, is theoretically appealing due to its adaptability, simplicity, and automatic and quick application in multimodal image registration. However, issues with accuracy and expensive/complex computing requirements have prevented this registration technique from being used in clinical settings.

13.10.1 Advantages of 3D Superimpositions

There could be a chance of errors in CBCT-derived cephalograms due to the errors that could occur while CBCT scanning, but various literature reported the accuracy of CBCT-derived or traditional cephalograms is the same.

1. 3D superimposition images show the most precise way to assess the changes. Surface comparison in 3D is more reliable and precise than 2D cephalometric evaluations as it can easily determine the location, magnitude, and direction of changes, providing a comprehensive quantification of structures in three dimensions.
2. Software-based craniofacial structure superimpositions are better than traditional superimposition methods because they remove the errors that are relative to the identification of landmarks.
3. 3D superimpositions based on software allow the user to open the two scans for registration at the same time to register the common landmarks easily.

13.10.2 Disadvantages of 3D Superimpositions

1. Very little evidence is available in the literature for 3D superimposition techniques and various other registration structures.
2. It is difficult to determine consistent directional tendencies because different craniofacial structures grow in different tendencies. Thus, vectorial analysis tools can help in the future for displacement directions.
3. The gold standard method for anatomical structure is yet not recognized. Thus, there is a need for universal software with the capability of control variables. It could differ the measurement outcomes depending on the definition of a plane and the number and thickness of sections.

4. A great amount of 3D CBCT superimposition data quantitatively could make it difficult for operators to articulate the landmarks and have very few points for registration and quantitative analysis.

13.11 Summary

3D superimposition has revolutionized diagnosis, treatment planning, and prediction. Although it is sensitive technique and prone to errors. The medicinal applications of this technology have immense promise. The use of 3D superimposition of craniofacial components has shown to be very advantageous for orthodontics and craniofacial surgery, as compared to traditional 2D imaging approaches. This method allows for a comprehensive evaluation of the craniofacial components across time, independent of whether the alterations are due to natural growth or medical interventions. Each of the three primary methods for 3D cephalometric superimposition, namely, landmark-based, surface-based, and voxel-based, has distinct advantages and disadvantages.

Landmark-based superimposition mainly focuses on recognizing certain anatomical landmarks that align and compare the 3D information, offering critical insights into changes in craniofacial morphology. However, this method may be time-consuming and thus prone to mistakes, especially in landmark recognition. Surface-based superimposition thus leverages the examination of the structure of the craniofacial features to compare the treatment before and after, offering the credibility of evaluations but also the vulnerability to changes in image quality. On the other hand, voxel-based superimposition is automatic and depends on intensity values to align and compare the data sets, affording it a stable and consistent approach for analyzing bone and tissue alterations.

Despite the advantages of 3D superimposition, a few challenges remain, such as the demand for standardized reference structures and software tools, as well as the interpretation of huge amounts of quantitative data. Nevertheless, improvements in imaging technology and software algorithms continue to increase the accuracy and efficiency of 3D superimposition techniques, opening the route for more accurate diagnosis, treatment planning, and evaluation in dentofacial orthopedics and adjacent domains.

References

1. Lee JH, Kim MJ, Kim SM, Kwon OH, Kim YK. The 3D CT superimposition method using image fusion based on the maximum mutual information algorithm for the assessment of Oral and maxillofacial surgery treatment results, Oral Surg Oral med Oral Pathol. Oral Radiol. 2012;114:167–74. https://doi.org/10.1016/j.tripleo.2011.06.003.
2. AlSamak S, Gkantidis N, Bitsanis E, Christou P. Assessment of potential orthodontic mini-implant insertion sites based on anatomical hard tissue parameters: a systematic review. Int J Oral Maxillofac Implants. 2012;27:875–87.
3. De Vos W, Casselman J, Swennen GR. Cone-beam computerized tomography (CBCT) imaging of the oral and maxillofacial region: a systematic review of the literature. Int J Oral Maxillofac Surg. 2009;38:609–25. https://doi.org/10.1016/j.ijom.2009.02.028.
4. Gkantidis N, Schauseil M, Pazera P, Zorkun B, Katsaros C, Ludwig B. Evaluation of 3-dimensional superimposition techniques on various skeletal structures of the head using surface models. PLoS One. 2015;10:e0118810. https://doi.org/10.1371/journal.pone.0118810.
5. Buschang PH, LaPalme L, Tanguay R, Demirjian A. The technical reliability of superimposition on cranial base and mandibular structures. Eur J Orthod. 1986;8:152–6. https://doi.org/10.1093/ejo/8.3.152.
6. Afrand M, Ling CP, Khosrotehrani S, Flores-Mir C, Lagravère-Vich MO. Anterior cranial-base time-related changes: a systematic review. Am J Orthod Dentofacial Orthop. 2014;146:21–32.e6. https://doi.org/10.1016/j.ajodo.2014.03.019.
7. Huzurbazar S, Kuang D, Lee L. Landmark-based algorithms for group average and pattern recognition. Pattern Recognition. 2019;86:172–87. https://doi.org/10.1016/j.patcog.2018.09.002.
8. Jiang Y, Song G, Yu X, Dou Y, Li Q, Liu S, Han B, Xu T. The application and accuracy of feature matching on automated cephalometric superimposition. BMC Med Imaging. 2020;20:31. https://doi.org/10.1186/s12880-020-00432-z.
9. Han G, Li J, Wang S, Wang L, Zhou Y, Liu Y. A comparison of voxel- and surface-based cone-beam computed tomography mandibular superimposition in adult orthodontic patients. J Int Med Res. 2021;49:300060520982708. https://doi.org/10.1177/0300060520982708.

10. Nada RM, Maal TJ, Breuning KH, Bergé SJ, Mostafa YA, Kuijpers-Jagtman AM. Accuracy and reproducibility of voxel based superimposition of cone beam computed tomography models on the anterior cranial base and the zygomatic arches. PLoS One. 2011;6:e16520. https://doi.org/10.1371/journal.pone.0016520.
11. Cevidanes LH, Motta A, Proffit WR, Ackerman JL, Styner M. Cranial base superimposition for 3-dimensional evaluation of soft-tissue changes. Am J Orthod Dentofacial Orthop. 2010;137:S120–9. https://doi.org/10.1016/j.ajodo.2009.04.021.
12. Björk A. Prediction of mandibular growth rotation. Am J Orthod. 1969;55:585–99. https://doi.org/10.1016/0002-9416(69)90036-0.
13. Björk A, Skieller V. Growth of the maxilla in three dimensions as revealed radiographically by the implant method. Br J Orthod. 1977;4:53–64. https://doi.org/10.1179/bjo.4.2.53.
14. P. Zheng, B. Belaton, R. Zaharudin, A. Irani, and Z. Rajion, Computerized 3D craniofacial landmark identification and analysis, eJCSIT (2011);1.
15. Lagravère MO, Major PW, Carey J. Sensitivity analysis for plane orientation in three-dimensional cephalometric analysis based on superimposition of serial cone beam computed tomography images. Dentomaxillofac Radiol. 2010;39:400–8. https://doi.org/10.1259/dmfr/17319459.
16. Sinko M, Kamencay P, Hudec R, Benco M. 3D registration of the point cloud data using ICP algorithm in medical image analysis. In: 2018 ELEKTRO. IEEE; 2018.
17. Chen Y, Zhao J, Deng Q, Duan F. 3D craniofacial registration using thin-plate spline transform and cylindrical surface projection. PLoS One. 2017;12:e0185567. https://doi.org/10.1371/journal.pone.0185567.
18. G. Swennen, F. Schutyser, and J.-E. Hausamen, Three-dimensional Cephalometry, a color atlas and manual. 2005.
19. DeCesare A, Secanell M, Lagravère MO, Carey J. Multiobjective optimization framework for landmark measurement error correction in three-dimensional cephalometric tomography. Dentomaxillofac Radiol. 2013;42:20130035. https://doi.org/10.1259/dmfr.20130035.
20. Hwang JJ, Kim KD, Park H, Park CS, Jeong HG. Factors influencing superimposition error of 3D cephalometric landmarks by plane orientation method using 4 reference points: 4 point superimposition error regression model. PLoS One. 2014;9:e110665. https://doi.org/10.1371/journal.pone.0110665.
21. Dot G, Rafflenbeul F, Salmon B. Voxel-based superimposition of cone beam CT scans for orthodontic and craniofacial follow-up: overview and clinical implementation. Int Orthod. 2020;18:739–48. https://doi.org/10.1016/j.ortho.2020.08.001.
22. Kanavakis G, Häner ST, Matthey F, Gkantidis N. Voxel-based superimposition of serial craniofacial cone-beam computed tomographies for facial soft tissue assessment: reproducibility and segmentation effects. Am J Orthod Dentofacial Orthop. 2021;159:343–351.e1. https://doi.org/10.1016/j.ajodo.2020.04.022.
23. Hajeer MY, Ayoub AF, Millett DT. Three-dimensional assessment of facial soft-tissue asymmetry before and after orthognathic surgery. Br J Oral Maxillofac Surg. 2004;42:396–404. https://doi.org/10.1016/j.bjoms.2004.05.006.
24. Lo Giudice A, Ronsivalle V, Zappalà G, Leonardi R, Campagna P, Isola G, Palazzo G. The evolution of the cephalometric superimposition techniques from the beginning to the digital era: a brief descriptive review. Int J Dentistry. 2021;2021:6677133. https://doi.org/10.1155/2021/6677133.
25. Audette MA, Ferrie FP, Peters TM. An algorithmic overview of surface registration techniques for medical imaging. Med Image Anal. 2000;4:201–17. https://doi.org/10.1016/s1361-8415(00)00014-1.
26. Besl PJ, Jain RC. Invariant surface characteristics for 3D object recognition in range images. Computer Vision Graphics Image Process. 1986;33:33–80. https://doi.org/10.1016/0734-189X(86)90220-3.
27. Thirion. Extremal points: definition and application to 3D image registration. In: 1994 Proceedings of IEEE Conference on Computer Vision and Pattern Recognition. IEEE; 1994. p. 587–92.
28. Campbell RJ, Flynn PJ. Eigenshapes for 3D object recognition in range data. In: Proceedings 1999 IEEE Computer Society Conference on Computer Vision and Pattern Recognition (Cat. No PR00149); 1999.
29. Johnson AE, Hebert M. Surface matching for object recognition in complex three-dimensional scenes. Image Vis Comput. 1998;16:635–51. https://doi.org/10.1016/S0262-8856(98)00074-2.
30. Ghoneima A, Cho H, Farouk K, Kula K. Accuracy and reliability of landmark-based, surface-based and voxel-based 3D cone-beam computed tomography superimposition methods. Orthod Craniofac Res. 2017;20:227–36. https://doi.org/10.1111/ocr.12205.
31. Häner ST, Kanavakis G, Matthey F, Gkantidis N. Valid 3D surface superimposition references to assess facial changes during growth. Sci Rep. 2021;11:16456. https://doi.org/10.1038/s41598-021-95942-3.
32. Cevidanes LH, Bailey LJ, Tucker GR Jr, Styner MA, Mol A, Phillips CL, Proffit WR, Turvey T. Superimposition of 3D cone-beam CT models of orthognathic surgery patients. Dentomaxillofac Radiol. 2005;34:369–75. https://doi.org/10.1259/dmfr/17102411.
33. Yatabe M, Prieto JC, Styner M, Zhu H, Ruellas AC, Paniagua B, Budin F, Benavides E, Shoukri B, Michoud L, Ribera N, Cevidanes L. 3D superimposition of craniofacial imaging-the utility of multicentre collaborations. Orthod Craniofac Res. 2019;22(Suppl 1):213–20. https://doi.org/10.1111/ocr.12281.
34. Maes F, Collignon A, Vandermeulen D, Marchal G, Suetens P. Multimodality image registration by maximization of mutual information. IEEE Trans Med Imaging. 1997;16:187–98. https://doi.org/10.1109/42.563664.

35. Cevidanes LH, Heymann G, Cornelis MA, DeClerck HJ, Tulloch JF. Superimposition of 3-dimensional cone-beam computed tomography models of growing patients. Am J Orthod Dentofacial Orthop. 2009;136:94–9. https://doi.org/10.1016/j.ajodo.2009.01.018.
36. Pluim JP, Maintz JB, Viergever MA. Mutual-information-based registration of medical images: a survey. IEEE Trans Med Imaging. 2003;22:986–1004. https://doi.org/10.1109/tmi.2003.815867.
37. Pennec X, Cachier P, Ayache N. Understanding the "Demon's Algorithm": 3D Non-rigid Registration by Gradient Descent. Berlin, Heidelberg: Springer; 1999.
38. C. Brun, N. Lepore, Y. Y. Chou, X. Pennec, G. de Zubicaray, K. McMahon, J. Gee, and P. Thompson, A 3D statistical fluid registration algorithm. 2010.
39. Mai DD, Stucki S, Gkantidis N. Assessment of methods used for 3-dimensional superimposition of craniofacial skeletal structures: a systematic review. Peer J. 2020;8:e9263. https://doi.org/10.7717/peerj.9263.
40. Ghamri M, Kanavakis G, Gkantidis N. Reliability of different anterior Cranial Base reference areas for voxel-based superimposition. J Clin Med. 2021;10:5429. https://doi.org/10.3390/jcm10225429.
41. Kanavakis G, Ghamri M, Gkantidis N. Novel anterior Cranial Base area for voxel-based superimposition of craniofacial CBCTs. J Clin Med. 2022;11:3536. https://doi.org/10.3390/jcm11123536.
42. Häner ST, Kanavakis G, Matthey F, Gkantidis N. Voxel-based superimposition of serial craniofacial CBCTs: reliability, reproducibility and segmentation effect on hard-tissue outcomes. Orthod Craniofac Res. 2020;23:92–101. https://doi.org/10.1111/ocr.12347.
43. Ponce-Garcia C, Ruellas ACO, Cevidanes LHS, Flores-Mir C, Carey JP, Lagravere-Vich M. Measurement error and reliability of three available 3D superimposition methods in growing patients. Head Face Med. 2020;16:1. https://doi.org/10.1186/s13005-020-0215-7.
44. Park JH, Tai K, Owtad P. 3-dimensional cone-beam computed tomography superimposition: a review. Semin Orthod. 2015;21:263–73. https://doi.org/10.1053/j.sodo.2015.07.007.
45. Naudi KB, Benramadan R, Brocklebank L, Ju X, Khambay B, Ayoub A. The virtual human face: superimposing the simultaneously captured 3D photorealistic skin surface of the face on the untextured skin image of the CBCT scan. Int J Oral Maxillofac Surg. 2013;42:393–400. https://doi.org/10.1016/j.ijom.2012.10.032.
46. Gerig G, Jomier M, Chakos M. Valmet: A New Validation Tool for Assessing and Improving 3D Object Segmentation. Berlin, Heidelberg: Springer; 2001.
47. Badiali G, Lunari O, Bevini M, Bortolani B, Cercenelli L, Lorenzetti M, Marcelli E, Bianchi A, Marchetti C. Existence of a neutral-impact Maxillo-mandibular displacement on upper airways morphology. J Pers Med. 2021;11:177. https://doi.org/10.3390/jpm11030177.
48. Nebbe B, Major PW, Prasad NG, Hatcher D. Quantitative assessment of temporomandibular joint disk status. Oral Surg Oral Med Oral Pathol Oral Radiol Endod. 1998;85:598–607. https://doi.org/10.1016/s1079-2104(98)90298-0.
49. Dai J, Wang X, Dong Y, Yu H, Yang D, Shen G. Two- and three-dimensional models for the visualization of jaw tumors based on CT-MRI image fusion. J Craniofac Surg. 2012;23:502–8. https://doi.org/10.1097/SCS.0b013e31824cd433.
50. Levitt MR, Vaidya SS, Su DK, Moe KS, Kim LJ, Sekhar LN, Hallam DK, Ghodke BV. The "triple-overlay" technique for percutaneous diagnosis and treatment of lesions of the head and neck: combined three-dimensional guidance with magnetic resonance imaging, cone-beam computed tomography, and fluoroscopy. World Neurosurg. 2013;79:509–14. https://doi.org/10.1016/j.wneu.2012.03.031.
51. Van den Elsen PA, Pol EJ, Viergever MA. Medical image matching-a review with classification. IEEE Eng Med Biol Mag. 1993;12:26–39. https://doi.org/10.1109/51.195938.
52. Maintz JB, Viergever MA. A survey of medical image registration. Med Image Anal. 1998;2:1–36. https://doi.org/10.1016/s1361-8415(01)80026-8.
53. Al-Saleh MA, Alsufyani NA, Saltaji H, Jaremko JL, Major PW. MRI and CBCT image registration of temporomandibular joint: a systematic review. J Otolaryngol Head Neck Surg. 2016;45:30. https://doi.org/10.1186/s40463-016-0144-4.

14 Craniofacial Imaging and Diagnosis of Temporomandibular Disorders Based on the Vienna Concept

Deepti Garg, Diwakar Singh, Sharvari Vichare, and Ritu Saneja

Abbreviations

TMJ	Temporomandibular joint
TMDs	Temporomandibular disorders
CMD	Craniomandibular disorder
CMR	Controlled mandibular repositioning
SCI	Sagittal condylar inclination
TCI	Transversal condylar inclination
CPV	Condylar position variator
CPM	Condylar position measurements
CMS	Craniomandibular structures
DJD	Degenerative joint disease
ThP	Therapeutic position
MLD	Mandibular lateral deviation
ICP	Intercuspal position
ID	Internal derangement
RP	Reference position
MRI	Magnetic resonance imaging
CBCT	Cone-beam computed tomography
TIM 1	Transversal induced mobility
TIM 2	Transversal induced motility

D. Garg (✉)
Center for Clinical Research, University Clinic of Dentistry, Medical University Vienna, Vienna, Austria

Clinical Division of Periodontology, University Clinic of Dentistry, Medical University Vienna, Vienna, Austria

D. Singh
Center for Clinical Research, University Clinic of Dentistry, Medical University Vienna, Vienna, Austria

Clinical Division of Prosthodontics, University Clinic of Dentistry, Medical University Vienna, Vienna, Austria

S. Vichare · R. Saneja
Department of Dentistry, All India Institute of Medical Sciences, Bathinda, Punjab, India

14.1 Introduction

Dental medicine revolves around the study of occlusion. The basis of occlusion is not simply the interdigitation of the teeth aligned in the jaws, but a combination of their positional relationship and the functional movement of the mandible [1]. The illness commonly referred to as Temporomandibular Dysfunction (TMD), has been one of the most contentious areas of dentistry for more than 50 years. The wide spectrum of conditions, such as tenderness in the temporomandibular joint (TMJ) and face area, dizziness, headaches, pain in the ear, hypertrophy of masticatory musculature, limited mouth opening, open or closed lock of the TMJ, occlusal wear, clicking sound in the joint, and other complaints, are included in Temporomandibular Disorders [2].

The American Academy of Orofacial Pain has defined Temporomandibular Disorders as: "a collective term embracing several clinical problems that involve the masticatory musculature, the temporomandibular joint (TMJ) and associated structures, or both" [3].

S. S. Rana et al. (eds.), *Applications of Three-dimensional Imaging for Craniofacial Region*, https://doi.org/10.1007/978-981-97-4608-8_14

Old ideas and concepts about treating TMD, head and neck pain, and migraines do not always hold up. Old ideas can be difficult to change, even though more knowledge has and is becoming available with more specific management of joint symptoms and muscle disorders. Years ago, splints and adjusting the bite were all that we were taught, and those ideas do not necessarily work for many patients, because muscle and joint disorders that have been developing for over one or more decades in these patients can become a large contributing factor in the diagnosis, management, and improvement in the patient's progress [4]. We need to know and understand how neuromuscular patterns affect these conditions and their relationships to the head, neck, joints, loss of range of motion, clenching and bruxing, and even headaches, migraines, occlusal wear patterns, tinnitus, etc. We also need to know and understand why these symptoms become more noticeable and pronounced in the fourth and fifth decade of their lives [4].

Functional diagnostics seems to be a standard requirement in modern dentistry but is by no means routinely applied. The masticatory organ is an extremely complex system of structural and functional connections, diagnostics is frequently neglected when dealing with its manifold disorders, while invasive therapy in the oral cavity is carried out without being based on solid diagnostic foundations. One reason for this is probably the fact that there is no unified scientific opinion regarding diagnostic methods. The diversity of opinion causes practising dentists to feel uncertain and even to be frightened away from utilizing systematic functional diagnostics in their daily practice. Without a diagnosis, any invasive therapy is hazardous. Searching for the causality of functional disorders requires systematic methods that can be adapted to the demands of the individual. The decision for therapy must be based on the foundation formed by a diagnosis. [5].

14.2 Diagnostic Process

The diagnostic process is the collection of records to find a diagnosis, and the consequence of the diagnosis is usually therapy. After the initial diagnosis, the patient's chief complaint should be discussed in detail. Exceptions to this rule are of course emergencies, which require immediate treatment. The patient's medical records and the information about the aspects of the talk should be obtained personally by the dentist. Particularly in cases of patients with functional disorders, this personal talk creates an atmosphere of trust which will be very useful during therapy. The occlusal index may be used as a tool to express the patient's subjective symptomatic condition, and this occlusal index is an organ-specific criterion of the patient's subjective functional condition [6, 7].

14.3 Systematic Analysis

Systematic analysis involves the following steps:

- The personal conversation.
- The small functional analysis (Fig. 14.1).
  - Clinical functional analysis.
  - Instrumental functional analysis.
- The large functional analysis (Fig. 14.2).
  - Clinical functional analysis.
  - Instrumental functional analysis.
  - Advanced radiological assessment.

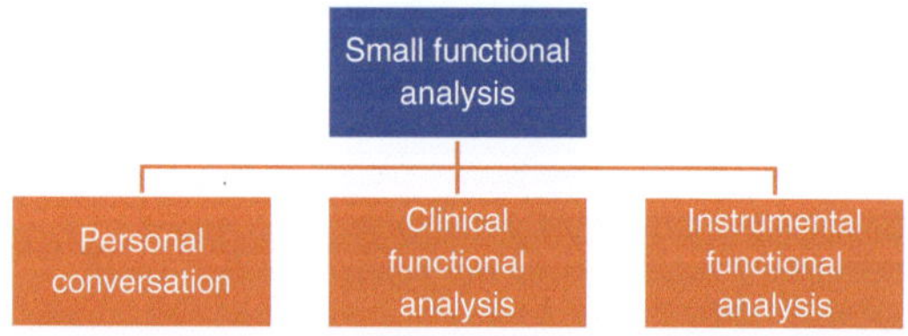

Fig. 14.1 Components of small functional analysis

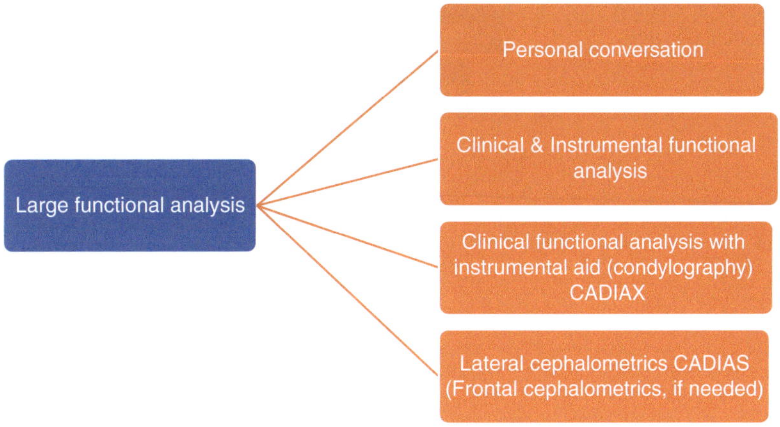

Fig. 14.2 Components of large functional analysis

14.3.1 Personal Conversation

Patients want to be listened to and understood. It sounds simple, but only the very best of doctors ever fully attain that goal in treating these patients. Patients expect professional competence. They expect the treating doctor to be a scholar and knowledgeable about all the recent innovations in the field of study. Patients want to be kept informed. When there is no one else to refer to, and the patient is on the verge of addiction to pain medication, the *caring* role of the doctor becomes larger than the *curing* role.

A screening history is to identify the subclinical signs and symptoms that the patient may not relate to. This may include a series of questionnaires [8].

14.3.2 Clinical Functional Analysis (Fig. 14.3)

14.3.2.1 Step 1. Muscle Palpation

The primary driving force behind all bodily movements is provided by muscles, which contract to cause movement of the affected body part [9]. The needs of mandibular function are met by numerous head and neck muscles through a complicated interplay of the different muscle groups. The prime movers are four pairs of muscles together known as muscles of mastication. They are as follows:

- The medial (inferior) pterygoid.
- The masseter.
- The lateral (superior) pterygoid.
- The temporalis.

The muscle palpation should be carried out simultaneously, uniformly, and symmetrically. This initial palpation confirms which side is more sensitive to pain and pressure. In addition, the patient may inform the examiner of instances of pain during palpation. Palpation includes the functional groups of the true masticatory muscles, the floor of the mouth and the tongue, the cervical and shoulder musculature, cranial and facial muscles, and manual examination of the cranio-mandibular system.

To determine muscle tenderness, digital palpation is the most widely accepted method.

The middle finger's palmar surface is primarily used for muscle palpation, with the forefinger and index finger used for checking the surrounding areas. The targeted muscles are compressed with gentle yet strong pressure in a tiny circular motion with the fingers. Preferably a single strong thrust lasting one or two seconds is given. Confirming the patient if it hurts or is just uncomfortable during palpation. The level of discomfort must be determined and noted for the muscle evaluation to be most beneficial. On palpation, the patient's response can be categorized as follows:

0—No pain or tenderness on palpation.

1—Slight discomfort on palpation (tenderness or soreness).

Fig. 14.3 Clinical functional analysis

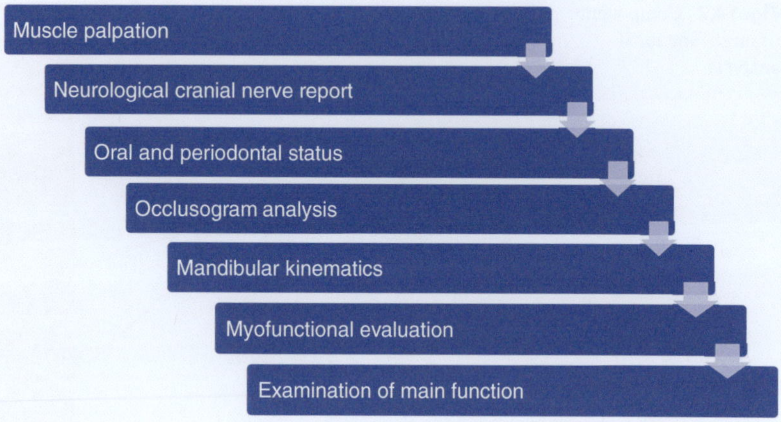

2—Definite discomfort or pain.

3—Eye tearing or patient deny for palpation again.

Each muscle's level of tenderness or pain is noted on an examination form. The myofascial pain trigger points that are hypersensitive should also be found during a complete muscle assessment. The examiner palpates each muscle's complete body to find trigger points. In a muscle having trigger points, generalized muscle discomfort might not exist. While recording examination findings, it is important to distinguish between trigger point pain and generalized muscle pain as the diagnosis and treatment for both is completely different. When trigger points are identified, an effort should be made to identify any pain referral patterns. After 4 to 5 seconds of pressure on the trigger point, the patient is questioned about if they feel any pain radiating from the area. On the examination form, the areas are noted. Certain pain problems can frequently be recognized and diagnosed using the pattern of transferred pain [10]. Once trigger points are identified, it is important to investigate whether there is a consistent pattern of pain referral associated with them. For 3 to 4 seconds, pressure is applied to the trigger point, and the patient is asked if he feels pain radiating in any direction, the following areas are noted on the examination sheet [10].

The sensitivity to muscle palpation is a very important part of the diagnostic protocol and helps us to locate the exact area of concern which includes the following

- The shoulder and neck region.
- Temporalis (anterior, middle, and posterior part).
- Lateral pterygoid muscles (helps in anterior repositioning if needed).
- Medial pterygoids (helps in transversal repositioning if needed).
- Masseter deep and superficial heads (as each head has its muscle vector).
- Digastricus (anterior and posterior belly of the muscle).
- Suprahyoid and infrahyoid group of muscles.
- Sternocleidomastoid (palpation at insertion and its origin and on both heads).
- Omohyoid muscle, has to be palpated with slightly more force as compared to other intra-oral structures.

14.3.2.2 Step 2. Slavicek Diagnostic Sheet (Fig. 14.4)

The diagnostic sheet allows us to understand the complexity of the patient. If the occlusal index is high, then we need pre-therapy which can be physiotherapy, postural management, or CMR therapy before planning for any kind of definitive treatment plan [11, 12] (Fig. 14.4).

14.3.2.3 Step 3. Occlusal Analysis (Fig. 14.5)

The occlusal factors' etiologic contribution is arguably the most debated. Occlusal influences should, like all other components, be viewed as one of several contributing reasons rather than as the only cause. [12–14] The severity of the

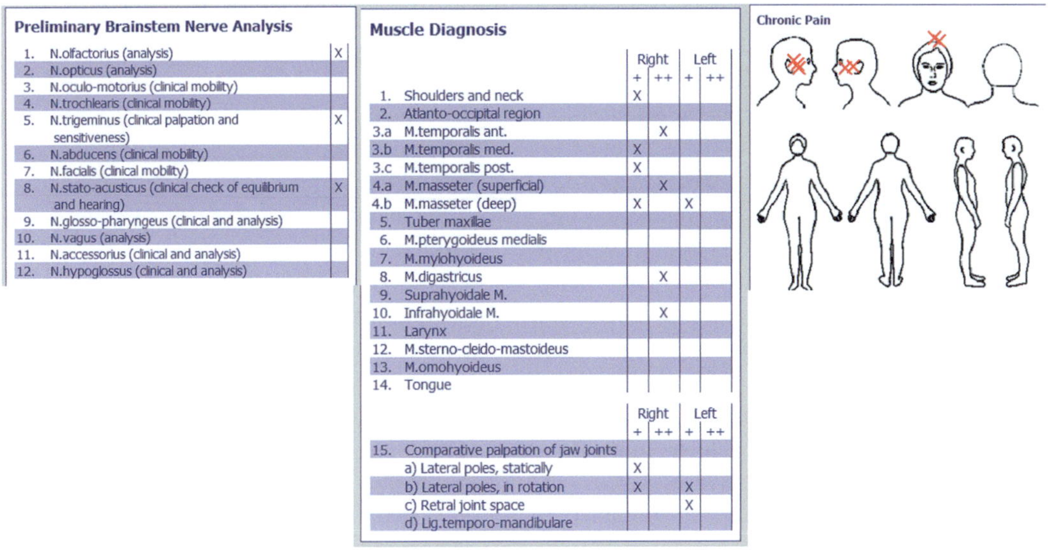

Preliminary Brainstem Nerve Analysis

1.	N.olfactorius (analysis)	X
2.	N.opticus (analysis)	
3.	N.oculo-motorius (clinical mobility)	
4.	N.trochlearis (clinical mobility)	
5.	N.trigeminus (clinical palpation and sensitiveness)	X
6.	N.abducens (clinical mobility)	
7.	N.facialis (clinical mobility)	
8.	N.stato-acusticus (clinical check of equilibrium and hearing)	X
9.	N.glosso-pharyngeus (clinical and analysis)	
10.	N.vagus (analysis)	
11.	N.accessorius (clinical and analysis)	
12.	N.hypoglossus (clinical and analysis)	

Muscle Diagnosis

		Right		Left	
		+	++	+	++
1.	Shoulders and neck	X			
2.	Atlanto-occipital region				
3.a	M.temporalis ant.		X		
3.b	M.temporalis med.	X			
3.c	M.temporalis post.	X			
4.a	M.masseter (superficial)		X		
4.b	M.masseter (deep)	X		X	
5.	Tuber maxillae				
6.	M.pterygoideus medialis				
7.	M.mylohyoideus				
8.	M.digastricus		X		
9.	Suprahyoidale M.				
10.	Infrahyoidale M.		X		
11.	Larynx				
12.	M.sterno-cleido-mastoideus				
13.	M.omohyoideus				
14.	Tongue				

		Right		Left	
		+	++	+	++
15.	Comparative palpation of jaw joints				
	a) Lateral poles, statically	X			
	b) Lateral poles, in rotation	X		X	
	c) Retral joint space			X	
	d) Lig.temporo-mandibulare				

Fig. 14.4 Slavicek diagnostic sheets (Slavicek et al. 2002) [12]

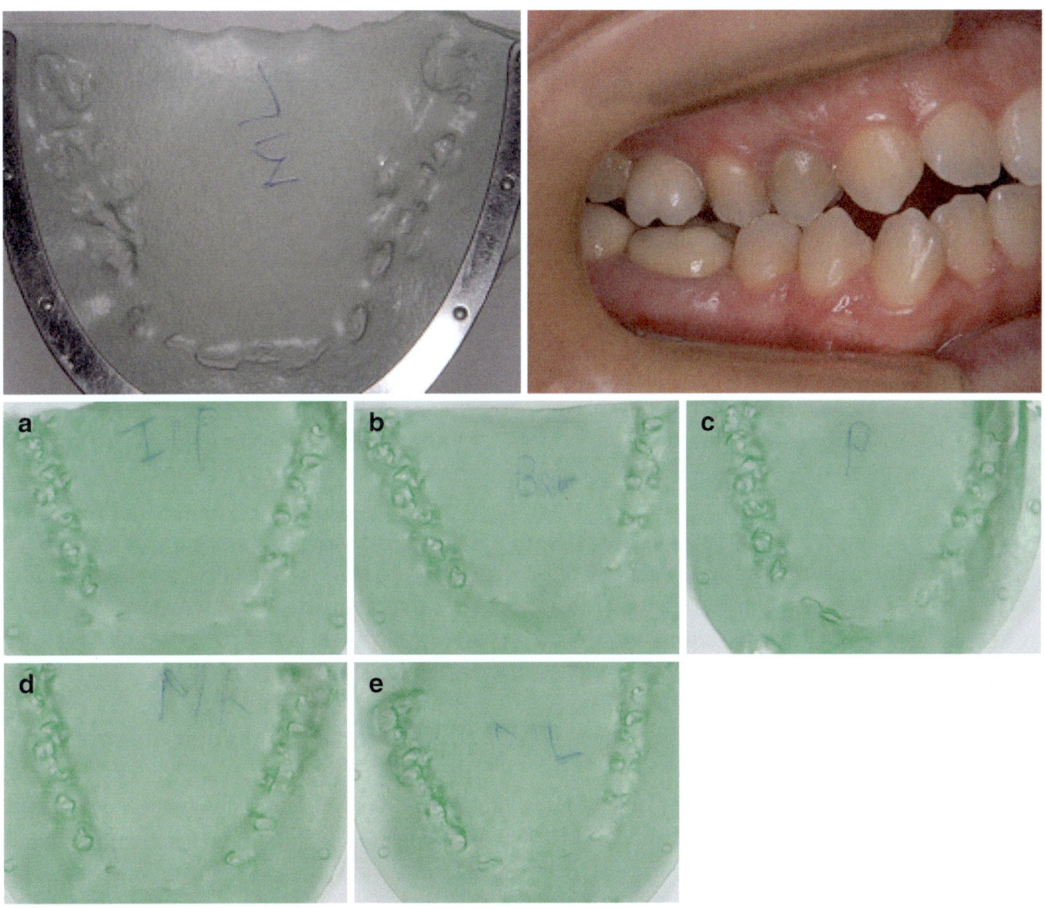

Fig. 14.5 Occlusogram wax with 0.3–0.4 mm of thickness, (**a**) ICP intercuspal position (**b**) ICP bruxing (**c**) ICP protrusion (**d**) ICP mediotrusion right (**e**) ICP mediotrusion left

dysfunction does not appear to be well predicted by the level of occlusal disharmonies. Another factor that has seldom been studied is the varying individual capacity of adaptation to occlusal disharmony. The first occlusal contact must be stable and take place simultaneously on as many teeth as possible. To effect a complete closure, the teeth must be squeezed after contact without causing any visible movement of the jaw. This is only possible if the teeth surfaces are in harmony with the instructions of the correctly placed condyles.

All conceivable mandibular positions and motions, including centric relation, intercuspal position, left and right laterotrusive movements, and protrusive movement, are investigated to confirm the contact pattern of occluding teeth. The occlusal contacts on the teeth can be found using a variety of methods. It is good practice to confirm by marking the contacts with wax or articulating paper. Occlusogram wax is 0.3 mm thick wax that can be used chairside and within minutes the clinician can see the occlusal interferences through the wax impressions and tears in the wax sheet.

For the ICP, we have to check for good occlusal support without possible anterior contacts, and for each movement, we have to look for possible interference either in mediotrusive or in the laterotrusive side, either there is good canine control or group function, etc.

The occlusal anatomy of the teeth controls the moves of the mandible's superior eccentric border. For the majority of patients, the mandible is guided or influenced by the anterior teeth during eccentric movements. The qualities of the guidance are carefully examined. The anterior teeth frequently give the rest of the dentition rapid instruction when they occlude during an eccentric mandibular movement. During the examination, the anterior guidance should be assessed for its efficacy in disoccluding the posterior teeth during eccentric movements.

The different movements are performed, and for each movement, a new sheet has to be used.

- *ICP Intercuspal Position*—After locating the musculoskeletally stable position, the mandible is closed to evaluate intercuspal occlusion.
- *ICP Protrusion*—The patient is instructed to slide the mandible forward from the intercuspal position till the mandibular anterior teeth have passed completely over the incisal edges of the maxillary anterior teeth or a distance of 6 to 8 mm.
- *ICP Laterotrusion*—The patient is instructed to move the mandible sideways until the canines pass beyond end-to-end relation or 6 to 10 mm, whichever comes first (i.e., canine guidance, group function).
- *ICP Mediotrusion*—When the mandible moves in a lateral direction, the neuromuscular system perceives, mediotrusive contacts as damaging, and reflex movement starts that attempts to disengage the teeth [15].

Brux Checker (Fig. 14.6)

According to Prof. Sato, atlas occlusion diagnosis by Brux Checker, Kanagawa dental college, and Research Institute of Occlusion Medicine, Kanagawa Japan [16],

- Brux Checker foils are single-sided color-coated.
- Foils are helpful for analysis and therapy planning.
- Foils are helpful for the diagnosis and treatment planning in the CMD therapy.
- For adjusting the occlusion in prosthetic restorations, occlusal interferences, e.g., bruxism, are registered by the attrition of the color-coating.
- In the analysis of the occlusal contact by Brux Checker, it is crucial to see the relation between mediotrusion and guidance.
- It can be made easily in a dental operatory with a dental vacuum machine.

14.3.2.4 Step 4. Mandibular Kinematics

The mandibular kinematics can be easily done on the dental routine dental chair; the goal of this measurement is to quantify the amount of natural mandibular movement and can be compared with manipulative or guided mandibular movement with the help of a simple ruler [17].

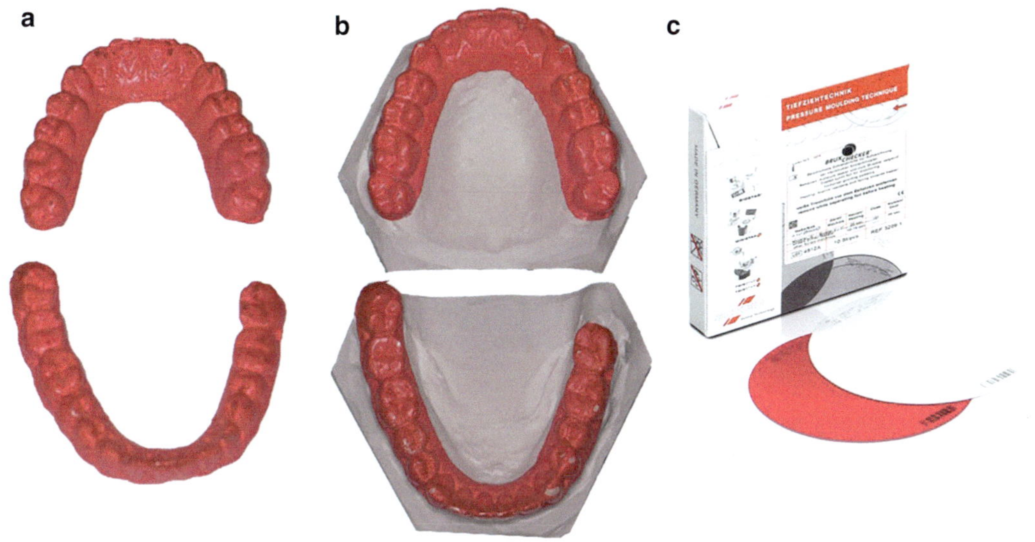

Fig. 14.6 The Brux Checker. (**a** and **b**) The fading of the red ink in the areas of contact during bruxism will determine the type of grinding pattern. (**c**) Brux Checker foils (0.1 mm). Sheets can be adjusted on the model using vacuum pressed machine (Sheu dental)

The movements measured are as follows:

- Maximum-Opening. The normal interincisal opening is between 53–58 mm. During function movement, symptoms are often accentuated hence leading to the assumption of restricted mouth movement. The patient is asked to open slowly until they experience pain. The distance between the incisal margins of the mandibular and maxillary anterior teeth is then measured. The most comfortable opening is this one. Next, the patient is instructed to fully open their mouth. It is noted that this is the largest opening. The maximum pleasant opening and the maximum opening are equivalent when there is no pain.
- Maximum-Protrusion.
- Maximum Mediotrusion Right.
- Maximum Mediotrusion Left.

14.3.2.5 Step 5. Myofunctional Evaluation

Myofunctional evaluation can be done by both quantitative and qualitative assessment. Evaluation involves checking for pattern of chewing and swallowing and basic tongue, lip, and jaw movement [18].

14.3.2.6 Step 6. Examination of Oral Function

Oral function examination involves speech assessment, swallowing, and chewing, details of which are beyond the scope of this chapter.

14.3.3 Instrumental Functional Analysis (Fig. 14.7)

Instrumental functional analysis is a term used in dentistry to describe examination techniques used to acquire a qualitative or quantitative assessment of the craniomandibular system's functional capacity using specialized tools and equipment. This instrumental functional analysis focuses on different aspects, especially the following:

- Kinematic aspects of the mandible—recording and analysis of mandibular movements (instrumental movement analysis) for articu-

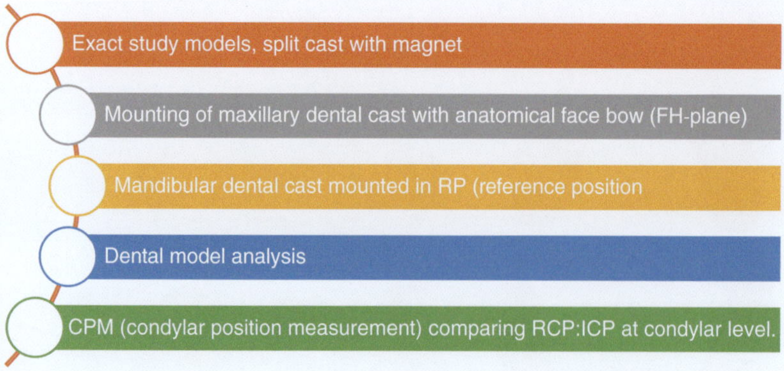

Fig. 14.7 Instrumental functional analysis

lator programming and/or for assessment of the functional capacity of the craniomandibular system.

- Position of the condyles.
- Jaw relation (horizontal jaw relation recording) which can be registered with a mounted kinematic face bow.
- Activity of the jaw muscles during various postures and movements of the mandible during complex tasks such as chewing (electromyographic (EMG) activity of the masticatory muscles).

According to the German Society of Craniomandibular Function and Disorders, the Dental Instrumental Functional Analysis is divided into four parts: [19].

Part 1: Instrumental Movement Analysis.

Part 2: Condylar Position Analysis.

Part 3: Jaw Relation Recording.

Part 4: Surface Electromyography of the Masticatory Muscles.

The instrumental functional analysis includes the following:

1. Exact dental models, split cast, double pin in lower arch with split cast.
2. Hinge-axis location, condylography procedure.
3. Mounting of the maxillary dental cast with kinematic facebow (AO-plane).
4. Lower model mounting in RP.
5. Model analysis.
6. Programming articulator to individual values coming from patient's condylography.
7. Cephalometrics (frontal and lateral).

14.3.3.1 Step 1. Exact Study Cast with Slit Cast and Magnet

Stone casts poured from the patient's impression are mounted on the articulator using split cast mounting. The maxillary cast is divided horizontally into two halves generally, thereby making it easier to remove and replace the cast and allowing for mounting's accuracy check. The split cast technique offers the advantage of addressing the occlusion changes brought on by the processing method [20].

14.3.3.2 Step 2. Hinge-Axis Location and Kinematic Aspects of the Mandible

The method of recording graphically the movements of mandibular condyles in living subjects was first described in 1902 [21].

Diverse registration systems exist for recording mandibular movement, based on the following measurement principles:

1. Electromechanic.
2. Optoelectronic.
3. Ultrasound.
4. Magnetic [22].

The principle of electronic, three-dimensional measurement of mandibular movements dates back to 1985. They were the first to be able to eliminate the disadvantages of the mechanical axiography/condylography measuring system by using electronic aids (substituting a high-resolution electronic stylus for the mechanical analogue metering clockwork and replacing the registration etiquette with resistance foil) [23].

The advantages of this electronic procedure, in comparison with conventional mechanical registration systems, are summarized as follows:

- Measurement of dynamics can be viewed directly on a computer screen.
- Three-dimensional, (Times-curves) possibilities in sagittal, frontal, or horizontal projections and clicking of TMJ can verified.
- Display of space-time movement of the hinge axis.
- Calculation of speed progression.
- Possibility of programming conventional articulators (Reference SL, Girbach, SAM, Artex CR, and many more which can be chosen from Gammadental software).
- Possibility of further processing the data for documentation purposes or for statistical evaluation and research purposes.

The simultaneous, real-time and three-dimensional registrations of the movements of both condyles is a major advantage of computer-supported condylography systems [24].

14.3.3.3 Applications of Condylography Procedure

- For articulator programming.
- For determining deviations between the centric jaw relation and maximal intercuspation.
- For diagnosis of discus position in reciprocal clicking.
- For diagnosis of clinically undetected disorders of the articular movement sequence, e.g., "muscular incoordination," "loose ligaments," etc.)
- For documentation of functional data.
- To collect measurement values for functional geometric examinations.
- To determine mandibular mobility near the condyles.

Using electronic condylography is especially indicated, if further diagnostic possibilities are called for, perhaps within the scope of an ongoing therapy for a dysfunctional patient. It is emphasized that condylography is not to be used alone, but should be utilized as a diagnostic detail within an overall diagnostic working procedure [25].

Additional research demonstrated that noninvasive methods are of great importance for the diagnosis of functional disturbances of the stomatognathic system. A comparison of computerized condylography with magnetic resonance imaging in the diagnosis of TMD was in accord in 70% of the patient groups of disk displacement with reduction and disk displacement without reduction. MRI can detect a large number of morphological alterations where the condylography produces no results. However, condylography is a better option for determining the dysfunctional dynamic [25, 26].

For an improved understanding of the functional disturbances of the stomatognathic system, a combination of both methods seems appropriate.

14.3.3.4 Step 3. Dental Casts Mountings (Fig. 14.8)

Dental cast mounting involves mounting the maxillary cast with the help of either anatomical facebow or kinematic facebow and mandibular cast mounting at the reference position.

1. Mounting with Anatomical Facebow.

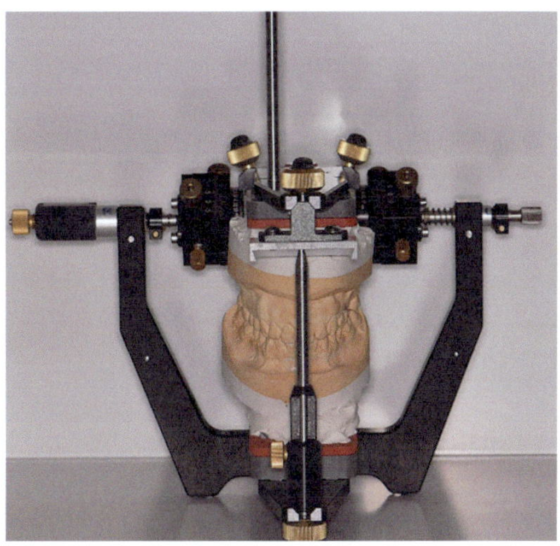

Fig. 14.8 SL articulator (Gamma Dental, Austria)

After initial consultation, it is easily determined if the patient is a routine case with simple orthodontics or just to change a single unit crown or initial diagnosis. Then, the maxillary split cast models are mounted with anatomic facebow in Frankfurt horizontal plane, and the mandibular dental cast is mounted in reference position (RP) or centric relation.

2. Mounting with Kinematic Facebow (Fig. 14.9).

   The kinematic facebow is recommended in slightly complex cases; the maxillary cast is mounted with a kinematic facebow in the axis-orbital plane with a hinge axis.

14.3.3.5 Step 4. Mandibular Cast Mountings

The mandibular cast is articulated either on a reference SL articulator or in CPV (condylar position variation depending on the complexity of the patient).

14.3.3.6 Step 5. Model Analysis (Fig. 14.10)

On mounted casts, the difference between the two positions RP/ICP or CO/CR is measured at the condylar level with the help of CPM (condylar position measurements) device.

This step can be done either in the traditional way or CADIAS 3D software using static and dynamic occlusal protocols.

Dynamic Occlusal Analysis

3. Diagnostic equilibrium/Selective grinding protocol using pin model (Fig. 14.11).

   Using the selective grinding protocol, we can first see on dental models how much of the plaster we have to grind till there is an equilibrium in occlusion which is controlled by the incisal pin; this selective grinding procedure guides us if we should treat the patient by enameloplasty or by adding. However, this decision also depends on the internal situation of TMJ and disc assembly [27].

4. Digital occlusal selective grinding protocol using CADIAS 3D software [8] (Fig. 14.12).

   CADIAS 3D is a state-of-the-art software for virtual occlusion design and analysis. CADIAS 3D is a software module of Gamma Dental Software and available from version 8.0 and later. The software aims at supporting the clinical and diagnostic aspect of digital dentistry, which is widely neglected by typical dental CAD/CAM applications [28].

14.3.3.7 Step 6. Programming the Articulator with Condylography Protocol for Complex TMD Patients Based on the Vienna Concept [28–30] (Fig. 14.13)

Condylography with CADIAX 4 Gamma Dental, Austria. Initially the mechanical hinge-axis loca-

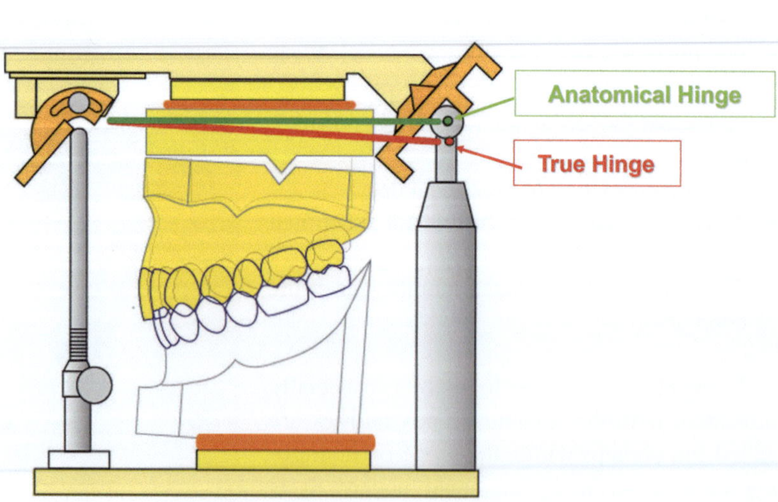

Fig. 14.9 Difference between the anatomic mounting and the mounting in the hinge axis (Image from Prof Sadao Sato/VieSID)

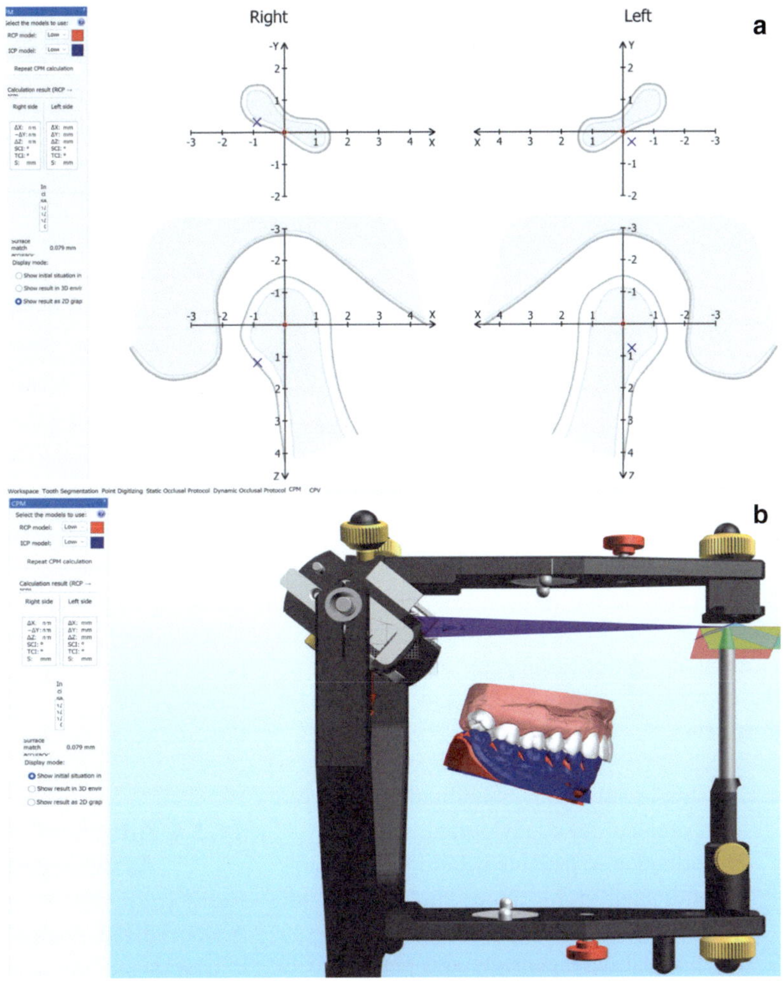

Fig. 14.10 Digital occlusion analysis to measure the discrepancy in two different positions at (**a**) condylar level and (**b**) occlusal level

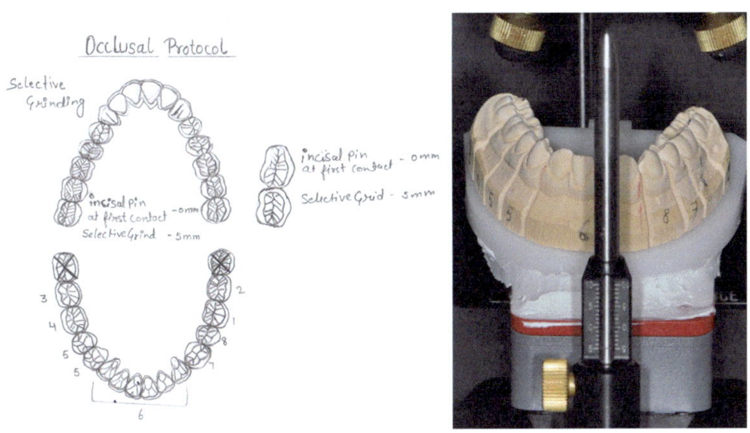

Fig. 14.11 (**a** and **b**) Schematic diagram showing diagnostic occlusal protocol for selective grinding using pin models and dental model equilibrium on articulator using incisal pin

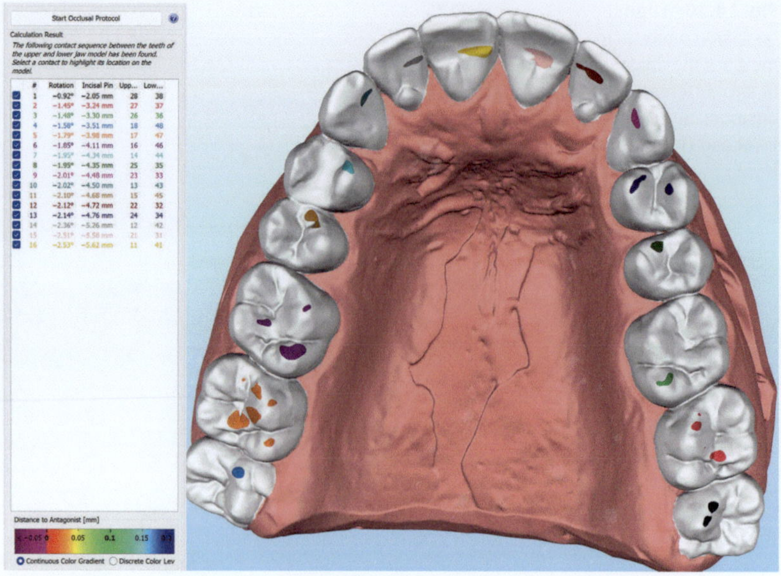

Fig. 14.12 Selective grinding: Virtual dynamic occlusal analysis using CADIAS 3D

tion is done followed by the electronic hinge-axis location and series of movements depending on the complexity of the patient and the need for treatment.

1. For simple full mouth rehabilitation, there is a short protocol for condylography.
2. For orthodontic patients needing orthodontic repositioning, few more movements are needed.
3. For internal derangements and patients with degenerative joint disease, there is a different condylography protocol.

14.3.3.8 Step 7. Cephalometrics (Lateral and Frontal)

Lateral cephalometric analysis Fig. 14.14 (Table 14.1).

The vertical and anteroposterior relationship between the maxillary and mandibular jaw, facial asymmetry, and sagittal skeletal traits can be studied using cephalometric analysis. The cephalogram can be recorded in several locations, such as centric occlusion, at rest, and first contact, to measure these parameters.

Frontal cephalometric analysis—Frontal cephalometrics is recommended for mandibular lateral displacement (MLD) cases. The amount of deviation from the midline can be assessed in posteroanterior cephalograms.

Chap. 11 provides an insight into the use of three-dimensional cephalometry.

14.3.4 Advanced Radiological Assessment

Advanced radiological assessment refers to the utilization of sophisticated imaging techniques, such as computed tomography (CT), magnetic resonance imaging (MRI), and cone-beam computed tomography (CBCT) to thoroughly evaluate tissue morphology and their spatial relationships more accurately [35].

CBCT provides detailed 3D images of the temporomandibular disorders, surrounding structures, and dental anatomy, which can be invaluable for diagnosing various TMJ disorders and planning appropriate treatment and has become the gold standard imaging modality for assessing degenerative bony changes of the condyle-disc complex, such as flattening, erosion, osteophytes, subchondral sclerosis, and subchondral cysts [36–39]. CBCT offers a great advantage of low radiation dose over CT [35]. MRI is a useful tool for evaluating discs and soft tissues with few con-

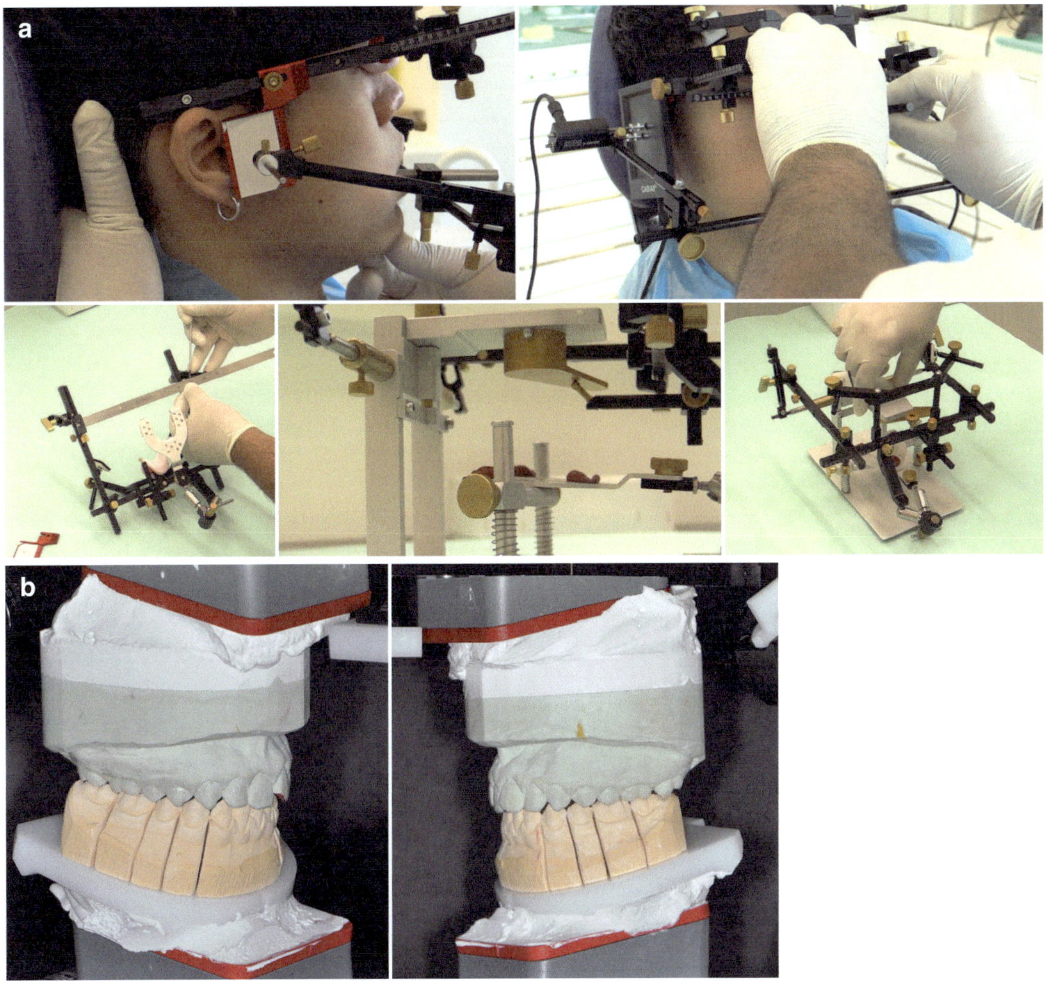

Fig. 14.13 (**a**) Condylography: facebow transfer (**b**) Mounting of models using kinematic face bow

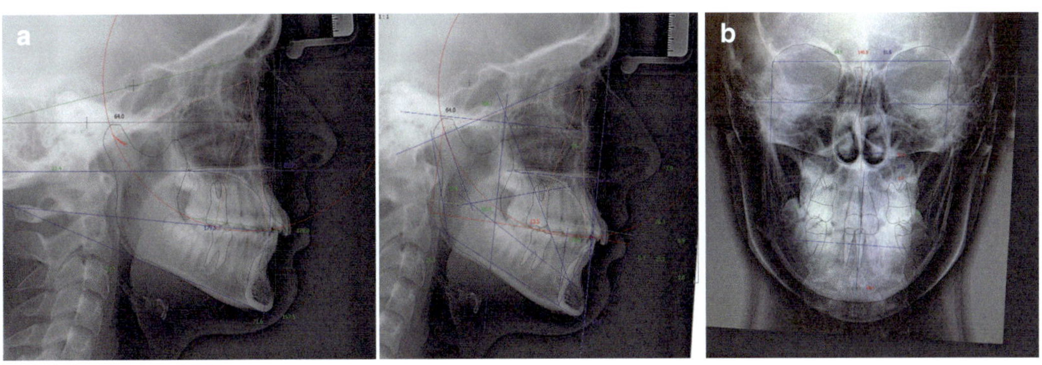

Fig. 14.14 Cephalometrics (**a**) Lateral (**b**) Frontal

Table 14.1 Cephalometric analysis used in the diagnostic process [31–34]

Sr. No.	*Parameter*	*Norm*
Sato analysis		
	Denture frame analysis	
1.	FH-MP	25.9^{0}
2.	PP-MP	24.6^{0}
3.	OP-MP	13.2^{0}
4.	OP-MP / PP-MP	54.0%
5.	AB-MP	71.3^{0}
6.	A'—P'	50.0 mm
7.	A'—6'	23.0 mm
8.	A' -6'/A'—P'	50.0%
9.	U1—AB (degree)	31.7^{0}
10.	U1—AB (mm)	9.5 mm
11.	L1—AB (degree)	25.4^{0}
12.	L1—AB (mm)	6.2 mm
13.	Inter molar angle	174^{0}
14.	FH—PP	1.3^{0}
	Upper occlusal plane	
1.	Mx—OP (A)	80.2^{0}
2.	Mx—OP (P)	76.6^{0}
3.	FH—OP (A)	7.7^{0}
4.	FH—OP (P)	11.3^{0}
Kim analysis		
1.	ODI	72^{0}
2.	APDI	81^{0}
3.	Combination factor	153.0^{0}
Rickett's analysis		
	Dental analysis	
1.	Molar relation right	1.5 mm
2.	Molar relation left	1.5 mm
3.	Molar width	54.0 mm
4.	Canine distance	27.5 mm
5.	Dental midline	0.0 mm
	Transversal analysis	
1.	Maxilla—mandible width right	10.0 mm
2.	Maxilla—mandible width left	10.00 mm
3.	Maxilla—mandible midth	0.0^{0}
4.	Molar—jaw relation right	9.5 mm
5.	Molar—Jaw relation left	9.5 mm
6.	Tooth—Jaw relation	0.0 mm
7.	Maxillary width	65.0 mm
8.	Mandibular width	86.0 mm
9.	Facial width	133.0 mm
	Symmetry	
1.	Postural symmetry	0.0^{0}

(continued)

Table 14.1 (continued)

	Atemwege, nasal	
1.	Nose width	33.0 mm
2.	Nose height	50.5 mm
	Occlusal plane	
1.	Occlusal plane shifting	0.0 mm
Slavicek analysis		
	Skeletal measurement	
1.	Facial axis	90.0^{0}
2.	Facial depth	89.0^{0}
3.	Mandibular plane	24.0^{0}
4.	Facial taper	68.0^{0}
5.	Mandibular arc	29.0^{0}
6.	Maxillary position	65.0^{0}
7.	Convexity	0.0 mm
8.	Lower facial height (by R. Slavicek)	45.2^{0}
9.	Lower facial height to point D	50.3^{0}
	Dental measurement	
1.	Interincisal angle	131.3^{0}
2.	Upper incisor protrusion	5.6 mm
3.	Upper incisor inclination	26.4^{0}
4.	Upper incisor vertical	Mm
5.	Lower incisor protrusion	0.9 mm
6.	Lower incisor inclination	22.3^{0}
7.	Upper molar position	18.0 mm
	Occlusal plane	
1.	Occlusal plane—Axis orbital plane (Slavicek)	--------^{0}
2.	Idealized occlusal plane—Axis orbital plane	--------^{0}
3.	Distance: Occlusal plane—Axis (DPO)	40.9 mm
4.	Radius of curve of Spee	-------mm
5.	Lip embrasure	0.0 mm
6.	Occlusal plane xi distance	−1.4 mm
	Functional measurement	
1.	Sagittal condylar inclination (right)	------^{0}
2.	Sagittal condylar inclination (left)	------^{0}
3.	Sagittal condylar inclination	------^{o}
4.	Relative condylar inclination	------^{0}
5.	Relative condylar inclination 6	------^{0}
6.	Relative condylar inclination 7	------^{0}
7.	Relative condylar inclination 8	0
8.	Anterior guidance (S—AOP)	0
9.	Relative anterior guidance	0
	Esthetic measurement (lip relation)	
1.	Esthetic plane	−2.3 mm

traindications in patients with pacemakers, or claustrophobia patients, which occurs in 1–15% of patients undergoing MRI [40, 41].

In the field of dentistry, MRI and CBCT are the most widely used diagnostic imaging techniques for the craniofacial complex. CBCT is optimum for viewing skeletal and dental tissues, whereas MRI is the standard for viewing masticatory muscles, ligaments, and the cartilaginous disc of TMJ. Due to differences in pixel voxel size, identification of anatomical structure, image orientation, and field of view (FOV), multimodality image registration between CBCT and MRI is challenging. However, for optimum diagnosis, treatment planning, and evaluation of treatment outcome, this registration is desirable.

14.3.4.1 Cone-Beam Computed Tomography (CBCT) of TMJ (Fig. 14.15)

CBCT examinations helps in determining the osseous changes of the condyle which eventually help in diagnosing the pathology [42]. This includes flattening of the condylar head, an osteophyte (marginal bony outgrowth), erosion (seen as an interruption or absence of the cortical lining), subchondral sclerosis (increased bone density including generalized sclerosis), subchondral cysts (round or oval-shaped osteolytic areas beneath the cortical bone), or combinations of two or more osseous changes.

CBCT is an important diagnostic aid for degenerative joint disease before treatment is recommended to know the amount of the destruction of condylar head and eminence. The goal of the treatment is to have positive remodeling of the condyle by unloading the joint [43]. Chap. 2 provides further insight into the use of CBCT in TMDs.

14.3.4.2 MRI Magnetic Resonance Imaging

MRI is the gold standard for confirming the internal derangements of TMJ. 3-Tesla MRI machine allows better visualization of the structures of TMJ as compared to 1.5 Tesla machine [44]. On MRI scans, joint effusion, disc configuration, and internal derangement can be assessed.

Disc configurations can be categorized as biconcave, flattened, folded, or convex when the MRI is recorded in the closed mouth position [45]. Internal derangements are classified as normal when the thin intermediate zone is stationed between the condyle and the articular eminence in the open-mouth position and the posterior band is situated above the apex of the condylar head in the closed-mouth position. Abnormal conditions and their descriptions are given below. MRI scans also help in diagnosing joint effusion cases and can be classified according to the T2 signal intensity in the joint space and the articular surface [46]. Chap. 3 gives a detailed explanation of the use of MRI for TMJ imaging.

Reducible Joint Luxation (Disc Displacement with Reduction) (Fig. 14.16)

Disc dislocation with reduction can be described as when the posterior border of the disc is thinned and the collateral ligament and superior retrodiscal lamina become elongated; the disc subsequently glides anteriorly through discal space. The disc is returned to normal position with condyle during jaw movements [47].

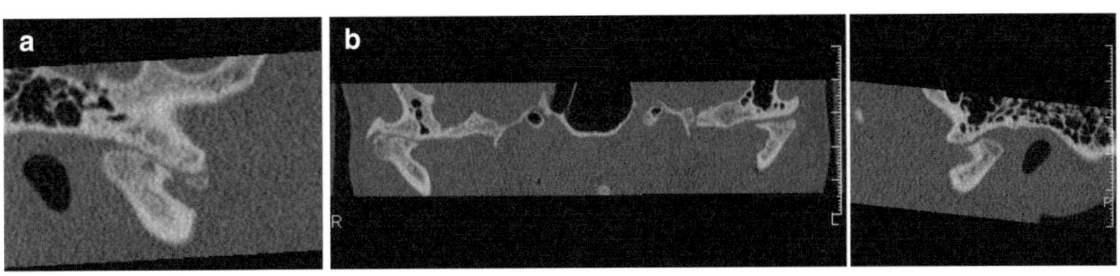

Fig. 14.15 CBCT showing the (**a**) right and (**b**) left arthritic joints in patients with degenerative joint disease

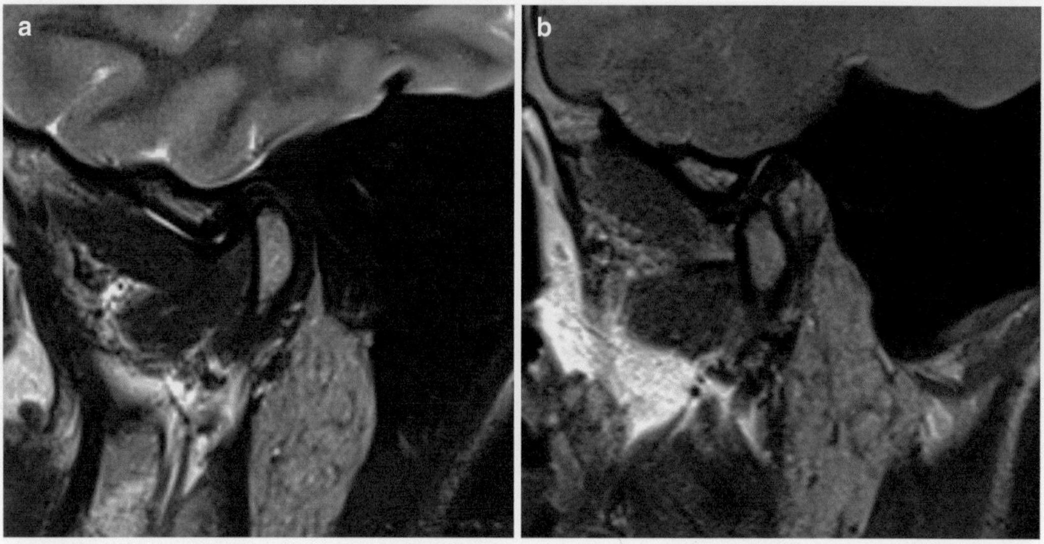

Fig. 14.16 MRI section showing reducible joint luxation (**a**) Closed mouth position (**b**) Open mouth position

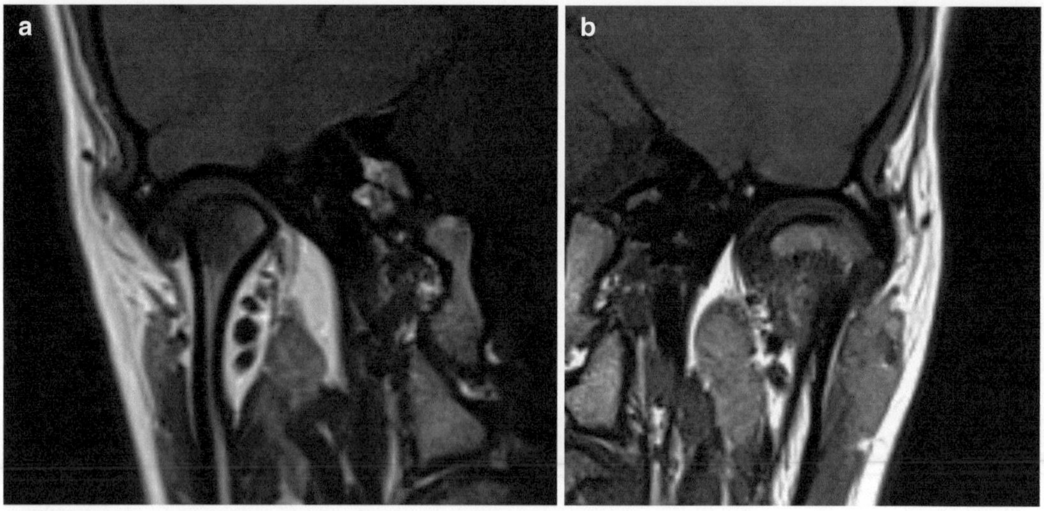

Fig. 14.17 MRI section showing transversal disc displacement (**a**) medial displacement (**b**) lateral displacement

Transversal Disc Displacement (Lateral and Medial Disc Displacement)(Fig. 14.17)

Lateral and medial disc displacement are two categories of sideway displacement of the disc without displacement of the anterior component. The same can be well appreciated in the coronal plane.

Non-reducible Joint Luxation (Fig. 14.18)

Patients experiencing frequent disc dislocations with reduction have chances of elongation of inferior retrodiscal lamina and the discal collateral ligaments in the future, with due course superior retrodiscal lamina loses its elasticity. If the condyle moves forward, then the disc does not return to its normal position [48].

Degenerative Joint Disease (DJD) (Fig. 14.19)

In high-resolution MRIs, the DJD can be seen, but CBCT is recommended if we see extreme

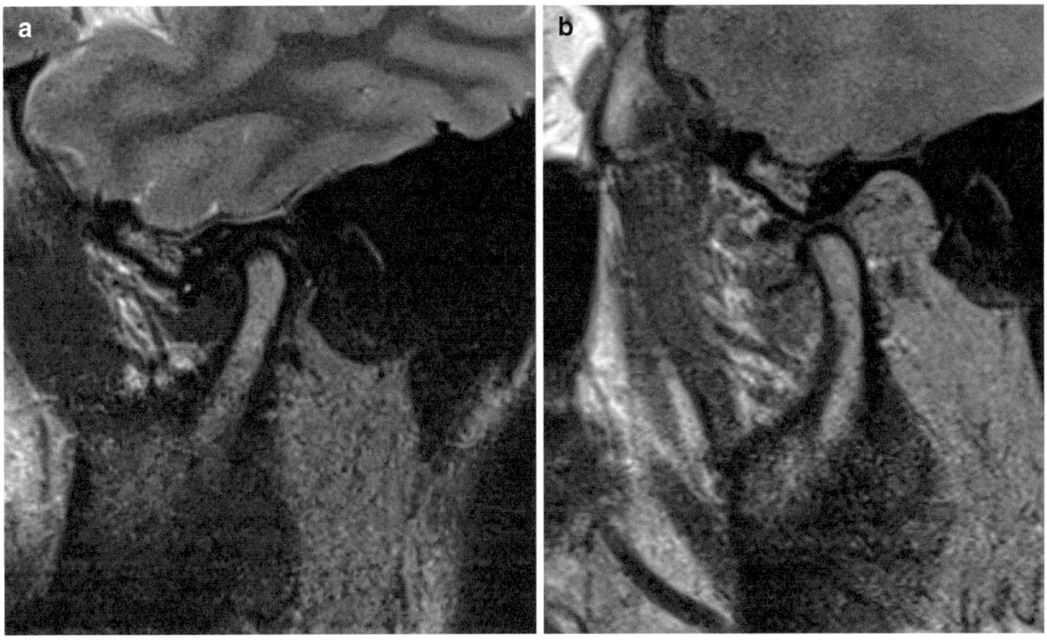

Fig. 14.18 MRI section showing non-reducible joint luxation (**a**) Closed mouth position (**b**) Open mouth position

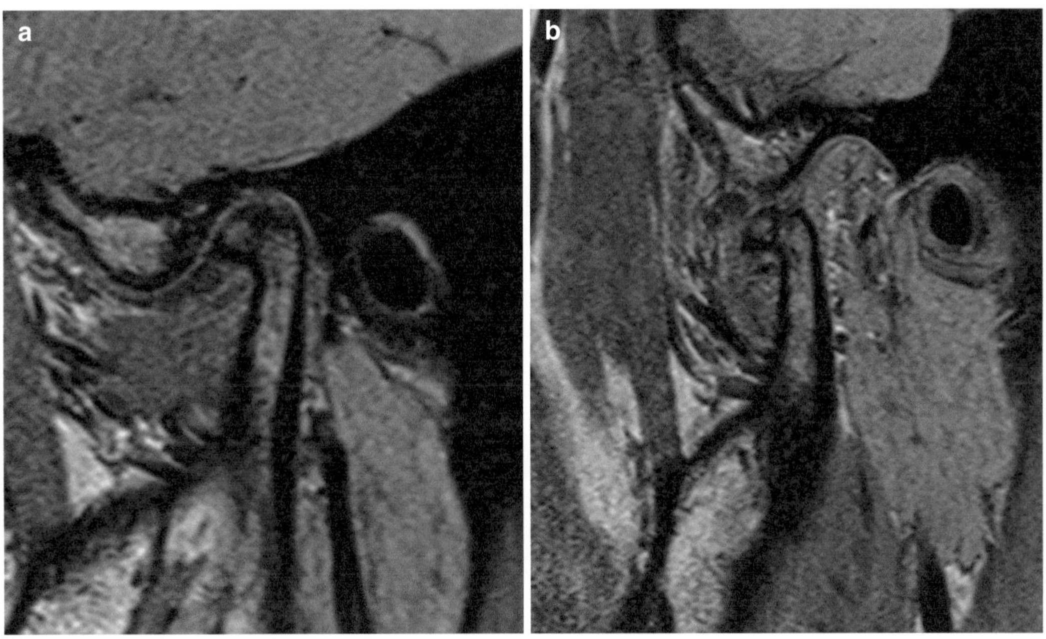

Fig. 14.19 MRI section showing degenerative joint disease (**a**) Closed mouth position (**b**) Open mouth position

flattening and irregular bony margins of condyles in panoramic X-rays, in MRIs, or in routine TMJ radiographs [49].

14.4 Final Diagnosis

At the end of all the diagnostics, we must come to a conclusion about which type of patient we are dealing with and how to begin with the treatment.

1. Simple patient not responding to neuromuscular treatment approach.
2. Patient with a tendency to internal derangement.
3. Patient with reducible joint luxation simple type only anterior disc displacement without transversal component.
4. Patient with reducible joint luxation anterior disc displacement with a transversal component with medial or lateral disc displacement.
5. Patient with acute non-reducible joint luxation.
6. Patient with chronic non-reducible joint luxation.
7. Patient with degenerative joint disease.
8. Patient needing treatment with an interdisciplinary treatment approach (physiotherapist, osteopath, sleep apnea or patients with postural problems, tinnitus, etc.)

This full functional diagnostic protocol will give us exact coordinates and the exact values of each individual for sagittal condylar inclinations (SCI), transverse condyle inclination (TCI), the Bennett angle, etc., and with the help of lateral cephalometric, we can plan the VDO vertical dimension of occlusion and do the repositioning orthodontically [50].

For the complex TMDs, we have to follow the method of controlled mandibular repositioning (CMR) which guides us to reposition the condyles against the articular disc if needed based on the condylography data and the sensitivity of the muscle palpation.

14.5 Treatment Modalities

14.5.1 Prosthodontics: Full Mouth Rehabilitation

Full mouth rehabilitation of patients typically requires intricate articulator settings and tabular form based on an individual patient. Patients practice instructed mandibular movements before actual condylography. The patient is instructed to perform all excursive movements at a specific time. The reference position is chosen when the mandible is in a maximally retrusive position from where lateral movements are possible without dental contacts and applied force. During the examination, all the movements of the mandible are observed by the operator and registered and assessed in the Gamma Dental Software.

The sagittal condylar inclination and the Bennett angle (Transversal condylar inclination) are anatomically driven values that cannot be changed, but the occlusal plane inclination and cusp inclinations can be changed according to the patient's needs which prevents unwanted interferences, muscle avoidance patterns, and the chippings of restorations, natural teeth, or ceramics. This concept allows us to plan a stable functional occlusion with the least possible interferences [51].

Here we see in the image the programming for condylar housing for Bennett inserts in white for TCI and yellow and white SCI inserts following the SCI path (Fig. 14.20). In the anterior part, we see the anterior teeth and posterior teeth sequential table from flat to steep (color coding); depending on SCI and TCI, we can select the inclinations (Fig. 14.21).

14.5.2 TMDs in Patients with and without Pain

Once the therapeutic position (ThP) has been estimated from the occlusal index and condylography curves, orthodontic repositioning can be achieved.

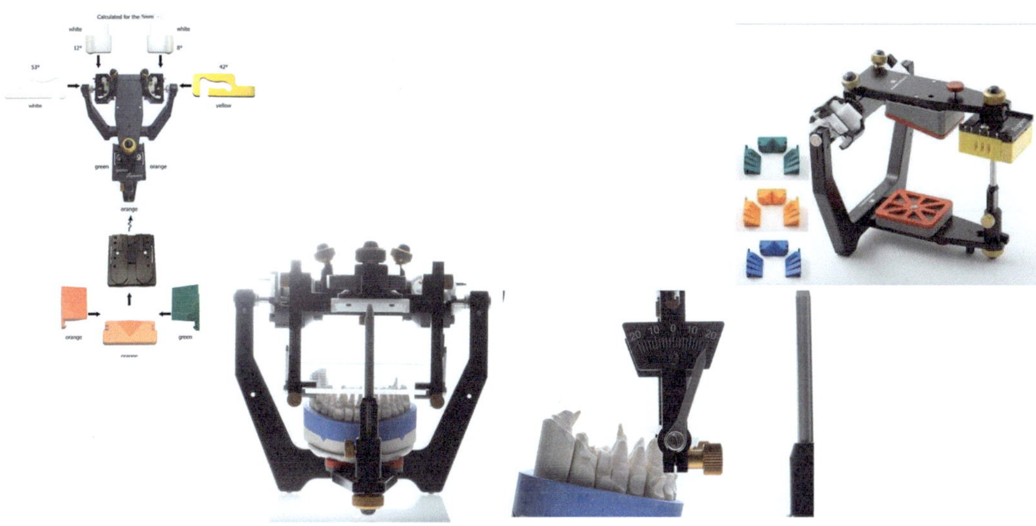

Fig. 14.20 Graphical form for articulator setting showing occlusal plane establishment with the help of occlusal table based on the condylar inclination of each side individually

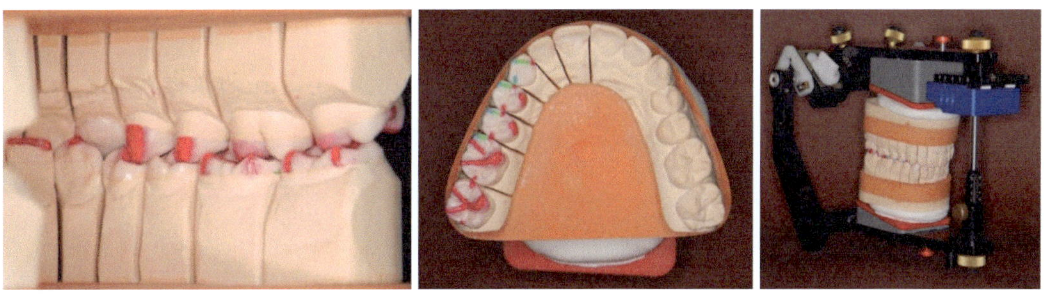

Fig. 14.21 Wax-up: Sequential wax-up concept

However, in the group of patients having pain with TMD, the goal is initially to relieve pain before going for orthodontic treatment. Graphical overlays can be established in calculated ThP, and later the orthodontic treatment can be initiated.

14.5.3 Complex TMDs (with Internal Derangement or DJD and Pain)

After diagnosis, the mandibular cast is mounted at condylar position variation (CPV), and controlled mandibular repositioning (CMR) is required, based on Dr. Alain Landry's protocol (Fig. 14.22).

The controlled mandibular repositioning (CMR) concept of functional diagnosis is very effective in treating internal derangements [52].

The major advantage of this CMR method is that the joints can be treated individually depending upon the conditions of the TMJs. (For example, the above patient has muscular problem only on the right side, but on the left side, there is reducible joint luxation, both condylar housings are independently programmed) as measured by the patient's condylography (Fig. 14.23).

The coordinate values from the condylography data help us to calculate the therapeutic position from the movements done during the condylography procedure.

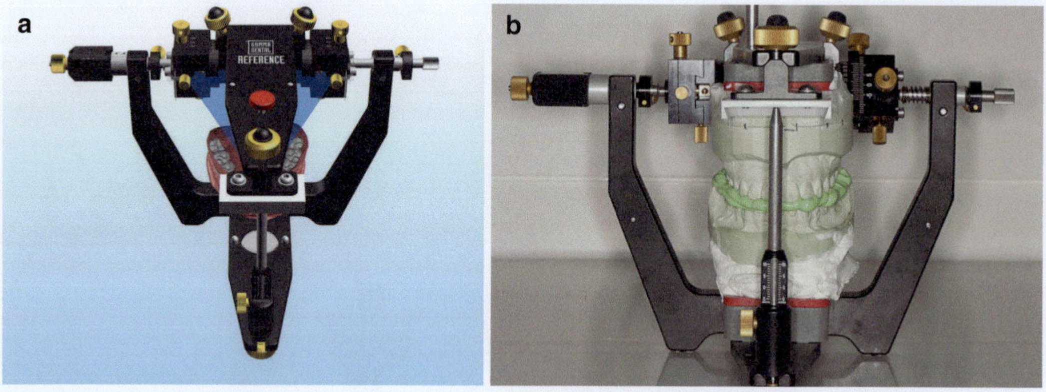

Fig. 14.22 (**a**) The virtual CPV, (**b**) analogue condylar position variator which is used to individually reposition the condylar housing independently of two joints

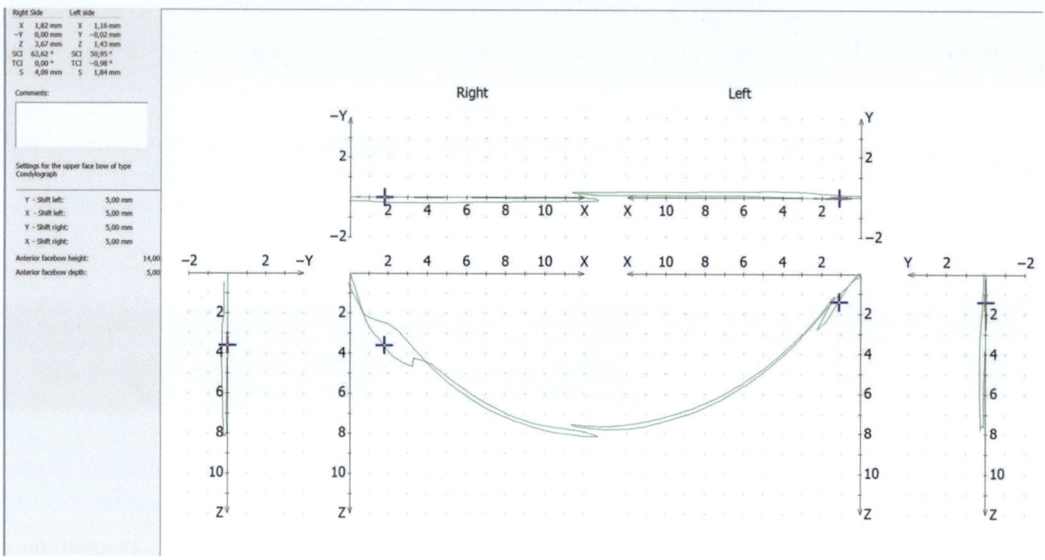

Fig. 14.23 Condylography tracing in open-close movement representing the luxation/cling during the movement for each joint, respectively, and which can be analyzed for individual joint

The condylography movement is as follows:

- Free and guided protrusion-retrusion, open-close, mediotrusion right, and mediotrusion left.
- Functional movements: Speech, bruxing, swallowing, and mastication.
- CPM: Condylar position measurements (fine measurements at condylar level).
- TIM, Tim 1, and Tim 2 for the ligaments and for the clicking/luxation in the joint.

14.6 Summary

Because of the dynamic relationship between head and neck posture, jaw position and dental occlusion, and its ultimate disturbance that is seen in TMJ dysfunction, headache, and head—and neck-related discomfort, it becomes necessary to provide an appropriate and comprehensive diagnosis to achieve treatment protocol for optimum results. In general Medicine and Dentistry, the right diagnosis is the key to the success of treatment. Depending on the complexity of the problem, one has to be flexible, and if needed, an interdisciplinary treatment approach may be required by referring the patient for psychological help or to an osteopath/physiotherapist.

The take-home message is we have to differentiate the type of patient as each group of patients has a different treatment approach, and therefore, we cannot treat all TMDs with a universal treatment protocol.

Acknowledgments This chapter is dedicated to our mentors in the journey of occlusion medicine from whom we can learn and teach this concept worldwide. We are grateful to our mentors Prof Rudolf Slavicek for the basic functional diagnostic part, Prof Sadao Sato for the treatment of complex TMDs with Craniofacial Orthodontics, Prof Rausch Fan for complex Ortho-Perio patients, Prof Eva Piehslinger for complex Prosthodontics, FMR patients, Dr. Alain Landry founder of CMR for treating all types of TMDs with a conservative approach, and Gamma Dental, Klosterneuburg, Austria, for playing a key role in functional diagnosis.

References

1. Sicher H. Zur Mechanik des Kiefergelenkes Stomatol. 1929;27:27–33.
2. Sicher H. Functional anatomy of the temporomandibular articulation. Austral J Dent Apr–Oct. 1951;55:73–85.
3. Ronald. Intraoral orthotic therapy. Dent Clin N Am. 1997;41(2):309–24.
4. McNeill C. Management of temporomandibular disorders: concepts and controversies. J Prosthet Dent. 1997;77(5):510–22.
5. Dawson PE. Evaluation, diagnosis, and treatment of occlusal problems. 2nd ed. Saint Louis: Mosby; 1989.
6. Litvak H, Malament KA. Prosthodontic management of temporomandibular disorder and orofacial pain. J Prosthet Dent. 1993;69:77–84.
7. Eversole LR, Machado L. Temporomandibular joint internal derangement and associated neuromuscular disorder. J Am Dent Assoc. 1985;110:69–79.
8. Patil N. Myofascial pain dysfunction syndrome. J Ind Prosthodont Soc. 2001;11:30–5.
9. Sicher H. Functional anatomy of the temporomandibular joint. In: Sarnat BC, editor. The temporomandibular joint. 2nd ed. Springfield; 1964. p. 28–58.
10. Shaber EP. Skeletal muscle: anatomy, physiology, pathophysiology. Dent Clin N Am. 1983;l27(3):435–42.
11. Wilkinson. The relationship between the disc and the lateral pterygoid muscle in the human TMJ. J Prosthet Dent. 1988;l60(6):715–24.
12. Slaviček M, Slavicek R, Fonograficzna "Gamma" F. The Masticatory Organ: Functions and Dysfunctions. GAMMA Medizinisch-wissenschaftliche Fortbildung-AG; 2002.
13. Ash MM, Ramfjord SP. Occlusion. 4th ed. Philadelphia: W.B. Saunders; 1995.
14. Jerolimov V. Association of horizontal and vertical overlap with prevalence of temporomandibular disorder. J Oral Rehab. 2002;29:588.
15. Alanen P. Occlusion and temporomandibular disorders (TMD): still unsolved question? J Dent Res. 2002;81(8):518–9.
16. Okeson JP. Management of temporomandibular disorder and occlusion. 4th ed. Missouri: Mosby; 1998.
17. Greven M, Ondera K, Sato S. The use of the BruxChecker in the evaluation and treatment of bruxism. J Craniomandib Func. 2015;7(3):34–5.
18. Dworkin. TMD and chronic pain; disease or illness? J Prosthet Dent. 1994;72:29–38.
19. Solberg WK. Temporomandibular disorders: data collection and examination. British Dent J. 1986;160:317.
20. Weinberg LA. Correlations of temporomandibular dysfunction with radiographic findings. J Prost Dent. 1972;28:519.
21. Nogueira SS, Russi S, Compagnoni MA, de Assis MF. A variation on split-cast mounting for complete denture construction. The J Prosthet Dent. 2004;91:386–8.
22. Campion CG. A method of recording graphically the movements of the mandibular condyles in living subjects. Br Dent J. 1902;23(1):713–6.
23. Edinger DH, Rall K, Schroeter P. Adding dynamic occlusion tocomputer-aided tooth restoration. J Gnathol. 1995;14:7–12.
24. Gsellmann B, Schmid-Schwap M, Piehslinger E, Slavicek R. Lengths of condylar pathways measured with computerized axiography (CADIAX) and occlusal index in patients and volunteers. J Oral Rehabil. 1998;25(2):146–52.
25. Piehslinger E, Celar A, Celar R, Jager W, Slavicek R. Reproducibility of the condylar reference position. J Orofac Pain. 1993;7(1):68.
26. Crow HC, McCall WD Jr, Mohl ND. Electronic technology for clinical prosthodontics. Curr Opin Dent. 1991 Apr;1(2):146–9.
27. Petrie CS, Woolsey GD, Williams K. Comparison of recordings obtained with computerized axiography and mechanical pantography at 2 time intervals. J Prosthodont. 2003;12(2):102–10.
28. Greven M. Comprehensive dental diagnosis and treatment planning for occlusal rehabilitation: a perspective. J Craniomandib Pract. 2016;9:215–7.
29. Celar AG, Tamaki K. Accuracy of recording horizontal condylar inclination and Bennett angle with the cadiax compact. J Oral Rehab. 2002;29:1076–81.
30. Clayton JA. A pantographic reproducibility index for use in diagnosing temporomandibular joint dysfunction: a report on research. J Prosthet Dent. 1985;54(6):827–31.

31. Ricketts MR, Roth HR, Chaconas JS, Schulhof JR, Engel AG. Orthodontic diagnosis and planning, Volume 1. Denver: Rocky Mountain, Data Systems; 1982. p. 42–143.
32. Celar AG, Freudenthaler J, Celar R, Jonke E, Schneider B. The denture frame analysis: an additional diagnostic tool. Eur J Orthod. 1998;20:579–87. https://doi.org/10.1093/ejo/20.5.579.
33. Kim YH, Caufield Z, Chung WN, Chang YI. Overbite depth indicator, anteroposterior dysplasia indicator, combination factor and extraction index. Int J MEAW. 1994;1(1):81–104.
34. Slavicek R, Sato S. Bruxism—a function of the masticatory organ to cope with stress [in German]. Wien Med Wochenschr. 2004;154:584–9.
35. Tamimi D, Kocasarac HD, Mardini S. Imaging of the temporomandibular joint. Semin Roentgenol. 2019;54:282–301. https://doi.org/10.1053/j.ro.2019.03.007.
36. Shetty US, Burde KN, Naikmasur VG, Sattur AP. Assessment of condylar changes in patients with temporomandibular joint pain using digital volumetric tomography. Radiol Res Pract. 2014;2014:106059. https://doi.org/10.1155/2014/106059.
37. Zain-Alabdeen EH, Alsadhan RI. A comparative study of accuracy of detection of surface osseous changes in the temporomandibular joint using multidetector CT and cone beam CT. Dentomaxillofac Radiol. 2012;41:185–91. https://doi.org/10.1259/dmfr/24985971.
38. dos Anjos Pontual ML, Freire JS, Barbosa JM, Frazao MA, dos Anjos PA. Evaluation of bone changes in the temporomandibular joint using cone beam CT. Dentomaxillofac Radiol. 2012;41:24–9. https://doi.org/10.1259/dmfr/17815139.
39. Alexiou K, Stamatakis HC, Tsiklakis K. Evaluation of the severity of temporomandibular joint osteoarthritic changes related to age using cone beam computed tomography. Dentomaxillofac Radiol. 2009;38:141–7. https://doi.org/10.1259/dmfr/59263880).
40. Tasaki MM, Westesson PL. Temporomandibular joint: diagnostic accuracy with sagittal and coronal MR imaging. Radiology. 1993;186:723–9. https://doi.org/10.1148/radiology.186.3.8430181.
41. Dill T. Contraindications to magnetic resonance imaging: non-invasive imaging. Heart. 2008;94:943–8. https://doi.org/10.1136/hrt.2007.125039.
42. Alexiou K, Stamatakis H, Tsiklakis K. Evaluation of the severity of temporomandibular joint osteoarthritic changes related to age using cone beam computed tomography. Dentomaxillofac Radiol. 2009;38:141–7. https://doi.org/10.1259/dmfr/59263880.
43. Dworkin SF. Le Resche research diagnostic criteria for temporomandibular disorders: review, criteria, examinations and specifications, critique. J Craniomandib Disord. 1992;6:301–55.
44. Hiltunen K, Peltola JS. A 5-year follow-up of signs and symptoms of TMD and radiographic findings in the elderly. Int J Prosthodont. 2003;16(6):631–5.
45. Arayasantiparb R, Tsuchimochi M, Mitrirattanakul S. Transformation of temporomandibular joint disc configuration in internal derangement patients using magnetic resonance imaging. Oral Sci Int. 2012;9:43–8. https://doi.org/10.1016/S1348-8643(12)00025-0.
46. Wänman A, Agerberg G. Mandibular dysfunction in adolescents. I. Prevalence of symptoms. Acta Odontol Scand. 1986;44:47–54. https://doi.org/10.3109/00016358609041297.
47. Parlett KPD, Tallents RH, Hatala MA. Temporomandibular joint axiography and MRI findings: a comparative study. J Prosth Dent. 1993;70(6):521–31.
48. Tognini. Comparison of ultrasonography and magnetic resonance imaging in the evaluation of temporomandibular joint disc displacement. J Oral Rehab. 2005;32(4):248.
49. Bertram SJ. Diagnosing TMJ internal derangement and osteoarthritis with magnetic resonance imaging. J Am Dent Assoc. 2001;132(6):753–61.
50. Barclay P, Hollender LG, Maravilla KR, Truelove EL. Comparison of clinical and magnetic resonance imaging diagnoses in patients with disk displacement in the temporomandibular joint. Oral Surg Oral Med Oral Pathol Oral Radiol Endod. 1999;88:37–43.
51. Sato S, Slavicek R. The masticatory organ and stress management. Intl J Stomat Occ Med. 2008;1:1–7.
52. Ecker GA, Goodacre CJ, Dykema RW. A comparison of condylar control settings obtained from wax interocclusal records and simplified mandibular motion analyzers. J Prosthet Dent. 1984;51(3):404–6.

Challenges for 3D Imaging for Craniofacial Applications

15

Payal Maken, Shailendra Singh Rana, Abhishek Gupta, and Harmeet Kaur

15.1 Introduction

Three-dimensional (3D) image analysis is performed for diagnosis and treatment planning. It replicates or describes the anatomic and physiological aspects precisely or displays the 2D (two-dimensional) or 3D anatomy accurately. 3D or 2D imaging is one of the most important tools of diagnosis for orthodontists and other specialties. It measures the size and evaluates the formation of craniofacial structures [1]. 2D imaging is frequently used for the visualization of craniofacial anatomy. However, 2D imaging does not give a detailed and localized structure [2]. Thus, 3D imaging developed in the 1990s gained importance in the medical field of dentistry, especially in orthodontics for orofacial surgical applications.

Volumetric images can be obtained from the 3D medical imaging modality. Most of the 3D diagnostic imaging technologies use radiological data such as " computed tomography (CT), cone-beam computed tomography (CBCT), micro-computed tomography (MCT), and magnetic resonance imaging (MRI), tune-aperture computed tomography (TACT)," etc. 3D imaging is composed of multiple 2D images which are stacked together using a reconstruction algorithm or a mathematical "back-projection" operation. These multichannel detector arrays detect the projected image signals which are passing through a patient. These are available for clinical practices to give a quality diagnosis and better treatment planning. This started in the twentieth century with innovation in the early 1970s by Godfrey Hounsfield [3] who invented computed axial tomography in 1979. These technological developments improve image quality at lower radiation doses and result in a wider range of applications of these modalities in medical research, academics, and clinical practice.

3D visualization is the foundation of modern radiology. 3D medical imaging uses 3D imaging modalities to provide an enhanced image of the anatomical structures of the body for medical analysis. This technology enabled healthcare professionals to access different angles, resolutions, and details to provide a more accurate anatomical view. The prevalence of chronic diseases, increasing population, demand for minimally invasive procedures, and better image quality provision are causing the expansion of 3D medical imaging. However, the market is facing

P. Maken
Shri Mata Vaishno Devi University,
Katra, Jammu & Kashmir, India

S. S. Rana
Department of Dentistry,
All India Institute of Medical Sciences,
Bathinda, Punjab, India

A. Gupta (✉)
Biomedical Applications Division,
CSIR-Central Scientific Instruments Organisation,
Chandigarh, India

H. Kaur
Department of Radiodiagnosis, All India Institute of
Medical Sciences, Bathinda, Punjab, India

S. S. Rana et al. (eds.), *Applications of Three-dimensional Imaging for Craniofacial Region*,
https://doi.org/10.1007/978-981-97-4608-8_15

many challenges as a result of high investment, unfavorable reimbursement policies, and a scarcity of skilled professionals.

3D imaging is advantageous for diagnosis and treatment planning for patients with craniofacial anomalies (CFA). The ideals and magnitude of the change are the factors to distinguish between patients with non-craniofacial anomalies and those with craniofacial anomalies. Technological advances are used by orthodontists and surgeons for treating CFA patients to improve the quality of the treatment. The deformities related to the facial and head bones in children are known as craniofacial anomalies [4]. These deformities are typically present at birth and can range in severity from mild to severe. One common craniofacial anomaly includes “cleft lip and palate (separation in the lip and the palate)”.

Numerous numbers of modalities can be utilized while studying craniofacial anomalies. 3D imaging has the potential to be used as a versatile tool for the valuation of outcomes in treatment planning or diagnosis. CT and CBCT are two of the preferred imaging methods for craniofacial applications. 3D imaging is widely used in craniofacial surgery for accurate and reproducible visualization of the anatomy. Morphometric analysis (It refers to the quantitative and mathematical analysis of the shape, form, and size.) [5] can be done by converting the voxel-generated models into coordinates. CT visualization of craniofacial bones is used as a gold standard for the analysis of skeletal variation. 3D models can be reconstructed in different planes using 2D images for better-improved viewing of anatomical or pathological features [6]. CT images provide enhanced image analysis capability compared to 2D radiographs. 3D data generated from CT can be used for custom-made 3D printing and also in regenerative therapy [7].

CBCT imaging has joined the armamentaria of digital imaging, radiography, and dental cast imaging which are replacing the traditional models. CBCT acquires images faster and with less radiation compared to CT. It employs a wider cone-shaped beam rather than a fan beam. It was developed in the 1990s at “Nihon University, School of Dentistry, Japan.” It has been now increasingly being used in dental and medical 3D imaging. It allows the visualization of the hard tissues because of its low radiation dosage. Airway visualization, dental implant planning, endodontic diagnosis, or reconstructions can be done using hard tissue images [8, 9]. CBCT is prone to artifacts because of restorations required for dental and the lack of contrast required for soft tissue segmentation. Contrast inconsistencies do not use the Hounsfield scale for bone and soft tissue differentiation. Surface scanning is used in the design and fabrication of craniofacial devices [10]. These devices captured images that are then registered to other medical images. It thus provides some accurate and visual models for designing and planning with medical models and surgical guides.

Magnetic resonance imaging produces intracranial soft tissue structure images without the use of radiation. It diagnoses the brain and spinal pathology of the craniofacial region. For example, MRI can be used to study brain morphology in patients with “Van der Woude Syndrome and cleft lip and palate [11] to assess the impact of these conditions on brain structure and surrounding soft tissues.” Its applications are expanding to include prenatal diagnosis [12]. The magnetic field required to generate the images interferes with the metal in the orthodontic appliances. Thus, MRI is not allowed to use on patients which require orthodontic appliances. However, advancements in MRI technology are attempting to alleviate this limitation [13].

One of the many advantages of 3D medical imaging is that information can be provided as needed and can be viewed instantly or can be retaken immediately if required. Some of the craniofacial applications of 3D imaging are provided in Sect. 15.2.6.

Craniofacial reconstruction was started using latest technologies in the early 1990s by Gronet et al. [14]. A patient’s anatomy was not only used for a 3D rendering on a digital display but also used for the developing a physical model for treatment planning.

15.2 Challenges of 3D Imaging

There are a certain number of challenges for 3D imaging in craniofacial applications which are concerning for radiologists. The challenges are categorized in some categories as indicated in Fig. 15.1. Researchers are working for minimizing the challenges as much as possible.

15.2.1 Challenges in Terms of 3D Imaging Modality

The challenges faced during 3D imaging in craniofacial applications may occure due to the different 3D imaging modalities such as CT, CBCT, x-rays, MRI, etc.

Computed Tomography: With the development of 3D imaging technology with time, 2D studies have been challenged. With regard to 3D technologies such as computed tomography, cone-beam computed tomography, MRI, etc., CT is often used to have precise measurements of cross-sectional areas which are further used for diagnosis and analysis. 3D reconstructions can also be used for volumetric measurements. Computed tomography is a commonly used 3D imaging modality in medicine. However, due to its drawbacks such as high cost and high radiation, it is not used for routine clinical assessments. Cone-beam computed tomography has overcome the drawback of high radiation exposure in a certain limit. Some of the challenges with computed tomography (CT) imaging are the following:

Exorbitantly Expensive: The average CT charge for imaging the abdomen, head, or chest costs very expensive which is a huge amount of price for an average pay scale employee for a health check-up. This will create a significant financial burden on the patients and even more if undergoing multiple CT examinations. This burden will be devasting for people without medical insurance.

High Dose of Radiation: A dose of radiation a patient receives from CT depends upon various factors such as scanner design, patient size, the volume of anatomy scanned, scanning protocol, quality of the x-ray beam, and technique used. Typical effective radiation doses in adults range from about 1.2 mSv for head CT to about 8 to 10 mSv for spine or heart CT as shown in Table 15.1. A normal abdominal CT scan delivers about 3.3 years of radiation with the same amount of background radiation in less than a minute. The values shown in a table can vary depending on the size of the patient and the imaging technology type used. Manufacturers of imaging

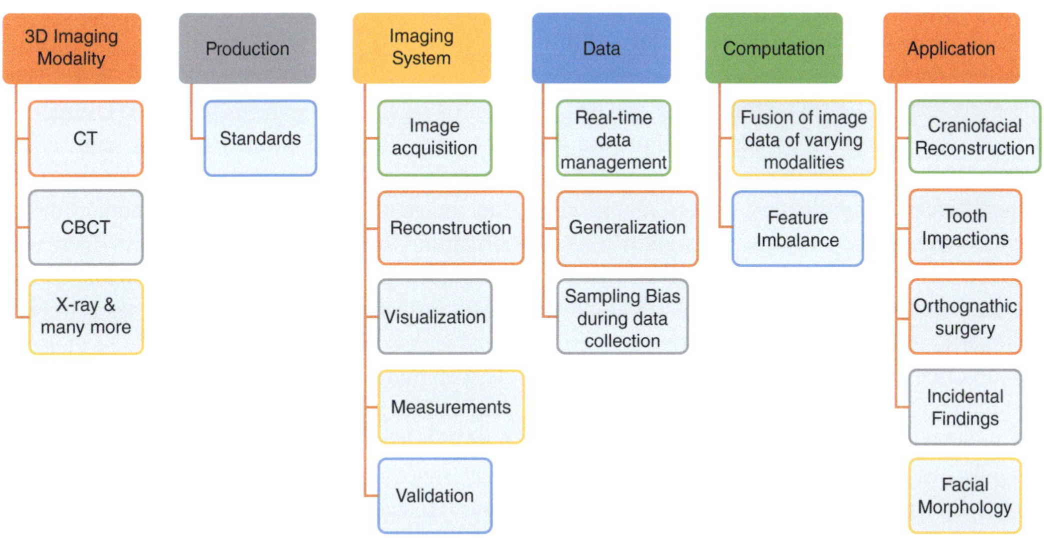

Fig. 15.1 Classification of challenges faced by 3D imaging during craniofacial applications

Table 15.1 Effective radiation doses comparison to background radiation in adults for various radiology procedures [15–21]

Region	Diagnostic procedure	Effective dose(mSv)	Time taken compared to natural background radiation
Abdominal	*Computed tomography*[16]	8	2.64 years
Chest	*CT—Chest*[16]	7	2.33 years
	CT—Lung cancer[17]	1.5	6 months
	Single chest x-ray[18]	0.02	~ 1 day
Dental	*Dental x-ray*[18]	0.004	Less than a day
	Panoramic x-ray[19]	0.02	Less than a day
	CBCT[19]	0.06–0.13	Less than a day
Heart	*Coronary computed tomography angiography (CTA)*[17]	12	4 years
Central nervous system	*CT—Brain*[20]	1.96	More than 6 months
	CT—Head[16]	2	Almost 8 months
	CT—Neck[21]	2.8	1 year
	CT—Spine[22]	6	2 years

technology are constantly working to reduce the radiation dosage exposure while also maintaining the quality of an image. These radiation doses are very high for a patient. CT is an expensive and high-dose procedure, with the radiation levels frequently increasing, and would be known to increase the likelihood of cancer. Even with the introduction of fluoroscopic, helical, or multislice techniques of imaging, the radiation doses have not decreased [22]. The radiation risks can be limited by reducing radiation exposure time, increasing the distance between source and body, using shielding for radiation absorption, having nonradioactive reagents as a substitution, etc.

Cone-Beam Computed Tomography: CBCT was developed and introduced in the market in the early 2000s. CBCT scanners are smaller in size and less costly compared to CT. For surgical tasks such as dental implants performed by dentomaxillofacial practitioners, CBCT along with application-specific software tools gives a solution for performing such tasks. Cone-beam volumetric imaging (CBVI) and cone-beam volumetric tomography (CBVT) are other terms that describe CBCT technology. Low-cost CBCT scanning has changed the dental practice's everyday approach as it is specially designed to have a 3D image of the maxillofacial region.

Quality assurance: There are some factors like noise, contrast resolution, scatter, and spatial which can affect the quality of the image and need to be minimized for quality assurance. Different attenuation of different tissues in x-rays results in contrast. The difference in signal or brightness between the structure of interest and its surroundings can also result in very minute contrast in radiographic images. This is because there is a relationship between the thickness, density, and radiographic contrast of tissues influences how distinct these differences appear in the images. For example, x-ray attenuation is highest in bone followed by the lowest in soft tissues and least in air. By changing the pixel values, to have the expected range of contrast depending on a particular clinical requirement and some image post-processing, one can enhance image quality. Inconsistent intensities (gray values) or distribution of signal results in image noise. Diffraction of x-ray photons from their original paths could result in scatter images, which then interact with the image detector, and produce nonuniformly structure intensities. Nonuniformly increased intensities of the diffracted x-ray photons can result in scattering in images which leads to poor contrast resolution images. Also, the scatter can be seen more in CBCT than in CT because of the single 2D image detector equipment used by CBCT [23]. The patients can also be a reason for scattering in images because of anatomical features. Executing artifact reduction algorithms with software tools of CBCT systems minimizes the scatter. The line pairs per millimeter (lp/mm) are measured as a spatial resolution. Very closed structures (fine details of the structure) are distinguished by spatial resolution. Structures and fine details which are positioned very close are distinguished using spatial resolution. To have a clear difference between different shades of gray in an image, a higher resolution is used. Smaller voxels with more exposure time result in a higher spatial resolution. However, scans with smaller FoV have a higher spatial resolution. The changes in an image that are unpredictable or organized but do not match the object's fluctuations in x-ray attenuation are known as radiographic noise. These all result in a "grainy appearance" of an image. It will destroy the display and result in an ambiguous structure. An increase in the exposure of time can decrease noise. The contrast resolution of an image is its ability to show subtle differences between tissues of different radiodensities. In other words, the image shows a clear distinction in various shades of gray. "Image noise, scatter, larger fields of view, reduced milliamperes, and other" settings of the x-ray generator all tend to reduce contrast resolution. An example of less or more contrast images is shown in Fig. 15.2.

Artifacts: A distortion in an image that is not related to the patient can be described as an artifact. Table 15.2 shows various components of artifacts that affect the quality of radiographic images. These distortions do not represent the corresponding patient's tissue region and are errors in a volumetric data set. The data or information loss in the images is due to artifacts that are produced automatically in the 3D images during their acquisition. CBCT images inherent more artifacts compared to CT units due to the use of a lower energy spectrum and cone-shaped beam geometry [29]. Many of the artifacts are the results of the discrepancies between mathematical assumptions and the physical imaging process during reconstruction algorithms. Some of the artifacts which may have been encountered in a volumetric imaging of the craniofacial region are shown in Fig. 15.2.

Beam hardening artifacts, which are due to the attenuation of the center than to the edges of the structure shown in Fig. 15.3a. Amalgam and cast metal restorations have higher atomic numbers resulting in a streak artifact shown in Fig. 15.3b. Scatter can also be a reason for streak artifacts. Partial volume averaging artifacts are a result of blurred tissue outlines, when an image voxel has more than one type of tissue and the gray value does not represent any specific tissue after the attenuation. If one voxel contains both soft and hard tissues, the end averaging the result of brightness values will be different tissues. This region thus will appear as a "step appearance." Ring or motion artifacts are also seen in images shown in Fig. 15.3c and d. It is usually caused due to the movement of the patient during the scanning process. It is the result of improper scanner calibration. To reduce the movement of the patient during scanning, the operator can educate the patient about the procedure, can use the headstand, and can have a shorter exposure time. Another artifact like Zipper artifact, a type of MRI artifact in shown in Fig. 15.3e, shows spurious bands of electronic noise extending across the image spoiling the image due to improper closure of MR scanner room door (red arrows). Fig. 15.3f displays wraparound artifact in axial

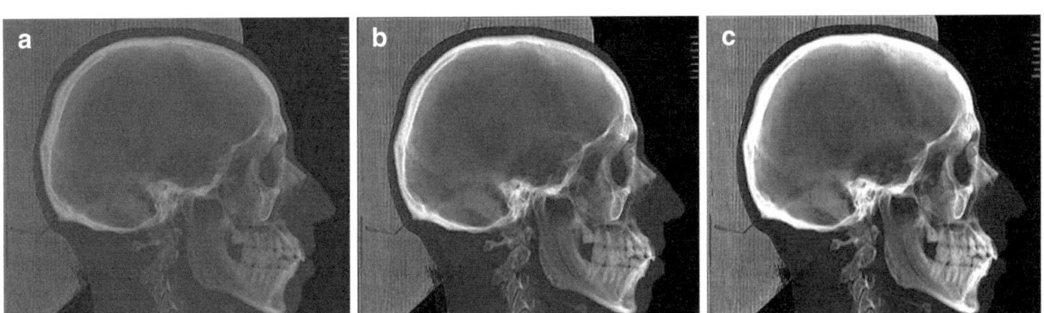

Fig. 15.2 (**a**) Low contrast image (**b**) Original image and (**c**) More contrast image

Table 15.2 Artifacts affecting the quality of medical images

S.No.	Artifact	Definition	Effects on images	Metric to measure	Solutions
1.	Noise [24, 25]	Noise can be seen as an aberrant granular pattern that deteriorates the quality of the image data	Quantum noise is the primary reason for the noise. It makes images unreadable or incapable of providing a correct diagnosis	Noise power spectrum	Controlling exposure factor could reduce noise.
2.	Scatter [23, 26]	Diffracted x-ray photons from their original pathways on contact with the image detector produce scatter in the images due to the nonuniformed increased intensities of the structures	Scatter decreases the contrast of the radiographs	Increased tissue volume, tube kilovoltage, matter density, and field size contribute to scattering radiations	"Close collimation, grids, or air gap technique"
3.	Spatial resolution [24, 27]	The image acquisition system ability to differentiate adjacent structures. It is the "measure of the smallest discernible details in an image"	Laser beam scattering during image reading, x-ray focal spot size, patient motion, exposure time, etc. can be a factor affecting the spatial resolution	Modulation transfer function (MTF)	"Decreasing field of view (FOV)"
3.	Contrast [27, 28]	The fractional difference between the region of interest and its surroundings in its signal or brightness is called radiographic contrast	Produces an unnatural image as it greatly affects the quality of an image for human visual perception as well as for image diagnosis	Histogram flatness measure (HFM) and histogram spread (HS)	Contrast can be adjusted by applying some post-image processing techniques—"histogram equalization, edge enhancement, grayscale processing, and noise reduction or change in pixel values"

MR T2-weighted image of the brain due to small field of view. Magnetic susceptibility artifact results in area of blooming obscuring details of upper alveolus on the right side due to metallic dental implant (green arrows) in axial MR FLAIR image shown in Fig. 15.3g. Therefore, precautions are always necessary and should be taken before the diagnostic image acquisition to have a true body part scanning. Tables 15.3 and 15.4 show some common CT and MR artifacts encountered in the craniofacial region, their reason of occurrence and corrections, respectively.

The rarity of experts: There are some laws and requirements which apply to orthodontic devices. The doctor should be aware of all these laws before purchasing any unit as a licensed dentist which is allowed to own and operate a device. CBCT systems are a variation of CT systems [30]. It is critical to have adequate training before operating which is provided by the manufacturer. The proper usage of the machine for patient positioning, various modes of image capturing are the part of hands-on training as provided by the manufacturer. This results in a good-quality image for treatment planning. The referring dentist should know the need for CBCT images and their use. The practitioner should be aware of all the risks associated with it. The dentist should be able to properly use the viewing software used for manipulating the CBCT data. He/she should have "sufficient knowledge of anatomy, its variations, incidental findings, or other pathological condi-

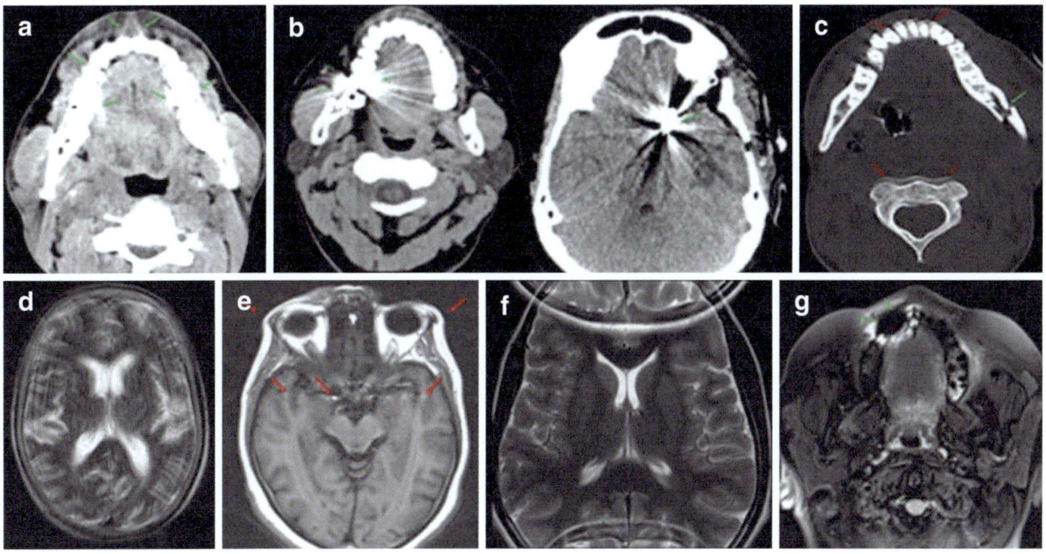

Fig. 15.3 Various artifacts encountered in craniofacial region. (**a**) Beam hardening artifact. Axial CT image soft tissue window at the oral cavity level reveals streaking bands at bone-soft tissue interface (green arrows). (**b**) Metallic streak artifact. (i) Axial CT image soft tissue window at the level of the lower alveolus shows streaking/white bands due to dental filling in right molar tooth (green arrows). (ii) Axial CT image brain soft tissue window reveals metallic streaking due to left ICA aneurysmal metallic clip (green arrow). (**c**) Motion artifact in an unconscious post-traumatic patient. Axial CT image bone window of the mandible shows blurred margins and distorted image representing movement of the patient during the scan (red arrows). Fracture mandible on left is also evident in this image (green arrow). (**d**) Motion artifact. Axial MR T2 image shows marked degradation of image quality due to excessive patient movement during the scan in a claustrophobic patient. (**e**) Zipper artifact. Axial MR T1-weighted image displays spurious horizontal bands spoiling the image due to improper closure of MR scanner room door (red arrows). (**f**) Wraparound artifact. Axial MR T2-weighted image of the brain shows wraparound artifact at the top and bottom of the image due to small field of view. (**g**) Magnetic susceptibility artifact. Axial MR FLAIR image shows area of blooming obscuring details of upper alveolus on the right side due to metallic dental implant (green arrow)

tions." It is the responsibility of the referring dentist to rule out any abnormalities and to report any important findings. Some practitioners due to the lack of good knowledge and practice choose to send the CBCT for further interpretation by an "oral and maxillofacial" radiologist specialist for a second opinion. Therefore, training is important for the whole team. Dawood et al. [31] stated that there is a need for training from specialists and manufacturers for complete knowledge. They will train on how to "operate the particular CBCT machine, radiation risks, imaging pitfalls, and the selection criteria." It should also include how to use the imaging viewing software tools which will help in the interpretation process of cross-sectional and 3D CBCT images. Radiologist experts who have very good knowledge about all imaging techniques are very uncommon. Automatic x-ray classification requires a great amount of time, effort, and expertise which are lacking currently. Pseudo-labeling, annotations, and activation maps often require subject matter experts, which are frequently lacking. Knowing where to look is more important in medical tasks than simply bucketing, which can lead to algorithms learning incorrect patterns. The solution is to have access to a group of subject matter experts. Hiring interns who can perform tasks such as labeling and learning to use tools to build models is also a good idea.

X-rays: X-rays present many advantages in medicine. It is recognized as an important tool for various examinations. They are noninvasive to diagnose disease and also to monitor therapy. Some of the risks associated with x-ray imaging are the following:

Table 15.3 Common CT artifacts encountered in the craniofacial region, their reason of occurrence and corrections

Sr. No	CT Artifacts	Reason	Correction
1.	Motion artifact	Patient movement during scan acquisition: – Voluntary – Involuntary (cardiac/respiratory pulsations)	– Immobilize or sedate the patient for voluntary movements – Use of head stand – Reduce scan time and breath holding for involuntary movements – Cardiac gating may be used for cardiac pulsations
2.	Beam hardening artifact	Occurs when radiographic beam containing polychromatic energies passes through a dense object gets hardened by selective attenuation of lower energy photons. It appears as follows: – *Streaking artifact*: Multiple dark/spurious streaking bands observed between two dense objects, commonly seen at posterior fossa due to presence of bones and soft tissues in same slice (Fig 15.3(a).) – *Cupping artifact*: Attenuation of beam at the center than to the edges of the structure	– By using dual energy imaging – Increasing tube voltage for better penetration of high density objects – Use of metallic filters to harden the beam before it reaches the patient
3.	Metallic streak artifact	Metals like amalgam, cast metal restorations, and jewelry (like nosepin, earrings, etc.) have high atomic numbers resulting in a dark and bright streaks which degrade the image quality Major causes are as follows: – Photon starvation – Beam hardening	– Use of metal artifact reduction software that is based on iterative reconstruction – By using dual energy imaging
4.	Partial volume averaging	Occurs when an image voxel has more than one type of tissue densities and the gray value does not represent any specific tissue after the attenuation resulting in impaired spatial resolution and erroneous image appearance with blurred tissue outline	– Use of thin section reconstructions, especially in CT angiography studies – Use of small field of view, small voxels, and/or increased matrix sizes
6.	Ring artifact	Observed as artefactual rings on images due to faulty detector or impaired functioning of detectors	– Correct the technical fault
7.	Cone beam artifact	Appears similar to partial volume artifact, observed at edges of the image acquired by multislice scanners	– Use of cone beam reconstruction algorithm

Tissue effects: Cataracts, hair loss, and skin reddening tissue effects occur at relatively high levels of radiation and are rare for many types of imaging. The use of a CT scanner or any conventional radiography equipment does not result in a tissue effect, but the radiation dosage to the skin for long complex interventional fluoroscopy procedures can be high enough to have such effects [32].

Ambiguity: X-ray imaging provides a 2D projected view of the 3D anatomical structure, which may not useful for the radiologist in severe cases [32, 33]. X-ray imaging often overlapped the anatomical geometry which results in creating confusion to understand the real anatomical structure, as seen in Fig. 15.4. The real measurements are lost as it is obtained from projected measurements of 3D to 2D. Thus, image calibration is required to read the x-ray images.

15.2.2 Challenges in Terms of Production and Means of Data Transfer

Standards: The data standards are the important informatics component that are required for any information flow in national health information

Table 15.4 Common MR artifacts encountered in the craniofacial region, their reason of occurrence and corrections

Sr. No	MR artifacts	Reason	Correction
1.	Zipper artifact	Occurs as spurious bands across the image due to hardware or software problems either of MR scanner itself or shielding	– Shut the MR door during imaging – Keep electronic devices away from MR scanner – Radiofrequency shielding should be optimal
2.	Wrap around/ aliasing artifact	When field of view (FOV) is smaller than the body part being scanned, then the part of the body that lies beyond the edge of FOV projected onto the opposite side of the image	– Increase the field of view – Use antialiasing software – Saturation bands on areas outside the FOV should be used
3.	Magnetic susceptibility artifact	Occurs as hypointense spots causing distortion of the image due to local magnetic field inhomogeneities that may occur due to metals like dental implants, amalgam, or orthopedic metallic implants. *Note*: This artifact is sometimes helpful to make small lesions containing hemorrhage/blood products more conspicuous (blooming artifact)	– Keep paramagnetic and ferromagnetic substances away from the part being scanned wherever possible
4.	Gibbs/truncation artifact	Appears as multiple fine parallel lines immediately adjacent to high-contrast interfaces, such as CSF-spinal cord and skull-brain interface, due to the reconstruction of the image by a Fourier transform from a finite sampled signal	– Increase the matrix size – Use fat suppression sequence if fat is one of the interface-causing artifacts
5.	Phase-encoded motion artifact (CSF pulsation artifact)	Appears as ghost-like structure, usually in direction of short axis, due to tissue/fluid moving during the scan like the following: – CSF pulsation – Arterial pulsation – Respiratory/cardiac pulsations	– Cardiac/respiratory gating – Presaturation bands placed over moving tissues – Switching phase and frequency directions – Shorten the scan time
6.	Herringbone/ crisscross artifact	Appears as uniformly placed crisscross stripes that resemble a fabric with the herringbone pattern Etiology: – Fluctuating power supply – Discrepancy in radiofrequency pulses – Electromagnetic spikes by gradient coils	– Recheck the RF coils plug/ clean them – Ensure uninterrupted and unfluctuating power supply – Contact the field/service engineer

infrastructure. Various patient safety systems and clinics share integrated medical data information where data is collected and reused for various purposes efficiently. There is a need for some specific standards for medical data in terms of uniformity. Information or data sharing between clinical laboratories, pharmacies, and radiologists is not possible without any common data standards. The lack of standards prevented the reusing of clinical data due to patient safety and quality requirements. Despite the availability of numerous communications technologies for the transmission of medical image data, there is no way to move data for clinical care with patient safety from one computer to another. For the systems at the receiving end to comprehend and accept the medical image data or information, it is necessary to create data standards for "organizing, representing, and encoding [34]." No such standard means of transmitting or representing data could result in unnecessary work performed by healthcare providers. The federal government is working on the recommendation of common standards for various safety measures. Many of the data standards are already available. The medical imaging information and other related data are communicated and managed using Digital Imaging and Communications in

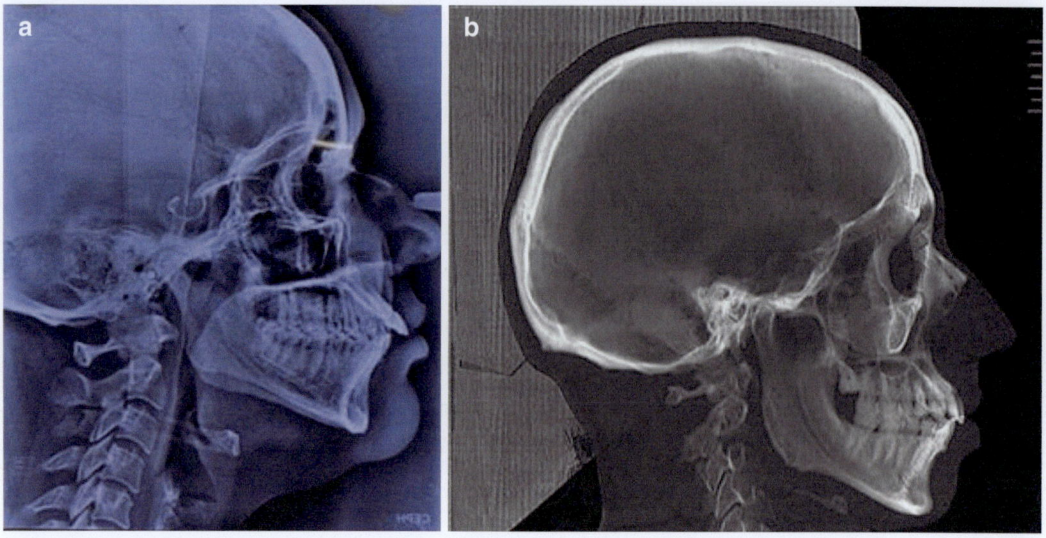

Fig. 15.4 (**a**) 2D lateral cephalogram (**b**) Lateral cephalogram derived for a CT

Medicine (DICOM) and picture archiving and communication system (PACS) international standards [35]. It saves multiple images per patient ID and stores metadata alongside the image pixels.

15.2.3 Challenges in Terms of the 3D Imaging System (CAD) [36]

Image Acquisition: It is one of the important phases in the research and development field. The analysis is based on the dataset acquired through image acquisition. The images acquired must be correct in terms of information content to compute the outcome without any bias. Thus, there is a necessity to strongly analyze and understand the errors to avoid any further impact. Various possible challenges associated with image acquisition are as follows:

Data collection: Diagnostic systems require a large amount of data from different patient cases. However, it is very difficult to acquire data from a clinic. Medical imaging datasets as compared to other domains are very difficult to find. A list of a few medical imaging datasets available for various medical applications is provided in Table 15.5. Medical imaging datasets for craniofacial applications are very rarely found online. Due to their proprietary nature, medical databases are hard to find online because they contain personally identifying information (IP), monetary value, and other aspects. In comparison to other fields, including self-driving cars with cameras that can capture images, the medical industry has fewer MRI and CT machines. One can always prefer to use retrospective data with anonymization. Data collection requires permission from "Institutional Ethics Committee (IEC)" [42] to follow certain rules and guidelines for data collection. Medical ethics are also an important step in data collection and research.

Standard posture: Some of the issues related to standing posture in imaging are that 2D radiographs are delicate in the symmetry and rotation of the head [43]. Deformities of the patient's skeletal may result in error-prone analysis. To increase or maintain the readability of the radiograph, ear rode and chin rest can be used to acquire a cephalogram. This could result in maintaining the standing posture. Figure 15.5 shows an example of a radiograph of a poorly positioned patient. In such cases of incorrect data acquisition, the patient can be recommended to repeat the radiograph. To have an automatic system, a patient's biological movement is also a challenge that should be understood by clinicians to have a robust system for diagnosis.

Table 15.5 List of a few medical imaging datasets available online for medical applications

S.No.	Dataset Name	Type	Format	Size	Link
1.	Kaggle [37]	Head computed tomography	Png	200 CT slices	https://www.kaggle.com/datasets/felipekitamura/head-ct-hemorrhage
2.	Computed Tomography Images for Intracranial Hemorrhage Detection and Segmentation [38]	Computed tomography	NIfTI	75 CT scans in nifty format are available out of 82 scans	https://doi.org/10.13026/4nae-zg36
3.	CQ500 Dataset [39]	Head computed tomography	DICOM	491 scans	https://www.v7labs.com/open-datasets/cq500
4.	Kaggle—Brain Tumour Classification [40]	Brain-MRI	Jpg	375 files	https://github.com/sartajbhuvaji/brain-tumor-classification-dataset
5.	Kaggle [41]	CT and MRI brain scan images	Png and jpg	5004 files	https://www.kaggle.com/datasets/darren2020/ct-to-mri-cgan

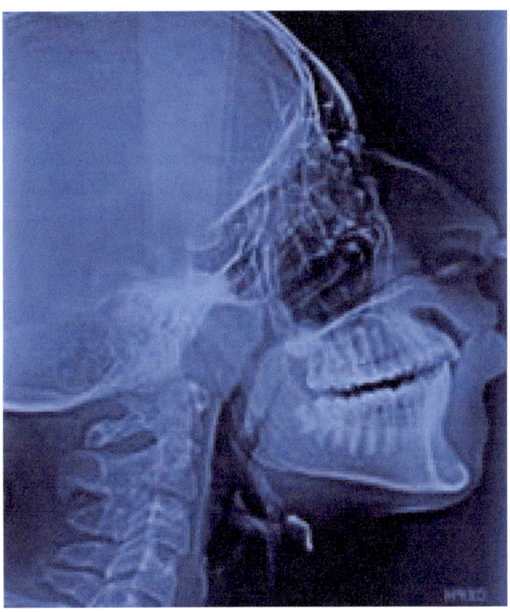

Fig. 15.5. Lateral cephalogram of a poorly positioned patient

Scanning protocol: To obtain a good quality image with high resolution, scanning protocol has an important impact on the information content. There is a need of designing an automatic system having a scanning protocol. The increase or decrease in the voxel or pixel size can affect the information in the images. The interpolation or extrapolation can be useful for getting the desired thickness of slices, but it will be predicted data. Therefore, it is required to give more radiation dosage for obtaining precise resolution [44]. This results in a trade-off between the required resolution of the image and radiation doses for the patient. This challenge must be taken cared of for designing a required automatic system with desired scanning protocol.

Variety of scanners: Numerous organizations produce a range of scanners with various preprocessing and scanning algorithms. The output of the data is influenced by these scanners in terms of visualization, pixel intensity, resolution, etc. For the same person, the data obtained from different scanners vary, although not statistically. Additionally, different equipment may produce varied quality of x-ray images [44]. Therefore, a variety of scanners should be required for developing an automatic diagnostic system. A list of a few CT/CBCT scanners is listed in Table 15.6.

Reconstruction: Image reconstruction from the raw input data is a challenging step. The factors which influence image reconstruction are as follows:

Reconstruction protocol: There are many protocols developed which can be used for convert-

Table 15.6 A list of various CT/CBCT scanners

S. No.	Scanner	Company Name	Type	Link
1.	Smart3D-X	LargeV instrument	CBCT	https://www.medicalexpo.com/prod/largev-instrument/product-122052-977866.html
2.	3D Accuitomo 170	Morita	CBCT	https://www.morita.com/america/en/products/diagnostic-and-imaging-equipment/cone-beam-ct-systems/3d-accuitomo-170/
3.	Aquilion S16	Toshiba	CT	https://lbnmedical.com/solution/toshiba-ct-scanner/toshiba-aquilion-s16/
4.	Pax-i3D	Vatech	CBCT	https://www.hospitalsstore.com/vatech-pax-i3d-cbct-machine/
5.	Giana HR 3D CEPH	NewTom	CBCT	https://www.hospitalsstore.com/newtom-giano-hr-cbct-machine/
6.	Aquilion lightning SP 80	Canon	CT	https://lbnmedical.com/solution/toshiba-ct-scanner/canon-aquilion-lightning-sp-80/
7.	Refurbished Siemens dual slice CT scan machine	Siemens	CT	https://dir.indiamart.com/impcat/siemens-ct-scan-machine.html

ing the 2D images or slices into 3D volumetric data. Every protocol developed differs in a parameter such as aggregation, approximation, and data prediction used for digital image formation. Raw data conversion into a specific image format such as jpeg, dicom, png, etc. also affects the quality of the image.

Visualization: Image visualization is a subjective theory, and it differs from person to person. Image quality is an important aspect for experts to plan and then diagnose properly. The preparation of the reference dataset or gold standard is a manual task. Image visualization may influence the accuracy/precision of gold standard dataset. The parameters which can affect the outcome of the visualization are suitable software, experts, or perception. A large amount of software available for 3D medical data visualization are listed in Table 15.7.

Measurements: Some of the measurement challenges are as follows:

Calibration: It is an important preprocessing step. The tools and software system need to be calibrated before operating to get adjusted to a new environment. If the calibration is not done properly, the linear measurements will not be obtained properly which results in an error. For example, an x-ray cephalogram requires manual calibration.

Manual Measurement: Manual measurements of ground truth is used to evaluate or validate the system. Data is considered a gold standard after measuring its "reliability, repeatability, and reproducibility" [55]. Blindly marking the data from more than one observer and more than one time will increase the data validation confidence. Data validation reliability can also get affected by other factors such as perception, imaging artifacts, noise, etc. A variety of scanners with different resolutions and fields of view could be used for measurements from sources such as x-ray and CT images. Such variations aid in the development of a robust dataset. A robust dataset is essential for designing an effective computer-aided diagnostic system.

Validation: Validation is the most important step for evaluating any designed system. If the process of validation is not adequate or the number of examples taken is insufficient, then the result may be erroneous. The validation process starts by comparing the results with the gold standard results or ground truth. The gold standards are generated by experts on anonymous patient data based on some true locations of landmarks in case of cephalometric analysis [56].

15.2.4 Challenges in terms of data

Some of the challenges that operators or practitioners face when dealing with 3D imaging related to data are as follows:

Table 15.7 A list of 3D imaging software

S. No.	Software	Applications	License	Link
1.	3D slicer [45]	*Clinical analysis*—2D, 3D, 4D visualization and simulation *Operations*—Export for 3D printing	Open source—BSD style	https://www.slicer.org/
2.	Dolphin [46]	• Fast 3D rendering • 3D airway analysis • Precise volume orientation • Volume stitching, etc.	Free and freely available	https://www.dolphinimaging.com/
3.	Simpleware ScanIP [47, 48]	• Import & visualization • Image processing & segmentation • Measurements & statistics • Surface model/mesh generation	Commercial	https://www.synopsys.com/simpleware/software.html
4.	NemoFAB [49]	• Image analysis • Cephalometric analysis • Treatment, management, • Visualization • Diagnostic • Treatment planning, etc.	Paid	https://www.medicalexpo.com/prod/nemotec/product-109911-814421.html
5.	Materialize mimics [50]	• Anatomy segmentation • Analyze anatomy, etc.	Paid	https://www.materialise.com/en/healthcare/mimics-innovation-suite/mimics
6.	InVivo 6 [51]	• Volume rendering • Implant planning • Orthodontic applications • Anatomage cloud • Endodontic visualization • Airway analysis • Case sharing • Accurate planning and many others	Perpetual and network	https://anatomage.com/invivo/ https://dexis.com/en-us/software-invivo-6
7.	3D doctor	• Convert DICOM to STL • Create a mesh model from the CT image • Create a mesh model from an MRI image • 3D surface rendering • Volume calculation	Paid	https://www.solidworks.com/partner-product/3d-doctor
8.	OsiriX [52]	*3D post-processing* – Multiplanar reconstruction (MPR), 3D rendering (MIP, volume rendering, and surface rendering)	Open source	https://www.osirix-viewer.com/osirix/osirix-md/
9.	On-demand 3D [53]	• Implant planning • Mandibular joint analysis • 3D visualization • Dental volume reformat (DVR) • Database manager (DBM)	Paid	https://dexis.com/en-us/ondemand3d
10.	NNT [54]	• Dental imaging • Surgery • 3D viewing • Dental implant simulation • Management	Paid	https://www.medicalexpo.com/prod/newtom/product-73766-525571.html

Real-time data management: Medical data is getting big or is growing in quantity due to an increase in the diversity of the data types resulting in big data. These big data in datasets are complicated to interpret and process using existing tools available. This arises a problem of "storage, analysis, and visualization." In the medical sector, three main types of digital data are clinical records, health research records, and organization operations records [57]. Radiologists should make progress in attaching big medical data to imaging. It can provide "personalized support, prognostic tools, optimized patient outcome, and clinical support" that were not previously possible [58].

Generalization: The images from the lab are significantly different from the real-time images. The real images are clearer and have a high resolution. These disparities in training and testing data can result in inconsistencies in actual models. The data generalization can be performed by modifying the images with noise, blur, and sharpness to simulate the real data.

Sampling bias during data collection: Data stitching and inadequate sampling could result in sampling bias. It can lead to incorrect model generation. For example, there were no COVID-positive patient x-ray images to compare with actual x-ray images. Merging these disparate datasets can result in data leakage, which is a significant challenge. Improper sampling can result in irrelevant patterns.

15.2.5 Challenges in Terms of Computation

Fusion of image data of varying modalities: It is the process of merging multiple images from different modalities to have a fused image with large information to be used for the clinical applications. Multimodality medical imaging has got increasing attention in recent years due to its significance in various fields. It refers to the simultaneous production of signals which are belonging to different medical imaging techniques, such as PET, SPECT, and MRI. Image fusion can be applied at three levels: pixel, feature, and decision level. Medical image fusion belongs to the pixel level. The fusion method performing without other fusion measures is called a block effect [59]. This challenge can be overcome by applying some fusion measures in the method such as "spatial frequency (SF), local variance (LV), and sum-modified-Laplacian (SML) [60]." The innovation in fusion methods for the medical image is relatively low because most of the work is the modification of the original methods. The problems in fusion methods such as color distortion, image feature information extraction etc. The most common mode of medical image modality fusion is MRI/CT; other modality fusions are still a challenge because of the compatibility of the algorithms [61].

Feature imbalance: There can be seen a shift in the algorithms to deep learning approaches for 3D imaging applications. Deep learning approaches differ in the features learning process which is learned as a training process [62]. This automatic feature learning process is referred to as representation learning. If features learned or extracted are not truly representative, it could give wrong results or measurements. Various physicians leverage clinical data (to be used as extracted features) about patients with medical images to have better results using deep learning methods. As balancing the extracted imaging features with various clinical features to prevent any clinical features from being drowned out is one of the major problems in 3D medical imaging using deep learning [47, 48].

15.2.6 Challenges in terms of application

There are several applications in craniofacial region using 3D imaging, and all applications are associated with one or two challenges to be solved. Some of the applications are listed below:

Craniofacial Reconstruction: 3D models reconstructed can be used to recognize the direction or position of the fractures, degree of dislocation, and the number of bone fragments efficiently. Reconstruction can be done by rebuilding the contours, positioning fabricating, and bending guides. Due to the length of model production with current additive manufacturing processes, a surgical delay may be a limitation. Solid models simulating "osteotomies and grafts, segmental jaw movements, and facilitating preoperative construction of templates, surgical devices, or guides" can be obtained from medical images in craniofacial reconstruction. Navigational technologies and mastication simulation have been developed in this domain of craniofacial reconstruction [63]. Standard data for the experiment, validation, and correct feature extraction (contours extraction) are challenges of craniofacial reconstruction. The need for a large dataset for correctly training the model using deep learning techniques is also a challenge.

Tooth Impactions: A condition in the tooth to not fully grow out from the gums are known as tooth impaction. Some reasons for a stuck or impacted tooth in tissue gum or bone are an overcrowded area; teeth getting twisted, displaced, or tilted during emerging; and a small jaw to fit the wisdom teeth. "Third molars and permanent maxillary canines" are common teeth impactions. The impacted tooth's position localization effect on the surrounding structures and angulation is often visualized using CBCT imaging [64]. CBCT imaging is useful in surgical planning and impacted canines' extrusion in the oral cavity. 3D imaging is useful for assessing using 3D visualization of the impacted canines with the proximity to the adjacent teeth, structures, pathology, and size of the follicular space [65]. 3D root structure visualization of a tooth with CBCT is significantly remarkable compared to 2D radiographic imaging. The technology improves the diagnosis and contribution to treatment modifications in many subjects. This application involves challenges related to the visualization of the data (x-ray or CT images). The quality of the image is a subjective matter, but it is a very important aspect as it helps the experts to plan and diagnose the tooth impaction condition properly. Also, the need of experts is important for understanding an applicable laws and requirements of the orthodontic device. Any licensed dentist should be well aware of all the laws and then can operate the device precisely.

Orthognathic Surgery: All information required in detail for volumetric reconstruction is provided using CBCT for orthographic surgery and treatment planning. A stereolithic model of the region of interest (ROI) can also be built using volumetric reconstruction. Lateral cephalometric imaging can be easily replaced by CBCT for skeletal and dental deformities diagnoses such as "hemifacial macrosomia and Treachery Collins syndrome." Oral and maxillofacial surgeons must be well aware of all the treatment complications, have a complete understanding of the types and causes, and should tell about these in advance to the patients who can have these complications [66]. So, there is a need for experts with complete knowledge of the surgery, imaging results, and anatomy.

Incidental Findings: Scanning a region of interest for diagnostic information can also reveal a variety of incidental findings. To interpret and evaluate the entire CBCT image dataset, clinicians need to have a detailed understanding of the anatomical structures to exclude any abnormalities. This application also requires experts with detailed knowledge of anatomy to identify incidental findings. The problems which are not related to the diagnosis and occur unintentionally during evaluation are called incidental findings [67]. Such findings should be communicated and discussed with the patient, as appropriate actions or recommendations could be made. Cha et al. [68] in their work have reported approximately around 25% to 54% of incidental findings on CBCT. They then measured the location, occurrence, and nature of various incidental findings in maxillofacial structures. The authors also evaluated the relationship between the findings and symptoms in orthodontic patients.

Facial Morphology in Three-Dimensional: Three-dimensional facial morphometry (3DFM) can be used as a supplement imaging procedure to other imaging procedures, particularly for lateral cephalometric analysis. In 3DFM, landmarks are placed on the face before being covered with semispherical reflective markers. The projective markers are illuminated using an ultraviolet stroboscope. Hand tracing and palpation are used for landmark locations. This application requires experts with anatomical knowledge and trainers to educate the practitioners about imaging device rules, regulations, and working understanding. Multiple facial angle analysis is necessary to obtain a whole mapping of the face [69]. This process is time-consuming and labor-intensive. It is not as accurate as other modern craniofacial imaging technologies.

15.3 Summary

With the advancements in medical imaging, 3D reconstruction or printing challenges are also increasing for designing, craniofacial surgery, or other medical specialties. 3D imaging is an evolving field for various craniofacial anomalies. Applications of 3D imaging in craniofacial surgery are driven by advances in technology. Factors like accuracy, cost, time, risks, or benefits should be considered in the treatment and planning of diagnosing craniofacial anomaly. There are many factors for the issues or challenges to be faced during craniofacial application using 3D imaging. All these factors are listed and specified in the classification of challenges along with their consequences and effects. The classification system is divided into categories like challenges in terms of computation, expertise, data, imaging system, production, and imaging modality. All these challenges are difficult to remove or overcome. Further, consideration and improvements could help in improving the results of the craniofacial applications using 3D imaging at some level.

References

1. Alshammery FA. Three dimensional (3D) imaging techniques in orthodontics-an update. J Family Med Prim Care. 2020;9(6):2626–30. https://doi.org/10.4103/jfmpc.jfmpc_64_20.
2. Hajeer MY, Millett DT, Ayoub AF, Siebert JP. Applications of 3D imaging in orthodontics: part I. J Orthod. 2004;31(1):62–70. https://doi.org/10.1179/146531204225011346.
3. Bhattacharyya KB. Godfrey Newbold Hounsfield (1919-2004): the man who revolutionized neuroimaging. Ann Indian Acad Neurol. 2016;19(4):448–50. https://doi.org/10.4103/0972-2327.194414.
4. Akram A, McKnight MM, Bellardie H, Beale V, Evans RD. Craniofacial malformations and the orthodontist. Br Dent J. 2015;218(3):129–41. https://doi.org/10.1038/sj.bdj.2015.48.
5. Goodwin AF, Larson JR, Jones KB, Liberton DK, Landan M, Wang Z, et al. Craniofacial morphometric analysis of individuals with X-linked hypohidrotic ectodermal dysplasia. Mol Genet Genomic Med. 2014;2(5):422–9. https://doi.org/10.1002/mgg3.84.
6. Kapila S, Conley RS, Harrell WE Jr. The current status of cone beam computed tomography imaging in orthodontics. Dentomaxillofac Radiol. 2011;40(1):24–34. https://doi.org/10.1259/dmfr/12615645.
7. Klammert U, Gbureck U, Vorndran E, Rödiger J, Meyer-Marcotty P, Kübler AC. 3D powder printed calcium phosphate implants for reconstruction of cranial and maxillofacial defects. J Craniomaxillofac Surg. 2010;38(8):565–70. https://doi.org/10.1016/j.jcms.2010.01.009.
8. Estrela C, Bueno MR, Azevedo BC, Azevedo JR, Pécora JD. A new periapical index based on cone beam computed tomography. J Endod. 2008;34(11):1325–31. https://doi.org/10.1016/j.joen.2008.08.013.
9. Grant GT, Liacouras P, Kondor S. Maxillofacial imaging in the trauma patient. Atlas Oral Maxillofac Surg Clin North Am. 2013;21(1):25–36. https://doi.org/10.1016/j.cxom.2012.12.002.
10. Sabol JV, Grant GT, Liacouras P, Rouse S. Digital image capture and rapid prototyping of the maxillofacial defect. J Prosthodont. 2011;20(4):310–4. https://doi.org/10.1111/j.1532-849X.2011.00701.x.
11. Nopoulos P, Boes AD, Jabines A, Conrad AL, Canady J, Richman L, et al. Hyperactivity, impulsivity, and inattention in boys with cleft lip and palate: relationship to ventromedial prefrontal cortex morphology. J Neurodev Disord. 2010;2(4):235–42. https://doi.org/10.1007/s11689-010-9060-5.
12. Munch EM, Cisek LJ Jr, Roth DR. Magnetic resonance imaging for prenatal diagnosis of multisystem disease: megacystis microcolon intestinal hypoperistalsis syndrome. Urology. 2009;74(3):592–4. https://doi.org/10.1016/j.urology.2009.02.071.
13. Proffit WR, White RP, Sarver DM, editors. Contemporary treatment of dentofacial deformity 2002.
14. Gronet PM, Waskewicz GA, Richardson C. Preformed acrylic cranial implants using fused deposition modeling: a clinical report. J Prosthet Dent. 2003;90(5):429–33. https://doi.org/10.1016/j.prosdent.2003.08.023.
15. McCollough CH, Bushberg JT, Fletcher JG, Eckel LJ. Answers to common questions about

the use and safety of CT scans. Mayo Clin Proc. 2015;90(10):1380–92.
16. https://www.webmd.com/cancer/radiation-doses-ct-scans.
17. https://19january2021snapshot.epa.gov/radiation/how-much-radiation-am-i-exposed-when-i-get-medical-x-ray-procedure_.html.
18. Li G. Patient radiation dose and protection from cone-beam computed tomography. Imaging Sci Dent. 2013;43(2):63–9. https://doi.org/10.5624/isd.2013.43.2.63.
19. Tan XM, Shah MTBM, Chong SL, Ong YG, Ang PH, Zakaria NDB, Lee KP, Pek JH. Differences in radiation dose for computed tomography of the brain among pediatric patients at the emergency departments: an observational study. BMC Emerg Med. 2021;21(1):106. https://doi.org/10.1186/s12873-021-00502-7.
20. Alzimami K, Jambi L, Mattar E, Alenezi A, Alfuraih A, Salah H, Bradley DA. Effective radiation doses in neck computed tomography scans. Radiat Phys Chem. 2022;200:110340. https://doi.org/10.1016/j.radphyschem.2022.110340.
21. Kadioglu O, Currier GF. Craniofacial 3D imaging current concepts in orthodontics and Oral and maxillofacial surgery. Cham: Springer International Publishing; 2019.
22. Wiest PW, Locken JA, Heintz PH, Mettler FA Jr. CT scanning: a major source of radiation exposure. Semin Ultrasound CT MR. 2002;23(5):402–10. https://doi.org/10.1016/s0887-2171(02)90011-9.
23. Stuart C. White MJP. Oral radiology: principles and interpretation. 2014.
24. V U SR, Bell D. Noise Radiopaedia 2011. [Updated 11 April 2022]. https://radiopaedia.org/articles/noise.
25. Murphy A CR, Jones J. Radiographic contrast: Radiopaedia.org; 2018 [updated 8 March 2022].
26. Yeung J MA, Park V. Spatial resolution (MRI): Radiopaedia.org; 2011 [updated 2 Apr 2020].
27. Tripathi AK, Mukhopadhyay S, Dhara AK, editors. Performance metrics for image contrast. 2011 International Conference on Image Information Processing; 2011.
28. Kumar M, Shanavas M, Sidappa A, Kiran M. Cone beam computed tomography—know its secrets. J Int Oral Health. 2015;7(2):64–8.
29. Tompe A, Sargar K. X-ray image quality assurance. In: StatPearls. Treasure Island (FL): StatPearls Publishing LLC; 2022.
30. Dawood A, Patel S, Brown J. Cone beam CT in dental practice. Br Dent J. 2009;207(1):23–8. https://doi.org/10.1038/sj.bdj.2009.560.
31. Luepker RV, Lakshminarayan K. Cardiovascular and cerebrovascular diseases. In: Detels R, Beaglehole R, Lansanga MA, Gulliford M, editors. Oxford textbook of public health. 5th ed. United Kingdom: Oxford University Press; 2011.
32. Gupta A, Kharbanda OP, Sardana V, Balachandran R, Sardana HK. A knowledge-based algorithm for automatic detection of cephalometric landmarks on CBCT images. Int J Comput Assist Radiol Surg. 2015;10(11):1737–52. https://doi.org/10.1007/s11548-015-1173-6.
33. Gupta A, Kharbanda OP, Sardana V, Balachandran R, Sardana HK. Accuracy of 3D cephalometric measurements based on an automatic knowledge-based landmark detection algorithm. Int J Comput Assist Radiol Surg. 2016;11(7):1297–309. https://doi.org/10.1007/s11548-015-1334-7.
34. Aspden P, Corrigan JM, Wolcott J. Health care data standards. In: Patient safety: achieving a new standard for care. Washington (DC): National Academies Press (US); 2004. https://www.ncbi.nlm.nih.gov/books/NBK216088/.
35. Yan L. DICOM standard and its application in PACS system. Medical Imaging Process & Technology. 2018;1:10.24294/mipt.v1i1.221.
36. Gupta A. Challenges for computer aided diagnostics using X-ray and tomographic reconstruction images in craniofacial applications. International Journal of Computational Vision and Robotics. 2020;10:360. https://doi.org/10.1504/IJCVR.2020.10029170.
37. Head CT—hemorrhage. 2018. https://www.kaggle.com/datasets/felipekitamura/head-ct-hemorrhage.
38. Hssayeni M. Computed tomography images for intracranial hemorrhage detection and segmentation. PhysioNet; 2020.
39. Chilamkurthy S, Ghosh R, Tanamala S, Biviji M, Campeau N, Venugopal V, et al. Development and validation of deep learning algorithms for detection of critical findings in head CT scans. Lancet. 2018;392(10162):2388–96. https://doi.org/10.48550/arXiv.1803.05854.
40. Sartaj Bhuvaji AK, Bhumkar P, Dedge S, Kanchan S. Brain tumor classification (MRI). kaggle; 2020.
41. CT and MRI brain scans. 2020. https://www.kaggle.com/datasets/darren2020/ct-to-mri-cgan.
42. Chenneville T, Menezes L, Bylsma LM, Mann A, Kosambiya J, Baxi R. Assessing institutional ethics committees in India using the IRB-RAT. Journal of empirical research on human research ethics : JERHRE. 2014;9(4):50–9. https://doi.org/10.1177/1556264614544101.
43. Kumar V, Ludlow J, Soares Cevidanes LH, Mol A. In vivo comparison of conventional and cone beam CT synthesized cephalograms. Angle Orthod. 2008;78(5):873–9. https://doi.org/10.2319/082907-399.1.
44. Katkar RA, Kummet C, Dawson D, Moreno Uribe L, Allareddy V, Finkelstein M, et al. Comparison of observer reliability of three-dimensional cephalometric landmark identification on subject images from Galileos and i-CAT cone beam CT. Dentomaxillofac Radiol. 2013;42(9):20130059. https://doi.org/10.1259/dmfr.20130059.
45. Fedorov A, Beichel R, Kalpathy-Cramer J, Finet J, Fillion-Robin JC, Pujol S, et al. 3D slicer as an image computing platform for the quantitative imaging network. Magn Reson Imaging. 2012;30(9):1323–41. https://doi.org/10.1016/j.mri.2012.05.001.

46. Power G, Breckon J, Sherriff M, McDonald F. Dolphin imaging software: an analysis of the accuracy of cephalometric digitization and orthognathic prediction. Int J Oral Maxillofac Surg. 2005;34(6):619–26. https://doi.org/10.1016/j.ijom.2005.04.003.
47. Saraf V, Chavan P, Jadhav A, editors. Deep learning challenges in medical imaging. Singapore: Springer Singapore; 2020.
48. Pettersen F, Høgetveit J. From 3D tissue data to impedance using Simpleware ScanFE+IP and COMSOL multiphysics—a tutorial. J Electr Bioimpedance. 2011;2:12–22. https://doi.org/10.5617/jeb.173.
49. Kumar M, Kumari S, Chandna A, Konark SA, Kumar H, et al. Comparative evaluation of CephNinja for android and NemoCeph for Computer for Cephalometric Analysis: a study to evaluate the diagnostic performance of CephNinja for cephalometric analysis. J Int Soc Prev Community Dent. 2020;10(3):286–91. https://doi.org/10.4103/jispcd.JISPCD_4_20.
50. Raluca Monica C, Tarcolea M, Vlasceanu D, Cotrut MC. Virtual 3D reconstruction, diagnosis and surgical planning with mimics software. Int J Nano Biomater. 2012;4:69–77. https://doi.org/10.1504/IJNBM.2012.048212.
51. Hosseinaee Z, Pellegrino N, Abbasi N, Amiri T, Simmons JAT, Fieguth P, et al. In-vivo functional and structural retinal imaging using multiwavelength photoacoustic remote sensing microscopy. Sci Rep. 2022;12(1):4562. https://doi.org/10.1038/s41598-022-08508-2.
52. Spiriev T, Nakov V, Laleva L, Tzekov C. OsiriX software as a preoperative planning tool in cranial neurosurgery: a step-by-step guide for neurosurgical residents. Surg Neurol Int. 2017;8:241. https://doi.org/10.4103/sni.sni_419_16.
53. Choi J, Yu H, Lee K, Park Y. Three-dimensional evaluation of maxillary anterior alveolar bone for optimal placement of miniscrew implants. Korean J Orthod. 2014;44:54–61. https://doi.org/10.4041/kjod.2014.44.2.54.
54. Bretaudeau C, Paredes F, Sergheraert J, Massa L, Sébastien L, Diebold M-H, et al. Dental implant placement in a patient with cystinosis. A case report. J Oral Med Oral Surg. 2018;24:138–42. https://doi.org/10.1051/mbcb/2018019.
55. Gupta A, Kharbanda OP, Balachandran R, Sardana V, Kalra S, Chaurasia S, et al. Precision of manual landmark identification between as-received and oriented volume-rendered cone-beam computed tomography images. Am J Orthod Dentofacial Orthop. 2017;151(1):118–31. https://doi.org/10.1016/j.ajodo.2016.06.027.
56. Neelapu BC, Kharbanda OP, Sardana V, Gupta A, Vasamsetti S, Balachandran R, et al. Automatic localization of three-dimensional cephalometric landmarks on CBCT images by extracting symmetry features of the skull. Dentomaxillofac Radiol. 2018;47(2):1–12. https://doi.org/10.1259/dmfr.20170054.
57. Akhtar U, Khattak AM, Lee S. Challenges in managing real-time data in health information system (HIS). Cham: Springer International Publishing; 2016.
58. Morris MA, Saboury B, Burkett B, Gao J, Siegel EL. Reinventing radiology: big data and the future of medical imaging. J Thorac Imaging. 2018;33(1):4–16. https://doi.org/10.1097/rti.0000000000000311.
59. Kim D, Ho Y-S, editors. A method for blocking effect reduction based on optimal filtering. Berlin, Heidelberg: Springer Berlin Heidelberg; 2005.
60. Tan W, Tiwari P, Pandey HM, Moreira C, Jaiswal AK. Multimodal medical image fusion algorithm in the era of big data. In: Neural computing and applications; 2020. https://doi.org/10.1007/s00521-020-05173-2.
61. Huang B, Yang F, Yin M, Mo X, Zhong C. A review of multimodal medical image fusion techniques. Comput Math Methods Med. 2020;2020:8279342. https://doi.org/10.1155/2020/8279342.
62. LeCun Y, Bengio Y, Hinton G. Deep learning. Nature. 2015;521(7553):436–44. https://doi.org/10.1038/nature14539.
63. Murphy RJ, Gordon CR, Basafa E, Liacouras P, Grant GT, Armand M. Computer-assisted, Le fort-based, face-jaw-teeth transplantation: a pilot study on system feasiblity and translational assessment. Int J Comput Assist Radiol Surg. 2015;10(7):1117–26. https://doi.org/10.1007/s11548-014-1114-9.
64. Kuijpers-Jagtman AM, Kuijpers MAR, Schols JGJH, Maal TJJ, Breuning KH, van Vlijmen OJC. The use of cone-beam computed tomography for orthodontic purposes. Semin Orthod. 2013;19(3):196–203. https://doi.org/10.1053/j.sodo.2013.03.008.
65. Lai CS, Bornstein MM, Mock L, Heuberger BM, Dietrich T, Katsaros C. Impacted maxillary canines and root resorptions of neighbouring teeth: a radiographic analysis using cone-beam computed tomography. Eur J Orthod. 2012;35(4):529–38. https://doi.org/10.1093/ejo/cjs037.
66. Kim YK. Complications associated with orthognathic surgery. J Korean Assoc Oral Maxillofac Surg. 2017;43(1):3–15. https://doi.org/10.5125/jkaoms.2017.43.1.3.
67. Lumbreras B, Donat L, Hernández-Aguado I. Incidental findings in imaging diagnostic tests: a systematic review. Br J Radiol. 2010;83(988):276–89. https://doi.org/10.1259/bjr/98067945.
68. Cha JY, Mah J, Sinclair P. Incidental findings in the maxillofacial area with 3-dimensional cone-beam imaging. Am J Orthod Dentofacial Orthop. 2007;132(1):7–14. https://doi.org/10.1016/j.ajodo.2005.08.041.
69. Ferrario VF, Sforza C, Poggio CE, Serrao G. Facial three-dimensional morphometry. AJODO. 1996;109(1):86–93. https://doi.org/10.1016/s0889-5406(96)70167-1.

Safety and Protection in 3D Craniofacial Imaging

16

Anurag Negi, Prateek Sihag, and Kaja Mohaideen.A

16.1 Introduction

Over the past decades, considerable progress has been made in the field of medical imaging, which has contributed immensely to patient care. For precise medical diagnosis and therapy, ionizing radiation used in medicine keeps growing tremendously. As per WHO estimates, medical radiation is responsible for 98% of anthropogenic radiation and accounts for 20% of the total population's exposure. Annually, there are over 3600 million diagnostic radiological examinations, 37 million nuclear medicine operations, and 7.5 million radiation treatments conducted worldwide. The sheer enormity of its use makes it important to understand and address the risks associated with ionizing radiation [1].

A. Negi (✉)
Department of Dentistry, AIIMS, Bibinagar, Telangana, India

P. Sihag
Department of Radiodiagnosis, AIIMS, Rajkot, Gujrat, India

K. Mohaideen.A
Department of Dentistry, AIIMS, Bilaspur, Himachal Pradesh, India

16.2 Ionizing Radiation-Associated Risks During Medical Imaging

Nonionizing radiation, in contrast to ionizing radiation, does not cause the excitation of electrons from atoms or molecules from living tissue, whereas ionizing radiation can alter the properties of these materials. Gamma and X-rays are ionizing radiation, while nonionizing radiation includes visible light, infrared, radio waves, and microwaves [2]. Interaction of ionizing radiations with the human body results in potential risks that are classified into stochastic and deterministic (or non-stochastic) effects. Malignancy induction, genetic mutations, and congenital abnormalities are examples of the former, which pertain to impacts that are random and stochastic. There seems to be no clear-cut threshold at which these effects will not happen, yet the likelihood of experiencing these effects rises as one's exposure to radiation increases [3].

Contrarily, deterministic or non-stochastic effects are distinguished by having the least value below which they will not manifest. These include skin erythema, cataract formation, hair loss, infertility, etc. In routine diagnostic imaging, it is the stochastic effects that are of main concern since exposure involved is usually well below threshold doses for deterministic effects to occur. The risk estimate for low-dose radiation used in diagnostic radiology is primarily derived

S. S. Rana et al. (eds.), *Applications of Three-dimensional Imaging for Craniofacial Region*, https://doi.org/10.1007/978-981-97-4608-8_16

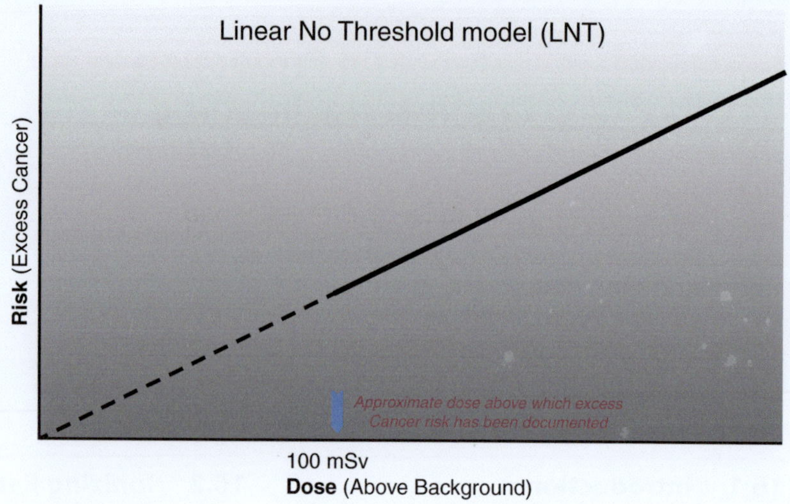

Fig. 16.1 Linear no-threshold model (solid line represents risk observed from a high level of radiation exposure, while the dashed line represents estimated risk from diagnostic range radiation exposure)

from data on survivors of high radiation exposure during the atomic bombings of Hiroshima and Nagasaki in 1945 and nuclear accidents like Chornobyl in 1986 due to a lack of data and strong statistical evidence [4]. Linear no-threshold models are used to calculate risk estimates for diagnostic radiation exposure. These models predict a small but substantial risk of developing cancer as a result of CT scanning and other ionizing radiation using medical imaging; especially in youngsters for a 1-year-old receiving an abdominal CT scan using this method, the expected lifetime risk is 0.18%. However, this risk estimate is theoretical and likely overestimates the actual danger; thus, the risk must be evaluated against the advantage of reaching an accurate diagnosis through the use of radiation-involved imaging technologies such as CT. Therefore, despite the lack of direct evidence of cancer genesis from low-dose radiation, the application of radiation protection principles needs to be strictly adhered to, by those involved in handling such types of equipment to minimize the risk if any. (Fig. 16.1) [5].

16.3 Units of Measurements of Radiation

The absorbed dose is the energy deposited by ionizing radiation into a substance per unit mass. The Gray (Gy) is the SI unit for this measurement, and it is defined as one Joule of energy absorbed per kilogram of matter. The biological consequences of ionizing radiation are linked to the class of radiation and the comparative radiosensitivities of the body organs. As a result, additional dosimetry values, equivalent dose, and effective dose which consider tissue sensitivity and type of radiation are used. The effective dose is a dosimetry quantity that accounts for the varying radiosensitivities of the body's organs and tissues. The equivalent dose takes into account the radiation type and is calculated by multiplying the absorbed dose by the radiation weighting factor (wR).

$$\text{Equivalent dose} = \text{Absorbed dose x } w_R$$

$$\text{Effective dose} = \text{Equivalent dose x } w_T$$

w_R. *Radiation weighting factor.*
w_T: *Tissue weighting factor.*

As we discuss the usage of X-rays (the radiation weighting factor for X-rays is 1) therefore, the absorbed dose and equivalent in our case will be numerically the same. Various tissues have different radiation sensitivities; the tissue weighting factor is utilized to account for the same. Therefore, Sievert (Sv) is used to avoid confusion brought on by the usage of the same unit. To give the reader an idea, the effective dose from a single chest X-ray is approximately 0.1 mSv (millisievert). The radiation dosage that is likely to result in the death of 50% of an exposed population within 30 days is lethal dose 50/30 and is in the range of 4000 and 5000 mSv delivered over a brief duration [6].

16.4 Principles of Radiation Protection

The revised recommendations issued by the International Commission on Radiological Protection (ICRP) in their publication dated 21 March 2007 anchored on three principles:

- *The Principle of Justification:* Any clinical situation that modifies the scenario of radiation exposure must have more benefits than harm.
- *The Principle of Optimization*: It emphasizes the need to minimize the likelihood of exposure, the individuals exposed, and the magnitude of doses, all within reasonable limits considering socioeconomic factors.
- *The Principle of Application of Dose Limits*: In situations involving planned exposure other than exposure of patients for medical reasons, the cumulative dose received from regulated sources by any individual should not surpass the acceptable thresholds set forth by the Commission.

The ICRP classifies exposure into three categories. Occupational exposure denotes the radiation exposure that workers encounter due to the nature of their profession. The employer bears the primary obligation for worker protection. Public exposure refers to radiation exposures of the general public that are not related to work or medicine. While natural sources are the most significant cause of exposure, it is crucial to also consider and control the smaller but more manageable exposures from human activities. The annual dose limit for occupational radiation workers is universally set at 20.0 mSv, but for pregnant radiation workers, it is reduced to 1.0 mSv as the developing embryo/fetus is considered a general public category. Patients are also exposed to radiation during diagnostic, interventional, and therapeutic procedures, which are referred to as medical exposure. This form of exposure is done on purpose and for the patient's benefit. Therefore, in medical exposure for the patient, application of a "dose limit" principle is inappropriate, as it may limit the benefit for the patient; so, only principles of justification and optimization apply [7].

16.4.1 Justification

Every procedure involving radiation needs to be justified because of health concerns and potential risks from radiation exposure that may result if such procedures are improperly applied. The objective of justification is to ensure that the advantages of radiation exposure outweigh the risks to individuals who may be exposed, hence avoiding the unneeded radiological procedure. Justification is a shared responsibility between the referring doctor and the imaging professional because, on the one hand, the referring clinician has a better understanding of the patient's clinical profile, whereas the imaging professional has a better understanding of the strengths and weaknesses of imaging modalities to answer the clinical question at hand.

A few relevant suggestions have been given at the International Conference on Radiation Protection in Medicine, Bonn, to enhance the implementation of justification: [8].

- Introduction and application of 3A's (appropriateness, awareness, and audit) as tools that are believed to aid and improve justification in practice.
- Formulation of evidence-based criteria aimed at enhancing the appropriateness of clinical imaging by engaging all parties concerned would facilitate the selection of the most suitable test for a particular clinical situation.
- Implement clinical imaging referral guidelines to support this decision-making process while considering local and regional disparities.

The American College of Radiology (ACR) has created evidence-based guidelines to assist referring physicians in selecting the most appropriate diagnostic or treatment approach for a given clinical problem [9]. Correspondingly, specific evidence-based guidelines for referral, optimization, and quality assurance (QA) in dental maxillofacial imaging using CBCT have also been published as a part of the SEDENTEXCT project in 2011(Table 16.1) [10]. The guidelines provided are not absolute constraints on clinical practice, and the clinician's judgment should be influenced by the individual clinical situation of each patient when making a referral. Nonetheless, a joint approach is required for justification, and a shared decision by referring clinician and radiologist at the level of an individual patient should be considered. While deciding upon justification of any medical exposure, the following factors need to be taken into account:

- Different radiological examinations deliver a wide range of radiation exposure to patients, with the risk being directly related to the amount of radiation received. (Table 16.2).
- The risk is notably greater for pediatric patients compared to adults.
- Possibility of a female patient being pregnant thereby the risks of exposure to the developing fetus.
- Whether alternative imaging methods that do not involve radiation, such as MRI or ultrasound, can be used to address the clinical question requires special consideration, especially in pediatric and pregnant patients.

16.4.2 Optimization

The "as low as reasonably achievable (ALARA) principle" in spirit refers to the optimization aspect of radiation protection. This principle suggests keeping ionizing radiation exposure low, considering socioeconomic factors. For example, on increasing radiation dose in certain examinations, higher quality images might be generated, but that might not always mean increased diagnostic advantage. The term "achievable" is important since it is important to mention that a medical radiation exposure lower than achievable can lead to poor diagnostic outcomes, which may require repeat exams. This principle involves multiple levels of workflow in radiology including the following:

- Design of the equipment: There shall be Automated Exposure Control (AEC) of X-rays in imaging procedures such as CT and fluoroscopy.
- Diagnostic reference levels (DRL): It represents a prescribed radiation dose for a specific imaging study that is not anticipated to be surpassed. Radiation doses administered to the patient during an examination are displayed on modern radiology equipment. This should be compared to the DRL for that study, and if it is found to be higher, an examination of the radiography method or equipment performance should be conducted. Having an average dosage less than a relevant DRL provides some assurance that patient doses in a given facility are reasonable, in line with other facilities and by the ALARA principle.
- Acquisition techniques: Selecting optimal parameters and strict collimation of radiation to the area of interest would enable the radiology technologists to produce diagnostic images at the minimal possible dose.
- Routine quality assurance tests of equipment and audits in the department to ensure adherence to ALARA.
- Use of equipment with newer technology which uses sophisticated technology and algorithms that can produce diagnostic-level images at lower doses than their predecessors [2].

16.4.3 Dose Limitation

Individuals' radiation exposure as a result of any relevant practices should be kept within particular dose limits, and doses above those limits are not regarded as appropriate, no matter how great the benefit is. Different countries' legislatures adhere to the recommendations for such dose limitations established by various scientific bodies. In India, recommendations by the Atomic Energy Regulatory Board (AERB) are followed, while the UK and Europe follow ICRP recommendations. Dose limits are applicable for only occupational exposure and public exposure. The restrictions vary due to the distinction between

Table 16.1 Adapted from evidence-based guidelines specific to CBCT use in dental-maxillofacial imaging for referral, optimization, and quality assurance (SEDENTEXCT project in 2011) [10]

S.no	Principles
1	History and clinical examination are a must before CBCT examinations and should not be carried out before doing them
2	CBCT examinations in each case must be justified and the benefits should overshadow the potential risks
3	CBCT examinations should provide additional information in conjunction with the preexisting information to assist in the management of the patient
4	CBCT examination must not be frequently repeated on a patient unless risks vs. benefits are analyzed
5	In the event of receiving a referral for CBCT from another dentist, it is essential to obtain a comprehensive clinical history and examination to substantiate the necessity of the CBCT examination
6	CBCT should be done only when the low-radiation conventional radiography is not adequate to diagnose the problem
7	A thorough radiological assessment of the entire DICOM dataset of a CBCT must be done
8	In situations where the assessment of soft tissue is necessary as part of the radiological evaluation, it is recommended to employ traditional medical computed tomography (CT) or magnetic resonance imaging (MRI)
9	CBCT equipment should offer volume size options (FOV) to adjust the radiation dose provided to patients based on clinical needs
10	A choice of resolution should also be available to ensure an adequate diagnosis with the lowest possible dose
11	An all-inclusive quality assurance program must be developed and executed for each CBCT facility, which encompasses equipment, techniques, and quality control procedures
12	The utilization of aids for precise positioning, such as light beam markers, should consistently be employed to guarantee accurate placement
13	A thorough examination of all new CBCT installations should be done before providing acceptance, to ensure radiation protection for hospital employees, patients, and the public
14	Routine tests of CBCT equipment should be done to ensure radiation protection of the facility users and patients
15	Guidelines on radiation protection in dental radiology (as per the European Commission document) should be followed for the protection of staff from CBCT
16	All individuals involved with CBCT operations must possess sufficient knowledge of radiation safety through appropriate training
17	Training and education of paramedics are required to effectively handle while adopting CBCT equipment
18	Dentists providing cone-beam computed tomography (CBCT) services should undergo supplementary theoretical and practical education for radio safety
19	Radiological report of dentoalveolar CBCT about the teeth, maxilla, mandible along with their supporting structures, and floor of the nose should be conducted by a radiologist or by a general dental practitioner equipped with specialized training
20	For non-dental-alveolar small FOV that do not fall within the aforementioned category, radiological reporting should be performed by a medical radiologist or a radiologist with specialized training

employment benefits for those working with radiation and unlike for the general public. The dose limits recommended by ICRP are provided in Table 16.3.

Dose limitation for pregnant personnel: To ensure the safety of the developing fetus of a pregnant staff member, the International Commission on Radiological Protection (ICRP) advises that the occupational exposure of pregnant women should adhere to the guidelines set for public exposure. This restriction is applicable during the entire duration of pregnancy, which commences upon the employee officially informing her employer in writing about her pregnancy. Subsequent to the notification, the working conditions for the pregnant worker must be arranged in a manner that restricts the additional radiation dose to the embryo or fetus to not exceed approximately 1 mSv throughout the remainder of the pregnancy [12].

Table 16.2 The effectiveness of common radiologic investigations of the craniofacial region

Type of radiologic investigation	Effective dose [Msv]
Radiographic examinations[a]	
Teeth	0.01
Skull	0.03–0.1
Cervical spine (two projections)	0.1–0.3
Computed tomography (CT) examinations[a]	
Skull	2–4
Spine	2–11
Based on dental CBCT unit type[a]	
Dentoalveolar (small and medium FOV)	0.01–0.67 (0.061)
Craniofacial (large FOV)	0.03–1.073 (0.087)

[a]Mean values of the effective dose of radiation during various X-ray examinations of the craniofacial region on standard patients with a body weight of 70 ± 5 kg, as adapted from BMU 2009 [11]

Table 16.3 Recommended annual dose limits (ICRP)

Organ	Occupational (mSv)/y	Public (mSv)/y
Effective dose		
Whole body	20[a]	1
Equivalent dose		
Eye Lens	20 mSv/year (averaged over 5 years) 50 mSv/year (in a single year)	15
Skin[b]	500	50
Extremities (hands and feet)	500	50

[a]With the further provision that the effective dose should not exceed 50 mSv in any single year
[b]Averaged over 1 cm^2 area of skin regardless of the area exposed

16.5 Practical Aspects of Radiation Protection

16.5.1 Protection of Staff

16.5.1.1 Design Safety

This pertains to the design of the facility and equipment type approval. In India, procurement and installation of X-ray-generating equipment for medical facilities is regulated by AERB. For all medical diagnostic X-ray equipment users, it is mandatory to obtain a License for Operation from AERB as per Atomic Energy (Radiation Protection) Rules 2004. These cover different aspects like notifying AERB of the purpose of using ionizing radiation by the employer, details of the site, design of the room housing the equipment, registration of radiation workers and radiation safety officer, QA examination of installed equipment's before it can be used, etc. In spirit, these regulations are intended to ensure the safe use of radiation equipment and need to be strictly followed. Details of these regulatory requirements are beyond the scope of this text, but anyone planning to install such equipment must be aware of and comply with these regulations [13, 14].

16.5.1.2 Operational Safety

Operational safety encompasses suitable operational protocols and the implementation of the principle of time, distance, and shielding. To ensure the operational aspect of radiation safety in the department, written operating procedures must be in place, as well as daily responsibilities for radiation protection and designated regulated areas. Worker exposure to high radiation doses (those that exceed 3/tenth of any dose limit) is likely to occur in controlled zones. This location must be prominently designated with warning signs, and access should be limited to required employees and the patient. The CT equipment room, X-ray machine room, and so on are examples. The following are the main components of operational safety:

- Ensuring that such equipment be handled only by qualified individuals.
- Application of principles of time, distance, and shielding.
  - *Time:* Reducing the amount of time spent near the X-ray source.
  - *Distance:* Because radiation exposure is inversely proportional to the square of the distance from the X-ray source (inverse square law), doubling the distance reduces exposure to 1/4th.
  - *Shielding:* Interposing a shielding material between the X-ray source and the operator, such as a Mobile Protective

Barrier, Lead Apron, or cubicle to stand behind, should be made if the operator's position is inside the equipment room. Employees working in the unprotected region of the controlled area must always wear personal protection equipment such as a lead apron, thyroid shield, protective gloves, and so on when the X-ray beam is activated. A 0.25 mm lead equivalent apron thickness would minimize the radiation dose by more than 90%. It is important to note that proper care and storage of lead aprons are of utmost importance since rough handling might lead to the development of cracks within the protective layer which would render it ineffective. The aprons should be hung properly on hangers with regular QA checks to ensure optimal protection [15, 16].

- *Usage of personnel monitoring devices*: For dental radiography, staff routine personal dosimetry is widely regarded as desirable, especially in centers with high workloads but not a mandatory requirement. Given the higher dose levels involved in 3D craniofacial imaging (CBCT, MDCT), there is a need for personal monitoring of radiation exposure. For this purpose, any type of monitoring device is available, but the most popular and commonly used is a thermoluminescent dosimeter (TLD) owing to its good sensitivity, reusability, and cost-effectiveness. To quantify deep and shallow dosages, TLDs are combined with filters that are installed in the badge holder. TLD badges are worn at the chest and, if a lead apron is used in an X-ray area, under the apron. When not in use, these should be stored in non-radiation areas to prevent erroneous readings. TLD badges are regularly sent at a specified interval to designated laboratories to measure radiation dose and generate dose reports. (Fig. 16.2) [17].
- *Preventive maintenance and periodic QA of equipment*: In India, AERB mandates periodic QA tests of equipment to improve imaging standards and reduction of unnecessary patient dose and hence dose to the staff. In India for dental equipment including OPG and CBCT, QA tests are required once every 5 years and, for other X-ray equipment, once every 2 years or after major equipment repair (like X-ray tube change or repair) tests are required [18].
- While general principles of radiation protection remain consistent, the regulatory requirements for installation and operating X-ray equipment might differ to some extent. Nonetheless, the employers and those involved in operating this equipment should keep themselves updated with the ongoing regulatory requirements of their respective countries.
- Excessive exposure: In India, in diagnostic radiology setup, if the dose received by any radiation worker exceeds dose limits prescribed by the Competent Authority (AERB), the employer should provide alternative work not involving radiation to the exposed person till further instructions are issued by AERB. Such investigation level dose limits

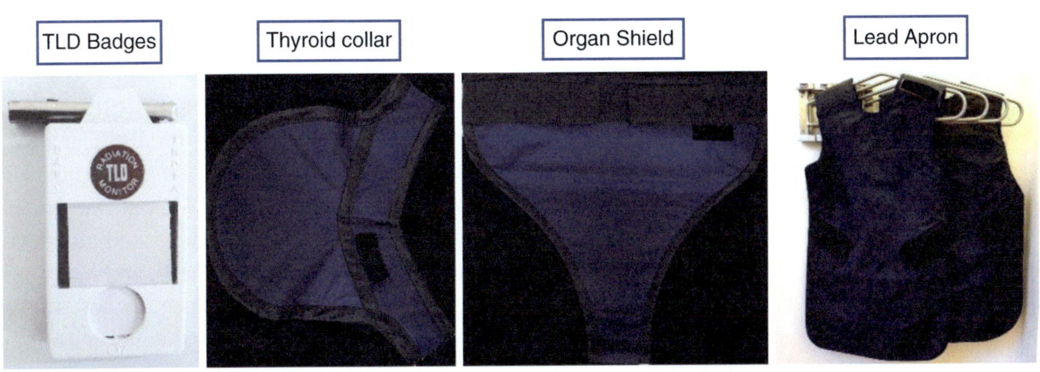

Fig. 16.2 Equipment for operational safety (Adapted from Department of Radiology, AIIMS Bilaspur)

provided by AERB are≥10 mSv per quarter (3 months) or ≥ 30 mSv per annum or ≥ 100 mSv for a block of 5 years. An investigation into cases of excessive exposure would usually include the following:

- Statement of exposed Individual and Radiation Safety Officer (RSO)/Head of the Institution to identify the probable cause of excess exposure.
- Review of work procedure and radiation safety practices followed by the exposed individual(s).
- Detailed radiation protection survey of the facility (including compliance with layout and design-safety requirements, licensing of ray facility).
- Analysis of the glow curve (amount of energy emitted relative to temperature during the procedure for dose measurement at the laboratory) of TLD.
- For exposures above >100 mSv, an estimation of the biological dose of the exposed individual(s) through chromosomal aberration (CA) test.
- Types of diagnostic procedures are carried out during the reporting period [19].

16.5.2 Patient Protection

The most significant considerations in patient protection are rationale and optimization, as previously addressed.

16.5.2.1 Supplementary Shielding

It serves as a means to safeguard vulnerable structures and parts not being examined especially in pregnant and pediatric patients. In the context of maxillofacial imaging, the thyroid gland, one of the more radiosensitive organs, is routinely exposed to dispersed radiation as a result of the examination and, on rare occasions, to the primary beam. Using a thyroid shield can limit exposure to skin-overlying thyroid by 33–84% in adults and 63–92% in children. To reduce exposure to the gonads and even embryos, the use of lead aprons has been advocated for patient reassurance. For female patients of child-bearing age, the possibility of pregnancy must be excluded before any kind of radiation exposure. For this, questioning the patient about the last menstrual period (LMP) or knowledge about being pregnant might help. In case of uncertainty, a pregnancy test may be done to rule out pregnancy [20].

16.5.2.2 Pregnant Patients

Imaging in pregnant women requires special consideration since the fetus's radiation risk is enhanced due to its tiny size and active cell cycle. The risk to the developing fetus is most pronounced during the initial 3 months of pregnancy, followed by a decrease during the middle trimester, and reaches its lowest point during the final trimester. The cumulative maximum "acceptable" fetal exposure for the duration of pregnancy, as per the National Council on Radiation Protection and Measurement, is 50 mGy (the majority of diagnostic radiological exams result in a dosage that is significantly lower than this threshold). Below this threshold, any adverse effect on the fetus is quite improbable. Nonetheless, US and MR should be the first imaging choices for pregnant patients. The choice to do a CT scan on a pregnant patient must take into account the possible benefit to both mother and child, as well as the risk-benefit ratio [21].

16.5.2.3 Pediatric Patients

It is crucial to use dose-efficient imaging methods, restrict CT to only definitive purposes, and educate healthcare professionals about the possible risk of low-dose radiation in the pediatric population as they are more susceptible to the adverse effects of radiation.

16.5.2.4 Dose Reduction Techniques

CT examinations, be it MSCT or CBCT, involve higher radiation exposure as compared to non-3D radiographic examinations. With advances in technology, improved scanning configurations and techniques have been devised, and many are under research, which can reduce the dose to the patient without compromising diagnostic formation. A few of the methods of dose reduction techniques are listed below:

- *Region-of-Interest Imaging*: By keeping the scan area practically minimal to cover the area of clinical interest, it is important to scan only that area that is of clinical interest (reduced FOV). This prevents adjacent body parts that are not necessary for diagnosis from being exposed to direct radiation.
- *Automatic Exposure Control (AEC)*: It is an advanced technique that is incorporated into most modern scanners wherein the tube current is automatically modulated to accommodate differences in attenuation due to patient anatomy, shape, and size.
- *Low-Dose Imaging*: Reducing exposure in CT by use of low mAs would result in increased noise in images thus produced. However, in certain examinations, the low dose can be utilized where images of the highest quality are not required and the information sought is optimally provided by the low-dose technique.
- *Short-Scan Imaging*: The minimization of scan duration and patient's radiation dosage is achieved by utilizing the short-scan angular range, which encompasses 180° plus the fan angle. This short-scan configuration/protocol is commonly found in the majority of dental CBCT scanners available in the market. Although this approach produces artefacts in off-middle planes and a relative reduction in image resolution, the overall image quality has been compared to the full rotation scan [22].
- *Optimization-Based Image Reconstruction*: Raw data generated after a scan has to be processed by the computers to generate diagnostic images of the scanned area. The filtered back projection was one such algorithm that was used in earlier machines. However, with advances in computing technology, most of the newer generation CT machines use an iterative reconstruction algorithm that can overcome noise associated with filtered back projection technique without increasing radiation dose. The adaptive-steepest-descent (ASD) projection-onto-convex-set (POCS) algorithm, along with a primal-dual algorithm devised by Chambolle and Pock (CP), has recently garnered considerable attention in the realm of cone-beam CT. This interest manifests in the extensive examination of these algorithms through simulation and real-data studies. These algorithms can help overcome artefacts associated with low-dose acquisition techniques described earlier [23–28].

16.6 MRI Safety

A brief mention of safety aspects in MRI craniofacial imaging would be relevant here since MRI scanners are associated with a unique set of risks owing to high-strength static magnetic fields, changing magnetic fields, and a high-powered radiofrequency coil system. Risks include projectile injury from the metallic object being pulled into the magnet, skin burns, peripheral nerve stimulation, acoustic injury, and malfunction of implants, viz., cardiac pacemakers, cochlear implants, etc. Due to this serious risk profile and increasing use of implants in medical fields, the US Food and Drug Administration published standards for MR imaging device safety terminology and mandated that all medical devices be labeled as "MR safe," "MR unsafe," or "MR conditional." (Table 16.4) A detailed screening and medical history of the patient is therefore required covering the presence of any implant,

Table 16.4 Table of terminologies and its definition by USFDA

Terminology	Definition by USFDA
MR conditional	"A medical device with demonstrated safety in the MR environment within defined conditions including conditions for the static magnetic field, the time-varying gradient magnetic fields, and the radiofrequency fields"
MR safe	"A medical device that poses no known hazards resulting from exposure to any MR environment. MR safe medical devices are composed of materials that are electrically nonconductive, nonmetallic, and nonmagnetic"
MR unsafe	"A medical device which poses unacceptable risks to the patient, medical staff or other persons within the MR environment"

surgical history, contrast media allergies, and presence of metallic objects (internal, fixed externally, or removable). For patients with implants, the decision for an MRI scan should only be taken after making sure that the implant is MRI-safe. Before scanning, appropriate clothing should be provided, and patients should remove hairpins, jewelry, and eye makeup (which can cause artefacts in head and neck imaging due to metallic residues) [29, 30].

Regarding the oral cavity, all the removable appliances made of metal should be removed before MRI. Dental fillings made of metal, titanium, gold, and amalgam do not need to be removed since they do not move and do not degrade the appearance of the oral and maxillofacial region. When deciding on an MRI for patients using orthodontic appliances, consideration should be given to the appliance composition and the area that will be imaged. Generally speaking, there is less image distortion and signal loss the farther away the orthodontic appliance is from the target area being scanned. Orthodontic appliances are typically constructed of stainless steel, which must be removed since it results in more picture distortion and signal loss than ceramic or titanium. To lessen image artefact, magnetic field interaction, and potential heat damage, the stainless steel orthodontic wires should also be removed. The ceramic and plastic brackets were MRI safe as they do not produce any artifacts, whereas the stainless steel brackets distort the cephalic organs such as orbits, frontal lobe, and pituitary gland. If the clinician is unaware of the type of orthodontic appliances worn, then it should be treated as MRI unsafe; hence the removal is advised before MRI [31–34].

16.7 Safe Use of Contrast Media

Exogenous contrast media are commonly used in head and neck CT and MRI imaging for problem-solving. It is critical to understand the dangers of using IV contrast material. The scope of this article does not allow for a thorough discussion of guidelines for the safe utilization of contrast media, but the readers are advised to seek additional information on the same. The main untoward effects linked to the use of IV contrast media are allergic reactions (varying from mild to severe anaphylactic), contrast-induced nephrotoxicity (for iodinated CT contrast media), and nephrogenic systemic fibrosis (Gd-based MRI contrast agents). Some of the risk factors for allergic reactions are a history of allergies, asthma, dermatitis, and urticaria. It is therefore important to identify those at risk and be ready to handle such clinical scenarios. To this end, an emergency drug kit should be always ready at the site, and the staff administering IV contrast media must be trained in identifying and managing allergic reactions. Patients with deranged renal functions are at risk of developing CIN and NSF. Those having or at risk of having renal disease should be identified by detailed history, presence of risk factors, and discussion with the clinician. Serum creatinine testing should be done in such patients beforehand, and the decision of the administration of contrast agents and type of contrast media should thereafter be based on existing guidelines and risk-benefit ratio [35–37].

16.8 Summary

It is the medical community's responsibility to maximize the benefits that ionizing radiation has to offer for patient care while keeping the risks to a minimum. With future scientific advances, understanding of radiation's effects on human health will be clearer, but till then with scientific evidence currently available we will have to treat carefully and follow the principles of optimization (ALARA), justification, and adherence to dosage limits to reduce radiation exposure. In addition, educating patients and healthcare workers about radiation protection, applying protocol-based workflow practices, and enforcing radiation protective strategies while keeping abreast with the latest recommendations and regulations by concerned scientific bodies would ensure minimizing the radiation-related health risks.

References

1. Ionizing radiation and health effects; 2024. https://www.who.int/news-room/fact-sheets/detail/ionizing-radiation-and-health-effects.
2. Allisy-Roberts P, Williams J. Farr's physics for medical imaging. 2nd ed; 2007. p. 1–207.
3. Dendy PP, Heaton B. Physics for diagnostic radiology. 3rd ed. CRC Press; 1999. p. 470.
4. Hendee WR, O'Connor MK. Radiation risks of medical imaging: separating fact from fantasy. Radiology. 2012;264(2):312–21.
5. Brenner D, Elliston C, Hall E, Berdon W. Estimated risks of radiation-induced fatal cancer from pediatric CT. AJR Am J Roentgenol. 2001;176(2):289–96.
6. NRC Web. 2024. Lethal dose (LD). https://www.nrc.gov/reading-rm/basic-ref/glossary/lethal-dose-ld.html.
7. ICRP. The 2007 recommendations of the international commission on radiological protection, vol. 37. ICRP Publication; 2007. p. 2–4.
8. Bonn Call for Action platform. IAEA; 2017. https://www.iaea.org/resources/rpop/resources/bonn-call-for-action-platform.
9. Subramaniam RM, Kurth DA, Waldrip CA, Rybicki FJ. American College of Radiology Appropriateness Criteria: advancing evidence-based imaging practice. Semin Nucl Med. 2019 Mar;49(2):161–5.
10. European Commission, Directorate-General for Energy, Cone beam CT for dental and maxillofacial radiology – Evidence-based guidelines, Publications Office, 2012, https://data.europa.eu/doi/10.2768/21874.
11. Allisy-Roberts P, Williams J. Chapter 2 - radiation hazards and protection. In: Allisy-Roberts P, Williams J, editors. Farr's physics for medical imaging. 2nd ed. W.B. Saunders; 2008. p. 23–47. https://www.sciencedirect.com/science/article/pii/B9780702028441500065.
12. ICRP. Pregnancy and medical radiation. ICRP Publication; 2000. p. 84.
13. Department of Atomic Energy. Radiation Protection Rules 2004. The Gazette of India: September 11, 2004 . Part-II-Section 3-Sub-Section (i). https://www.barc.gov.in/about/07.pdf.
14. Atomic Energy Regulatory Board. E-licensing of radiation applications (eLORA) system guidelines (2016). https://www.aerb.gov.in/images/PDF/DiagnosticRadiology/e-LORA-Diagnostic-Radiology-Guidelines.pdf.
15. Kim JH. Three principles for radiation safety: time, distance, and shielding. Korean J Pain. 2018;31(3):145–6.
16. Radiation Exposure of the Hand and Chest during C-arm Fluoroscopy-Guided Procedures - PMC. 2024. https://www.ncbi.nlm.nih.gov/pmc/articles/PMC3546211/.
17. Atomic Energy Regulatory Board, 2020. Personnel monitoring of radiation Workers in Radiation Facilities. https://aerb.gov.in/images/PDF/Personnel-monitoring-in-Radiation-Facilities-FINAL-JUNE-2020.pdf.
18. Radiological Safety Division, Atomic Energy Regulatory Board. Radiation Safety Training Module: Diagnostic Radiology; Radiation Protection in Diagnostic Radiology. https://www.aerb.gov.in/images/PDF/DiagnosticRadiology/RADIATION-PROTECTION-IN-DIAGNOSTIC-RADIOLOGY.pdf.
19. Radiological Safety Division, Atomic Energy Regulatory Board. Radiation Safety Training Module: Diagnostic Radiology Causes, Investigation and Prevention of Excessive Radiation Exposure in Diagnostic Radiology. https://www.aerb.gov.in/images/PDF/DiagnosticRadiology/EEI.pdf.
20. Horner K. Review article: radiation protection in dental radiology. Br J Radiol. 1994;67(803):1041–9.
21. Laura. NCRP report 174. Bethesda, MD: NCRP; 2015. https://ncrponline.org/publications/reports/ncrp-report-174/.
22. Thanasupsombat C, Thongvigitmanee SS, Aootaphao S, Thajchayapong P. Investigation of image quality on short-scan CBCT reconstruction. In: 2018 IEEE nuclear science symposium and medical imaging conference proceedings (NSS/MIC); 2018. p. 1–2. https://ieeexplore.ieee.org/document/8824758.
23. Chambolle A, Pock T. A first-order primal-dual algorithm for convex problems with applications to imaging. J Math Imaging Vis. 2011;40(1):120–45.
24. Sidky EY, Kraemer DN, Roth EG, Ullberg C, Reiser IS, Pan X. Analysis of iterative region-of-interest image reconstruction for x-ray computed tomography. J Med Imaging (Bellingham). 2014;1(3):031007.
25. Sidky EY, Chartrand R, Boone JM, Pan X. Constrained TpV minimization for enhanced exploitation of gradient sparsity: application to CT image reconstruction. IEEE J Transl Eng Health Med. 2014;2:1800418.
26. Bian J, Wang J, Han X, Sidky EY, Shao L, Pan X. Optimization-based image reconstruction from sparse-view data in offset-detector CBCT. Phys Med Biol. 2013;58(2):205–30.
27. Zhang Z, Han X, Kusnoto B, Sidky E, Pan X. Preliminary evaluation of dental cone-beam CT image from reduced projection data by constrained-TV-minimization. 2014.
28. Kusnoto B, Kaur P, Salem A, Zhang Z, Galang-Boquiren MT, Viana G, et al. Implementation of ultra-low-dose CBCT for routine 2D orthodontic diagnostic radiographs: cephalometric landmark identification and image quality assessment. Semin Orthod. 2015;21(4):233–47.
29. Health C for D and R. Testing and labeling medical devices for safety in the magnetic resonance (MR) environment. FDA; 2023. https://www.fda.gov/regulatory-information/search-fda-guidance-documents/testing-and-labeling-medical-devices-safety-magnetic-resonance-mr-environment.
30. Tsai LL, Grant AK, Mortele KJ, Kung JW, Smith MP. A practical guide to MR imaging safety:

what radiologists need to know. Radiographics. 2015;35(6):1722–37.
31. Dobai A, Dembrovszky F, Vízkelety T, Barsi P, Juhász F, Dobó-Nagy C. MRI compatibility of orthodontic brackets and wires: systematic review article. BMC Oral Health. 2022;22(1):298.
32. Mathew CA, Maller S, Maheshwaran null. Interactions between magnetic resonance imaging and dental material. J Pharm Bioallied Sci. 2013;5(Suppl 1):S113–6.
33. Poorsattar-Bejeh Mir A, Rahmati-Kamel M. Should the orthodontic brackets always be removed prior to magnetic resonance imaging (MRI)? J Oral Biol Craniofac Res. 2016;6(2):142–52.
34. Elison JM, Leggitt VL, Thomson M, Oyoyo U, Wycliffe ND. Influence of common orthodontic appliances on the diagnostic quality of cranial magnetic resonance images. Am J Orthod Dentofacial Orthop. 2008;134(4):563–72.
35. Beckett KR, Moriarity AK, Langer JM. Safe use of contrast media: what the radiologist needs to know. Radiographics. 2015;35(6):1738–50.
36. Nouh MR, El-Shazly MA. Radiographic and magnetic resonances contrast agents: essentials and tips for safe practices. World J Radiol. 2017;9(9):339–49.
37. Thomson KR, Varma DK. Safe use of radiographic contrast media. Aust Prescr. 2010;33:35–7.

17 Application of Three-Dimensional Scanning for In-Office Digital Manufacturing of Direct Printed Aligners

Abirami Rajasekaran, Shailendra Singh Rana, and Prabhat Kumar Chaudhari

17.1 Introduction

In the realm of digital orthodontics, the adoption of three-dimensional (3D) dental scanners and aligner therapy has a positive impact on the practicing capabilities of healthcare professionals in providing comprehensive orthodontic treatment [1].

3D dental scanning is the acquisition of digital dental data to facilitate diagnosis, treatment planning, appliance designing, progress monitoring, and patient education. It enables digital storage and transfer of data, streamlining both in-office workflows and remote handling for aligner manufacturing processes.

Aligners are removable orthodontic appliances that achieve planned tooth movement primarily through the shape-molding effect [2]. Its widespread adoption is attributed to patient preference and reduced clinical visits compared to the traditional braces; however, the preferential choice of an in-office workflow is related to the additional customization capabilities it endows the clinicians [1].

The introduction of biocompatible resins with appropriate force exertion characteristics paved the way for designing and directly printing aligners using additive manufacturing technology (also called "3D printing"). This eliminates 3D tangible dental models previously employed in the conventional manufacturing of thermoformed aligner workflow (Fig. 17.1a, b) [3].

A. Rajasekaran · P. K. Chaudhari (✉)
Division of Orthodontics and Dentofacial Deformities, Centre for Dental Education and Research (CDER), All India Institute of Medical Sciences, New Delhi, Delhi, India

S. S. Rana
Department of Dentistry, All India Institute of Medical Sciences, Bathinda, Punjab, India

S. S. Rana et al. (eds.), *Applications of Three-dimensional Imaging for Craniofacial Region*, https://doi.org/10.1007/978-981-97-4608-8_17

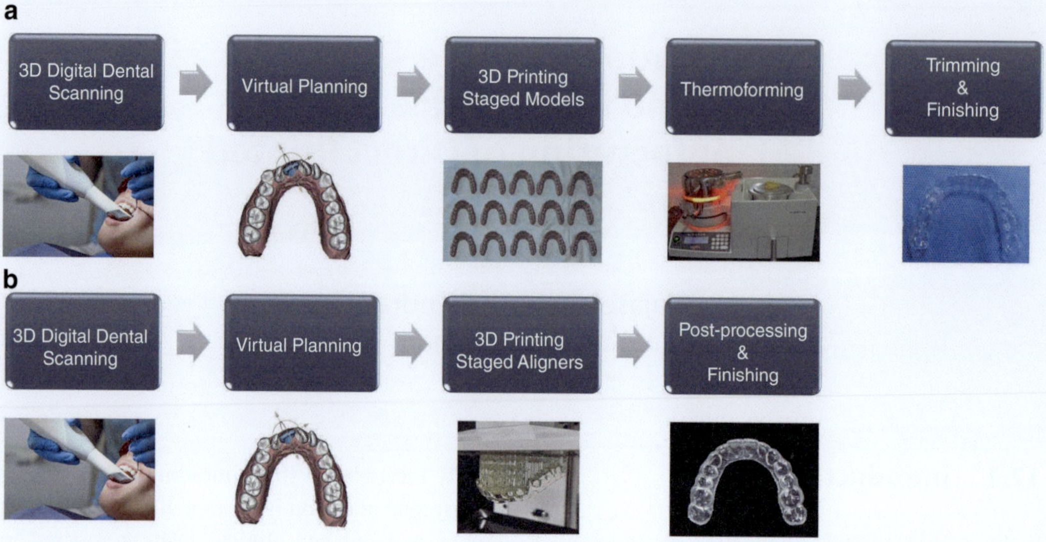

Fig. 17.1 Outline of the in-house aligner workflow: (**a**) Thermoformed aligners, (**b**) Direct 3D printed aligners

17.2 History

17.2.1 Evolution of Three-Dimensional Scanning in Aligner Manufacturing: From Impression Scanning to Intraoral Scanning

17.2.1.1 Pre-2010s

The early years of aligner therapy relied on traditional impression-based workflows. Orthodontists were mandated to submit their polyvinyl siloxane (PVS) impressions along with bite registration to the third-party outsourcing company (e.g., Align Tech for thermoformed aligner fabrication). Digitization of these impressions involved any of the two methods mentioned below:

(a) Direct CT scanning: PVS impressions were directly scanned using industrial computed tomography (CT) technology. This method involved mounting the impression on a rotating platform in front of an amorphous silicon x-ray sensor, which generated images referred to as "sinograms." Mathematical algorithms were employed to create reconstruction slices of 116 μ thickness. These slices were electronically stacked and inverted, and the resulting surface was smoothened to produce digital model of the dentition [4].

(b) Indirect scanning of positive replica: A dental model poured from the impression was scanned by destructive method or nondestructive methods like laser/white light scanning [4]. The destructive scanners had a rotating numerical-controlled machine cutter making passes over encased models, removing a thin layer with each pass [4, 5]. The nondestructive methods like white light scanning involved capturing the reflected interference patterns or moire patterns, while laser scanning involved capturing the scatter pattern and reconstructing using mathematical algorithms [4].

17.2.1.2 Post-2010s

By 2011, the iTero intraoral scanner (Cadent, San Jose, Calif.) was integrated into the aligner platform (Invisalign, Align Tech, Santa Clara, Calif.), thereby enabling the submission of direct 3D digital scans instead of physical impressions [6, 7].

Currently, aligner workflows utilize either direct intraoral scanning or indirect desktop scanning for both in-office and outsourced manufacturing. Majorly, their underlying principles are based on structured light technique, parallel confocal imaging, triangulation, accordion fringe interferometry, and three-dimensional in-motion video imaging [8, 9].

17.2.2 Evolution of Aligners: From Incremental Retainers to 3D-Printed Aligners

Aligner therapy represents a significant technological advancement based on Dr. Kesling's concept as incremental retainers [10, 11]. Initially, the workflow involved digital dental scans to create and 3D print staged models for the indirect manufacturing of aligners using thermoformable sheets like mono/multilayer polyurethane (PU) and polyethylene terephthalate glycol (PET-G, Fig. 17.1a) [12].

By 2012–2013, there was a pivotal shift indicating a process patent filing on direct manufacturing method indicating 3D printing the digitally designed staged aligners using biocompatible clear resins (Europen Patent EP2581062A2; US Patent US20130122448A1/US10383704B2) [13, 14]. This workflow ideology eliminated the need for physical models, thermoforming, trimming, and polishing (Fig. 17.1b).

The earliest documented works of direct 3D-printed aligners (DPA) appeared in the literature around 2019, with publications by Nakano et al. [15] and Jindal et al. [16] Nakano et al. developed and tested an acrylic-epoxy hybrid photopolymerizable resin (3D:1 M, Okamoto Chemicals, Japan) for aligner fabrication with thicknesses of 0.7 and 1.5 mm, but the properties were unmatched for clinical utility [15]. Jindal et al. utilized the dental clear long-term (LT) resin (Formlabs, Somerville, Mass., USA) for DPA manufacturing [16]; however, a critical comment [17] highlighted that this resin has been indicated for passive appliances (e.g., occlusal guard) rather than DPAs.

Contemporarily, Tera Harz TC-85 DAC (Graphy Inc., Seoul, South Korea) resin is gaining traction in clinical practice and research. It is a CE (Conformité Européenne) Class-IIa material with Korean and United States FDA (Food and Drug Administration) approval for DPA manufacturing [18, 19]. It is characterized to be a polymer based on "aliphatic vinyl ester–urethane with methacrylate functionalization" [20] demonstrating shape memory property [21].

17.3 Workflow of In-Office Digital Manufacturing of Direct 3D-Printed Aligners

The overall technical steps for DPA manufacturing using Tera Harz TC-85 DAC resin (Graphy Inc., Seoul, South Korea) can be majorly divided into two phases:

(a) 3D Data Acquisition and Virtual Planning (Fig. 17.2)
   - Digital dental scanning
   - Virtual planning

(b) 3D Printing and Post-processing (Fig. 17.3).
   - Print Preparation
   - 3D printing
   - Centrifugation
   - Post-curing
   - Ultrasonic cleaning
   - Boiling

17.3.1 3D Data Acquisition and Virtual Planning

Digital data of dentition and associated structures are acquired using separate recordings of the maxillary arch, mandibular arch, and maxillo-mandibular relationship. High-quality scans must ensure complete coverage of the teeth and gingiva devoid of bubbles or voids. Common output file formats include Standard Tessellation Language (STL), OBJect (OBJ), and PoLYgon (PLY).

The mesh quality of the scan files is checked and continued for virtual planning. The software interface allows the segmentation of individual teeth and verification of their local origin to define the long axis as well as the center of rota-

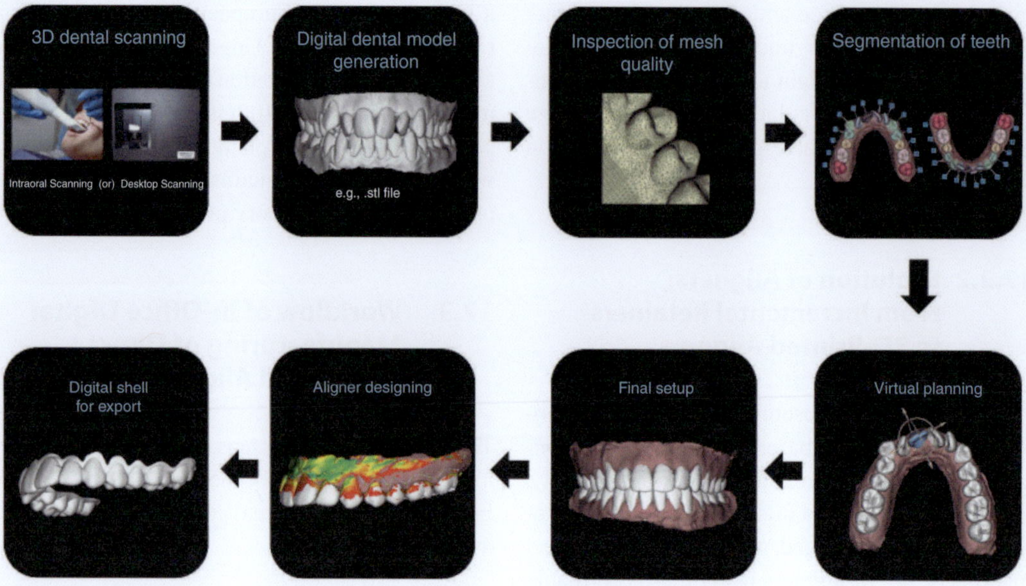

Fig. 17.2 Steps involved in 3D data acquisition and virtual planning

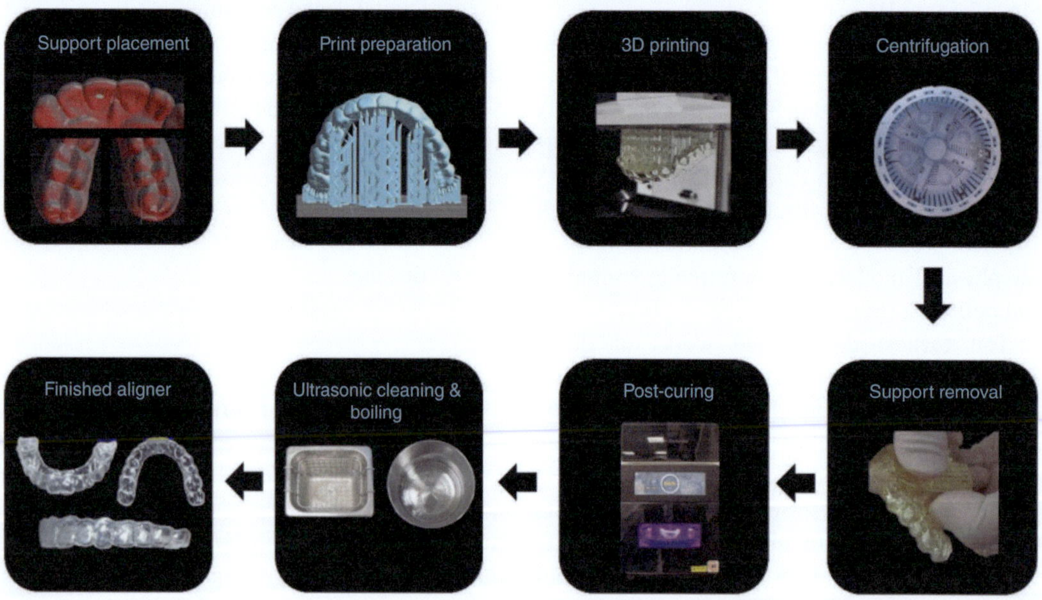

Fig. 17.3 Steps involved in 3D printing and post-processing

tion in three planes. Adjustments to virtual root length can be made, or the data can be integrated with the patient's tomographic scan information.

Based on the treatment plan, tooth movements are strategically sequenced and implemented as stages, also known as steps or layers. This process may involve considerations such as attachments, auxiliaries, interproximal reduction, and possible extractions. A final predicted setup with a comprehensive movement overview is documented, and specific movement limits per stage are established to create sequential sets. The total number of steps or stages is determined, followed by aligner preparation (along with an etching guide, in case of attachment placement). Aligner designing involves establishing the thickness, extension, type of trim line, marginal adaptation, offset, and block-outs. After labeling, the digital shells are exported in STL format.

The software to carry out virtual planning includes Maestro Dental Studio (AGE solutions, Pisa, Italy), Direct Aligner Designer (Graphy, Seoul, South Korea), OnyxCeph Aligner 3D (Image Instruments, Chemnitz, Germany), Blue Sky Plan (Blue Sky Bio, Libertyville, Illinois, USA), ArchForm (Sunnyvale, Calif., USA), and 3Shape Clear Aligner Studio (3Shape, Copenhagen, Denmark),

17.3.2 3D Printing and Post-Processing

The aligner STL files are imported for print preparation wherein the orientation angle and distance relative to the build plate are assigned and nesting is performed. The layers are verified thoroughly for island identification, and adequate supports of appropriate dimensions are placed. "Islands" refer to the small sections of the designed entity that are not connected to the main structure; thus it requires support (i.e., sacrificial material) during printing. The print layer thickness (z-resolution) is set according to the clinician's choice (preferably, 50 or 100 µ) and slicing is carried out. The resultant G-code file is transferred to the 3D printer via memory card, USB drive, LAN, USB cable, WiFi, or Bluetooth for launching the print job.

For 3D printing DPAs using TC-85 DAC (Graphy, Seoul, Korea), an open-source printer based on vat polymerization technology (wavelength 405 nm) is recommended. Machine leveling, platform calibration, optical path transparency, and z-axis motor lubrication are verified before printing. The vat is manually filled with liquid photopolymer and resin homogeneity is assessed. The print job is initiated based on calibrated exposure time, print delay time, and base curing parameters.

The examples for the vat polymerization-based 3D printers include (based on research papers and the manufacturer's catalog of calibrated printers) the following:

- Digital Light Processing (DLP): SprintRay Pro 95, 55 (SprintRay, Los Angeles, Calif., USA), Asiga Pro 4 k, MAX UV (Asiga, Sydney, Australia), MiiCraft 125(Young Optics Inc., Hsinchu City, Taiwan).
- Liquid Crystal Display (LCD): Uniz NBEE, SLASH 2 (Uniz, San Diego, Calif., USA), Phrozen Sonic XL 4 k (Phrozen Technology, Hsinchu, Taiwan).
- Stereolithography (SLA): Sindoh A1+ (Sindoh, South Korea).

Once the print job is complete, the aligners are removed from the build plate and centrifuged for 6 min. Centrifugation involves the removal of the excess resin from the 3D printed shells by spinning (Tera Harz Spinner, Graphy, Seoul, South Korea; ~500-600 rotations per minute) with internal heating function during operation. This eliminates the need for alcohol-based washing typically used after vat polymerization.

The support structures are removed by digital pressure or nippers, and cleaned specimens are exposed to a high-intensity light (ultraviolet, UV) and heat environment to achieve final properties. The manufacturer recommends a THC-2 post-curing unit (Graphy, Seoul, South Korea; wavelength, 405 nm; intensity, 2,80,000 mJ/cm^2—5 min based) system with a level 2 function for 20 min. The equipment has an additional feature of a nitrogen generator which in turn is connected to a compressor unit (with pressure > 7 bar).

After post-curing and polishing, the aligners are placed in an ultrasonic cleaner with ~80 °C for 2 min followed by immersion in boiling water (100 °C) for 1 min. Hazy aligners indicate incomplete polymerization, often due to deviation from the recommended post-curing workflow. Finally, ensure complete drying and store the aligners in either the aligner case or sealed opaque pouches.

17.4 Attributes

Direct 3D-printed aligners (DPAs) are in their early stages of development and present technical challenges, particularly in standardization [22]. However, their capability of enabling appliance customization remains a key advantage.

For a tooth-bonded auxiliary (e.g., button), an aligner cutout can be digitally designed to allow space and eliminate interference (Fig. 17.4a). Alternatively, for engaging elastics directly onto the aligner, the auxiliary can be integrated to the aligner shell (Fig. 17.4b).

Auto functions in the software interface (e.g., Direct Aligner Designer, Graphy, Seoul, South Korea) enable the configuration of scalloped, curved, or straight trim lines (Fig. 17.5a). The extent of the trim lines can be modified to create sectional aligners or a full arch aligner (Fig. 17.5b).

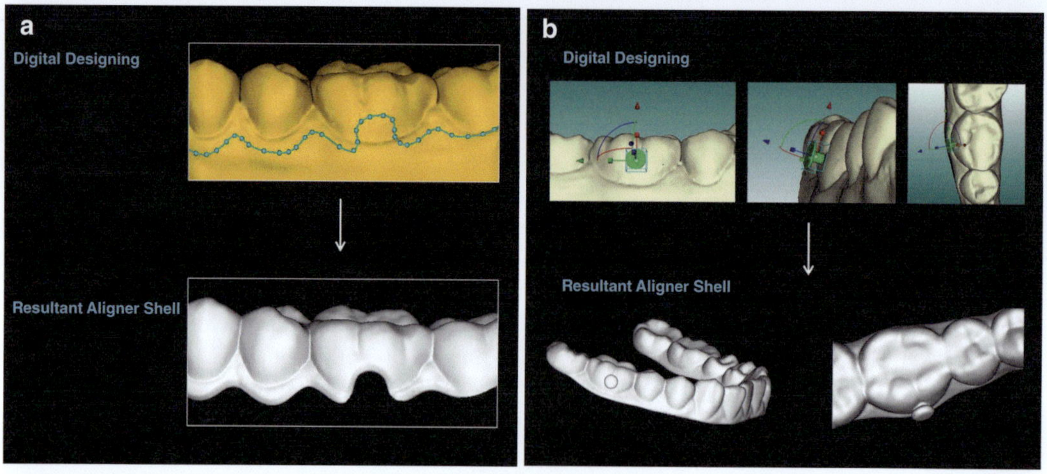

Fig. 17.4 Aligner design options for incorporating auxiliary—(**a**) Cutouts in aligner for bonded auxiliary, (**b**) Integrated auxiliary button

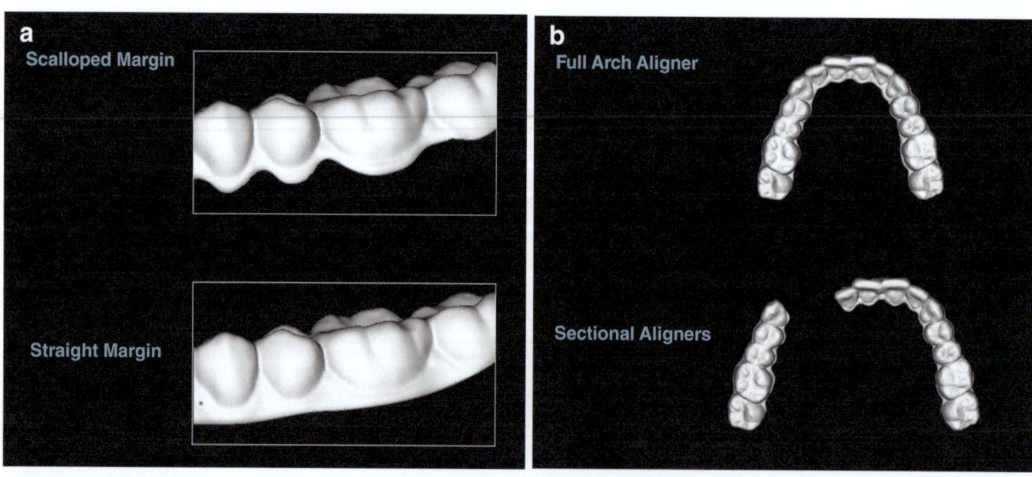

Fig. 17.5 Aligner trim line designs—(**a**) Scalloped or straight trim, (**b**) Sectional aligner trim line

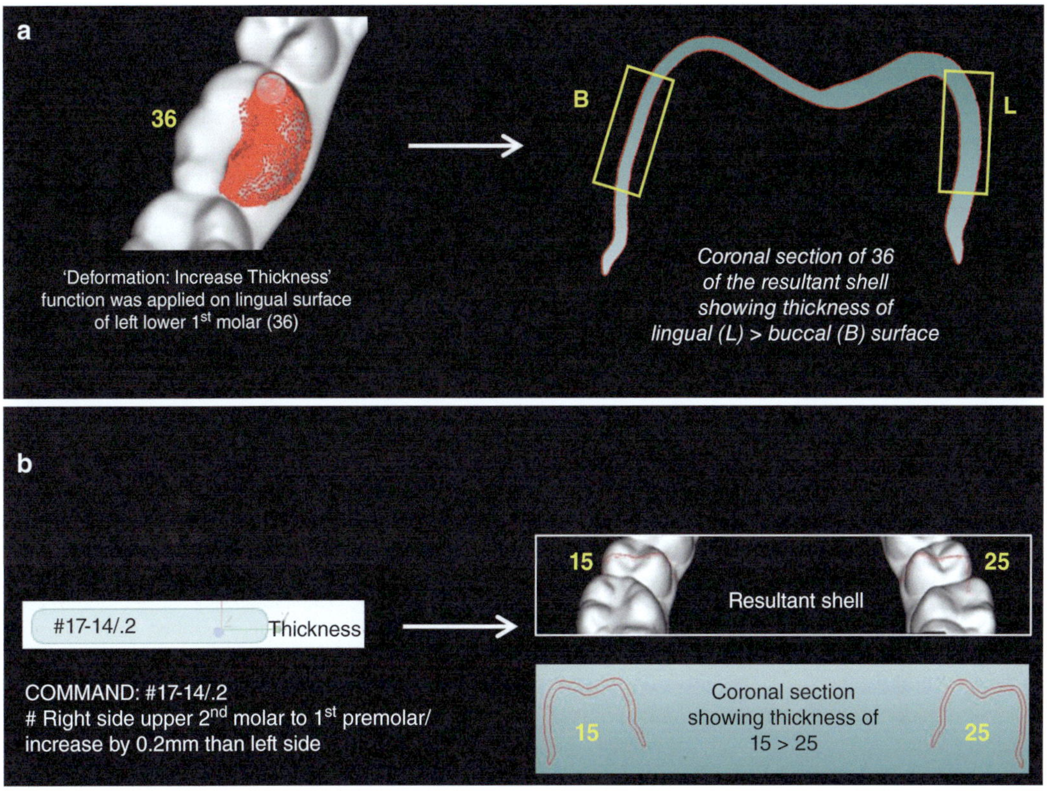

Fig. 17.6 Variable thickness designing of the aligner—(**a**) Over a surface of the tooth, (**b**) Over a section of the arch

The ability to assign and alter localized thickness at the surface of a tooth (Fig. 17.6a or section of an arch (Fig. 17.6b) can optimize the force exertion characteristics.

17.5 Current Evidence

The widely adopted TC-85 DAC (Graphy, Seoul, South Korea) resin is characterized to be an "aliphatic vinyl ester-urethane polymer, possibly with methacrylate functionalization" [20] that specifically complies with the structure of urethane dimethacrylate [23] (UDMA) derivative through the attenuation total reflection–Fourier-transform infrared spectroscopy (ATR-FTIR) [20]. The material has a cross-linked structure exhibiting temperature-dependent shape recovery and the reported glass transition temperature being ~69 °C [21].

Shirey et al. [24] evaluated two different photopolymers, namely, OD-Clear TF (3D Resyns, Barcelona, Spain) and Material X (EnvisionTec, Inc.; Dearborn, Mich). Clear-A resin (Senertek, Izmir, Turkey) and Luxcreo resin (Luxmark, Belmont, USA) have also been enlisted in the literature for DPA manufacturing [25].

Based on literature evidence, the material properties of TC-85 DAC were influenced by the type of 3D printer (LCD Vs DLP) [26] and the post-curing method (i.e., centrifugation Vs alcohol rinse) [27]. However, the print orientation (horizontal Vs vertical) [28] and post-curing environment (THC-2 unit with Vs without nitrogen) [27, 29, 30] did not significantly impact its properties. The beneficial effect exclusively linked to nitrogen (N_2) gas incorporation to the post-curing is proven to be statistically insignificant in terms of the degree of polymerization [27, 29], material thickness [30], and mechanical properties [29]. This could be attributed to N_2 exposure occurring after the initial polymerization of material during 3D printing, resulting in minimal discernible impact [29].

Based on the leaching characteristics, DPAs manufactured using TC-85 DAC were reported to be bisphenol-A free [31], however with a significant urethane dimethacrylate (UDMA) level of 50.91±5.6 μg/L (95%CI: 35.3-66.5) [23]. The potential cumulative toxicity due to the weekly change of the appliance demands further investigation.

An in vitro experiment involving multi-axis force/moment sensors indicated that increasing the thickness on the movement direction along with the opposite side of the adjacent anchor teeth could alter and improve the biomechanics with DPAs [32].

17.6 Conclusion

Direct 3D-printed aligners represent a promising innovative approach in orthodontics. Ensuring true biocompatibility and clinical utility necessitates strict adherence to the manufacturer's recommendations. However, at present this technology remains in its early stages of development; the software platforms, material characteristics, and technically sensitive printing/post-processing protocols are still to undergo refinement for efficient integration into the in-office workflow.

Acknowledgments The authors would like to thank the Science and Engineering Board, Government of India for funding the research project titled "3D printed aligners as a state-of-the-art smile designing appliance for its integration in Indian public hospital" (SERB-EEQ/2021/001073).

References

1. Jacox LA, Bocklage C, Edwards T, Mihas P, Lin F-C, Ko C-C. Understanding technology adoption by orthodontists: a quantitative study. Am J Orthod Dentofacial Orthop. 2022;161(3):364–74.
2. Upadhyay M, Arqub SA. Biomechanics of clear aligners: hidden truths & first principles. J World Fed Orthod. 2022;11(1):12–21.
3. Rajasekaran A, Chaudhari PK. Integrated manufacturing of direct 3D-printed clear aligners. Front Dental Med. 2023;3:1089627.
4. Kuo E, Miller RJ. Automated custom-manufacturing technology in orthodontics. Am J Orthod Dentofacial Orthop. 2003;123(5):578–81.
5. Wong BH. Invisalign a to Z. Am J Orthod Dentofacial Orthop. 2002;121(5):540–1.
6. Garino F, Garino GB, Castroflorio T. The iTero intraoral scanner in invisalign treatment: a two-year report. J Clin Orthod. 2014;48:98.
7. Our history. https://www.aligntech.com/about. Accessed 14 Apr 2024.
8. Kravitz ND, Groth C, Jones PE, Graham JW, Redmond WR. Intraoral Digital Scanners. J Clin Orthod. 2014;48:337.
9. Kim YJ, Jha N, Gupta S, Zvirin A, Qendro A, Zere E, Sokhi RK, Naveen KS, Sharan J, Sinha S, Anil S. Principles and applications of various 3D scanning methods for image acquisition for 3D printing applications in Oral health science. In: Chaudhari PK, Bhatia D, Sharan J, editors. 3D printing in Oral health science: applications and future directions. Cham: Springer International Publishing; 2022. p. 7–45. https://doi.org/10.1007/978-3-031-07369-4_2.
10. Kesling HD. The philosophy of the tooth positioning appliance. Am J Orthod Oral Surgery. 1945;31(6):297–304.
11. Boyd RL, Miller RJ, Vlaskalic V. The Invisalign system in adult orthodontics: mild crowding and space closure cases. J Clin Orthod. 2000;34(4):203–12.
12. Bichu YM, Alwafi A, Liu X, et al. Advances in orthodontic clear aligner materials. Bioact Mater. 2023;22:384–403.
13. Andreiko C, Kitching I. Direct manufacture of an orthodontic aligner. EP2581062A2, European Patent Office. https://patents.google.com/patent/EP2581062A2/en. Accessed 19 Apr 2024.
14. Kitching I. Direct manufacture of orthodontic aligner appliance. US10383704B2, United States https://patents.google.com/patent/US10383704B2/en. Accessed 19 Apr 2024.
15. Nakano H, Kato R, Kakami C, Okamoto H, Mamada K, Maki K. Development of biocompatible resins for 3D printing of direct aligners. J Photopolym Sci Technol. 2019;32(2):209–16.
16. Jindal P, Juneja M, Siena FL, Bajaj D, Breedon P. Mechanical and geometric properties of thermoformed and 3D printed clear dental aligners. Am J Orthod Dentofacial Orthop. 2019;156(5):694–701.
17. Panayi NC. Consider material properties when selecting a resin for 3-dimensionally printed aligners. Am J Orthod Dentofacial Orthop. 2021;159(6):706.
18. Tera Harz Clear, Graphy Inc. Certification number CE-MDD-0093/04/2020/01.
19. Clear TH, Graphy Inc. 510(k) Summary Report for Device K223355. https://www.fda.gov/medical-devices/510k-clearances/november-2022-510k-clearances. Accessed 19 Apr 2024.
20. Can E, Panayi N, Polychronis G, et al. In-house 3D-printed aligners: effect of in vivo ageing on mechanical properties. Eur J Orthod. 2022;44(1):51–5.

21. Lee SY, Kim H, Kim H-J, et al. Thermo-mechanical properties of 3D printed photocurable shape memory resin for clear aligners. Sci Rep. 2022;12(1):6246.
22. Eslami S, Kopp S, Goteni M, Dahmer I, Sayahpour B. Alterations in the surface roughness and porosity parameters of directly printed and Invisalign aligners after 1 week of intraoral usage: an in vivo prospective investigation. Am J Orthod Dentofacial Orthop. 2024;165(1):73–9.
23. Willi A, Patcas R, Zervou S-K, et al. Leaching from a 3D-printed aligner resin. Eur J Orthod. 2023;45(3):244–9.
24. Shirey N, Mendonca G, Groth C, Kim-Berman H. Comparison of mechanical properties of 3-dimensional printed and thermoformed orthodontic aligners. Am J Orthod Dentofacial Orthop. 2023;163(5):720–8.
25. Eliades T, Panayi N, Papageorgiou SN. From biomimetics to smart materials and 3D technology: applications in orthodontic bonding, debonding, and appliance design or fabrication. Jpn Dental Sci Rev. 2023;59:403–11.
26. Zinelis S, Panayi N, Polychronis G, Papageorgiou SN, Eliades T. Comparative analysis of mechanical properties of orthodontic aligners produced by different contemporary 3D printers. Orthod Craniofacial Res. 2022;25(3):336–41.
27. Šimunović L, Jurela A, Sudarević K, Bačić I, Haramina T, Meštrović S. Influence of post-processing on the degree of conversion and mechanical properties of 3D-printed polyurethane aligners. Polymers. 2023;16(1):17.
28. Camenisch L, Polychronis G, Panayi N, Makou O, Papageorgiou SN, Zinelis S, Eliades T. Effect of printing orientation on mechanical properties of 3D-printed orthodontic aligners. J Orofac Orthop. 2024;26:1–8.
29. Mattle M, Zinelis S, Polychronis G, et al. Effect of heat treatment and nitrogen atmosphere during post-curing on mechanical properties of 3D-printed orthodontic aligners. Eur J Orthod. 2024;46(1):cjad074.
30. Migliorati M, Drago S, Lagazzo A, et al. Effect of curing time and nitrogen generator usage on direct 3D-printed aligners thicknesses—an in vitro micro-CT study. Appl Sci. 2023;13(21):11952.
31. Grant J, Foley P, Bankhead B, Miranda G, Adel SM, Kim KB. Forces and moments generated by 3D direct printed clear aligners of varying labial and lingual thicknesses during lingual movement of maxillary central incisor: an in vitro study. Prog Orthod. 2023;24(1):23.
32. Pratsinis H, Papageorgiou SN, Panayi N, Iliadi A, Eliades T, Kletsas D. Cytotoxicity and estrogenicity of a novel 3-dimensional printed orthodontic aligner. Am J Orthod Dentofacial Orthop. 2022;162(3):e116–22.

18 Protection Over Innovation in Craniofacial Imaging

Debapreeti Mohanty, Pritam Mohanty, Shailendra Singh Rana, and Anjana Rajagopalan

18.1 Introduction

Anything made by the brain is called intellect. The term intellectual property (IP) refers to inventions that have a high commercial value and are therefore referred to as property. "Intellectual property rights" (IPR) are the legal privileges that an inventor or creator is allowed to safeguard their creations for a predetermined amount of time [1]. These legal rights grant the inventor/creator or his assignee the sole right to completely use their innovation for a finite amount of time [2].

Intellectual property (IP) is universally recognised as being crucial to the modern economy. The development of intellectual capital has been crucial to the economic growth of prosperous developing nations. These nations comprehend that innovation encompasses more than just high-tech products and that entrepreneurial orientation needs to be established at a young age to have the learning capabilities necessary for "catch-up" to transpire. Intellectual property rights are an effective tool for safeguarding financial, time, and labour investments. Both the cost of research and development (R&D) and the funding required to introduce a new technology to the market have increased dramatically [3]. Technology developers are facing ever-higher stakes, which means that, at least temporarily, information must be protected from unauthorised use to ensure that R&D and related costs are recovered and that there are enough profits to fund additional R&D expenditures [4].

In this new era, dentistry, especially the field of craniofacial imaging, is moving ahead to a more up-to-date technological point of view. Many innovations have been made in this field. Displaying a patient's anatomical reality has been the aim of imaging in both medicine and dentistry [5]. Craniofacial imaging has diagnostic uses in various departments of dentistry such as orthodontics, oral and maxillofacial surgery, etc. In this chapter, the main focus will be on the protection of IPs in the area of craniofacial imaging.

18.2 What Is IP?

IP denotes the ideas or a design formation utilizing brain power. A few types of intellectual property (IP) protection provided by the law that enable people to make money or become well-

D. Mohanty
Department of Conservative Dentistry and Endodontics, Institute of Dental Sciences, SOA University, Bhubaneshwar, Odisha, India

P. Mohanty (✉)
Department of Orthodontics, Institute of Dental Sciences, SOA University, Bhubaneshwar, Odisha, India

S. S. Rana · A. Rajagopalan
Department of Dentistry, All India Institute of Medical Sciences, Bathinda, Punjab, India

S. S. Rana et al. (eds.), *Applications of Three-dimensional Imaging for Craniofacial Region*, https://doi.org/10.1007/978-981-97-4608-8_18

known from their inventions are patents, copyrights, and trademarks. The IP system aims to create a conducive atmosphere for creativity and innovation by achieving a fair balance between the interests of inventors and the broader public good [6].

18.3 Types of IP

The definition of "intellectual property" has expanded significantly from its original use, which limited it to patents, trade names, and industrial designs. The ways that IPR advances technology are as follows: [1, 3, 4, 7].

1. It offers a procedure for dealing with unlawful use, piracy, and infringement.
2. Since all kinds of IP are disclosed, except trade secrets, it gives the general public access to a wealth of information.

A range of intellectual endeavours can be protected by IP, which includes the following:

1. Patent: An innovation is awarded an absolute undivided entitlement known as a patent. Generally speaking, a patent empowers the owner regarding decisions to be made regarding the utilization of his innovation by others. In return for this privilege, the patent holder publishes technical details about the innovation in the patent document for public consumption. Different countries adapt various types of processes for approval of a patent grant.
2. Industrial design: An industrial design is represented as the most appealing portion of an entity. A design can be drafted using colours, motifs, figures, etc. (can be two dimensional or three dimensional).
3. Copyright: The legal title that creators, including authors, painters, artists, designers, filmmakers, software engineers, and others, possess over their creative works is referred to as "copyright". Original creative expressions, such as literary, artistic, and dramatic works, are primarily protected by copyrights. It is still relevant for the duration of the author's life plus 60 years following their passing. In most nations across the world, protection is offered. Intellectual or creative works are protected by copyright. The moment the authorship develops the work, they acquire exclusive rights over the copyright. There is no need for a temporary application or any kind of symbolic representation to indicate registration.
4. Trademarks: A trademark is an insignia that gives a company's goods or services a sense of exclusivity. For their trademarks, the majority of businesses employ various taglines, memorable phrases, and signage. Having a trademark is not new; it has been practised for a very long time when creators would mark their works with a customary mark. By renewing the trademark every 10 years, it is possible to make its validity eternal for 10 years. It is territorial, and to assert rights, one must apply it to each nation separately. The branding that goods and services are sold under is protected by trademarks. Following registration, the mark's applicant is entitled to all rights associated with the mark. Typically, registration takes 12–18 months.
5. Trade secret: Trade secrets refer to the intellectual property rights of proprietary knowledge that may be sold or licensed. According to legal rights, prior authorization is required to put to use any trade secrets for business purposes, otherwise it is a punishable offence [6]..

18.4 Patents

Patent rights are constitutional. Generally speaking, the rules of the country or territory where a patent application was filed and granted are the only ones that grant exclusive rights [6].

Some advantages associated with patents are like prevention of duplication, the creation of a path for further discoveries, etc. [8] 20 years of protection for patents are granted, and within this period, no one else is allowed to produce the product other than the owner, and if anyone uses the patent, they must pay royalties to the owner, and the owner is allowed to obstruct rivals. After

Table 18.1 Websites for patent search across various countries

#	Search engine/database	URL
Government Organizations (Freely Available)		
1	USPTO (United States Patent and Trademark Office)	http://patft.uspto.gov/
2	EspaceNet (EPO; European Patent Office)	http://www.epo.org/searching/free/espacenet.html
3	Japan Patents (IPDL; Industrial Property Digital Library)	http://www.ipdl.inpit.go.jp/homepg_e.ipdl
4	Indian Patent Information Retrieval System (Indian Patent and Design Office)	http://ipindia.nic.in/
5	PatentScope (WIPO; World Intellectual Property Organization)	http://patentscope.wipo.int/search/en/search.jsf
Open Access		
6	Patent Lens	http://www.patentlens.net/patentlens/structured.html
7	Google Patent Database	https://www.google.com/?tbm=pts
8	Free Patents Online	http://www.freepatentsonline.com/search.html
9	IP.com Intellectual Property Library	http://ip.com/
10	Fresh Patents	http://freshpatents.com

20 years, the invention will be available in the public domain. Different types of patents are there as follows [9].

Utility patents can cover the following: a device, a manufacturing item, a composition of matter (such as a chemical compound), a kit for achieving a practical objective, a method or process for synthesis or production, or an advancement of any of the previously listed categories.

Design patents cover a novel decorative design of a manufactured item.

Plant patents protect any asexually reproduced unique and novel variety of plants. Table 18.1 shows various websites for patent search across various countries.

18.5 Patent Filing Process in India

The Office of the Controller General of Patents, Designs, and Trade Marks (CGPDTM), located in Mumbai, is in charge of all intellectual property. The patent office has its head office in Kolkata and its branch offices in Mumbai, New Delhi, Chennai, and Kolkata. Patents may be submitted electronically or in person at the patent office [10].

The Indian Patent Office (IPO), a division of the Controller General of Patents, Designs, and Trademarks (CGPDTM), is in charge of granting patents in India. It is a part of the Ministry of Commerce and Industry's Department of Industrial Policy and Promotion.

18.5.1 Locations for Patent Application Registration (WHERE)

Patents can be filed at the head office of the patent office or the branch office, depending on the situation, within whose territorial bounds the patent office is relevant, i.e.,

Either the residence or domicile of the applicant; OR.

Applicant's business location; OR.

The area from where the invention originated [10]. Different patent offices according to regional jurisdiction are listed in Table 18.2.

In the patent office, documents can be submitted either electronically (e-filing)(www.ipindiaonline.gov.in/online) or via mail or in person. In general, the process of obtaining a patent in India is charted out in Fig. 18.1.

Table 18.2 Patent offices in India according to regional jurisdiction

Office	Territorial Jurisdiction
Patent Office Branch, Chennai	The States of Andhra Pradesh, Karnataka, Kerala, Tamil Nadu, and the Union Territories of Pondicherry and Lakshadweep
Patent Office Branch Mumbai	The States of Maharashtra, Gujarat, Madhya Pradesh, Goa, and Chhattisgarh and the Union Territories of Daman and Diu and Dadra and Nagar Haveli
Patent Office Branch, New Delhi	The States of Haryana, Himachal Pradesh, Jammu and Kashmir, Punjab, Rajasthan, Uttar Pradesh, Uttaranchal, Delhi, and the Union Territory of Chandigarh
Patent Office, HO Kolkata	The rest of India

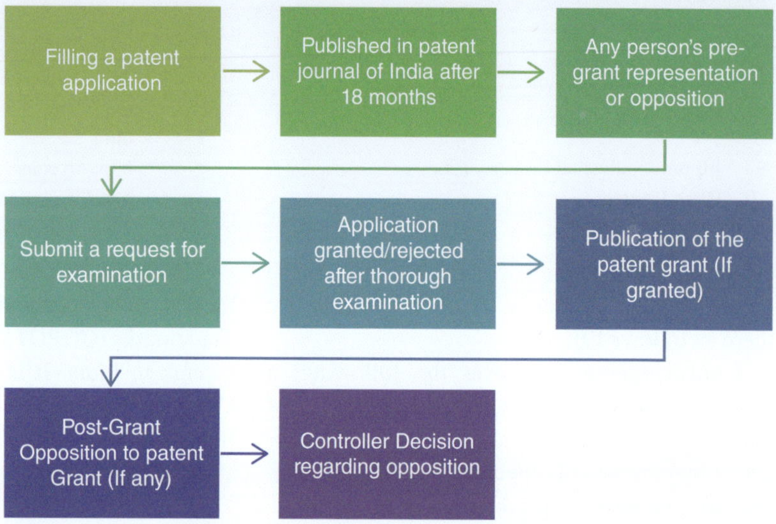

Fig. 18.1 Patent granting procedures

18.5.2 Documentation Regarding the Filing of Patent Application (WHAT)

Various documents are required to be kept ready before filing for a patent application. The list of documents tabulated in Table 18.3 is derived from Section 7. Rule 2(fa)/ 2(fb), Rule 7(1), 8, 10, 12, 13, 135. Form-1, 2, 3, 5, 26, 28. Section 6 of Biological Diversity Act, 2002 of Patent rules.

18.5.3 Patent Application Filing Eligibility (WHO)

Any of the following individuals may apply for a patent for an invention, either individually or jointly with another individual:

(a) Original and first inventor.
(b) Original and first inventor assignee.
(c) A legal representative of an expired original and first inventor.

18.5.4 Electronic Filing (E-Filling)

The Controller General of Patents, Designs, and Trade Marks' (www.ipindia.nic.in) official website offers a comprehensive platform for online submission of patent applications and related forms in a safe and verified electronic manner.

18.5.5 What Can Be Patented and What Cannot Be Patented?

There are some products and services that are considered "inventions" as per the interpretation

Table 18.3 Documents required for filing a patent application

Sl no.	Documents required for patent application
1.	Cover letter—enlisting the documents
2.	Application for patent grant (Form-1)
3.	Proof of rights by inventors in a relevant paragraph of Form-1.
4.	Provisional/complete specification in Form-2.
5.	Statement and undertaking in Form 3
6.	Statement and undertaking under Section 8 (1) in Form-3:
7.	Form 26 (original) Power of Attorney (if filed through attorney)
8.	Declaration of Inventor-ship in Form 5
9.	Submitting a request for examination in Form 18
10.	Stipulated statutory fees (in form of Demand draft/cheque)

of Section 2(1)(j) of the Patents Act but cannot be patented [1].

As per Section 3(f), any product/process that is simply an arrangement, rearrangement, or duplication of existing devices, each of which functions freely of one another in a way known to the public, shall not fall under the definition of an "invention" under the Patents Act and, thus, would not be patentable.

According to Section 3(i) of the Act, any process for the medicinal, surgical, curative, prophylactic diagnostic, therapeutic, or any other treatment of humans or any process that offers similar treatment for animals to free them from some disease boosts their economic value or that of their products shall not be considered an "invention" and, thus, would not be patentable.

Section 3(p) of the Act states that any invention that in effect is a traditional method or a compilation or duplication of the known aspects of traditionally known components shall not be considered an "invention" and, thus, would not be patentable.

The below-mentioned processes have been excluded to guide the patent officers concerning patentability of processes:

- Medicinal methods, for example, the process of giving medicine orally, via injectables, topically, or via a dermal patch.
- Surgical methods, for example, a no-stitch incision method for cataract surgery.
- Diagnostic methods.
- Curative methods, for example, a new method to clear plaque from teeth.
- Prophylactic methods, for example, vaccination methods.
- Therapeutic methods, for example, a new process for therapy.
- Any operation on the body that needs the surgeon's knowledge and expertise and consists of treatments like abortion, cosmetic treatment, embryo transplants, etc.
- Several notable medical patent developments have recently made headlines. One such example is given below:

Patent on the method for Automatic Detection of Anatomical Landmarks in Volumetric Data patent received by Gupta et al. (2019) assigned to the Council of Scientific and Industrial Research, New Delhi (IN); National Informatics Centre Department of Electronics and Information Technology, New Delhi (IN).

18.5.6 Difference Between a Research Manuscript and a Patent [4]

A valid patent can never be obtained at all if an application is not filed prior to any public disclosure of the invention. On the other hand, a paper's topic can be discussed informally and in public settings such as online, at conferences, and other venues.

18.5.7 Penalties for Wrong Claims [1, 11]

1. Violating secrecy provisions pertaining to specific inventions: In this instance, anyone found in violation of section 39 of the Patents Act, 1970, or failing to follow section 35's instructions in filing an application for a patent will be subject to a fine, imprisonment for a maximum of 2 years, or both.

2. Falsification of entries in the register, presenting fraudulent representations in an effort to mislead or manipulate a government official or agency, etc.: If someone, knowingly or unknowingly, makes a false entry in the Patent Register or writes a document falsely claiming to be a copy of an entry in such a register, they may be punished with a fine, 2 years in prison, or both.
3. Unauthorised claim of patent rights: A person may be fined up to infinity if they falsely state or claim that any product they sell is patented in India; if the product has the word "patent" or "patented" stamped, engraved, or otherwise applied to it; if the product bears any other word expressing or implying that the patent has been obtained in India; or if the product is the subject of an application for a patent in India. Incorrect use of the term "patent office": If someone uses the term "patent office" on his place of business, on any document he issues, or in any other way that gives the impression that his place of business or any document he issues is associated with or connected to the patent office, that person is guilty of an offence that carries a maximum of 6-month jail sentence, a fine, or both.
4. Refusal or failure to provide information: In any case, if the individual fails to provide information that is false and that he either knows or does not believe to be true, as required by the central government under section 100(5) of the Patents Act, 1970, or refuses to provide information about how patents operate that is required to be provided according to section 146 of the Patents Act, 1970.

18.5.8 Patent Lifecycle and Expiry [1, 4]

1. The patents that are granted against non-dividing applications or applications for patent addition have a 20-year expiration period from the date of filing. The expiration date should be determined from the provisional filing date, even in cases where the patent application was submitted with a provisional specification and the entire specification was filed within a year of that date.
2. Regarding patents awarded in opposition to divisional patent applications: 20 years pass after the day the patent application is filed, either with a complete specification or a provisional one.
3. For patents obtained in opposition to patents of addition, the principal invention's patent expires when the patent for the addition expires.

18.6 International Patent Filing Procedures

It is possible to file an international patent application in many nations. Three methods are available: [12].

1. Direct: Submit individual patent applications simultaneously in each country where a patent is required (for some countries, regional patents are available).
2. Paris Convention: After submitting the initial patent application in one of the Member States of the Paris Convention for the Protection of Industrial Property, the applicant may submit additional patent applications in the other Member States of the Paris Convention within 12 months of the initial application's filing date, with the benefit of claiming the original application's filing date in all subsequent applications.
3. Patent Cooperation Treaty: Submit a PCT application immediately or during the Paris Convention's 12-month window following the filing date of a first application that is accepted by all PCT Contracting States

18.6.1 What Is PCT?

An international agreement known as the Patent Cooperation Treaty (PCT) has been ratified by over 155 countries. It is supervised by the World Intellectual Property Organisation (WIPO).

The PCT allows for simultaneous patent protection of an innovation in many different countries by filing a single "international" patent application as opposed to multiple separate national or regional patent applications.

In what is referred to as the "national phase", national or regional patent offices continue to have authority over the issuance of these international patents.

18.6.2 Steps Regarding Patent Filing Process (PCT Procedure) (HOW)

The PCT process entails the following: (Fig. 18.2).

Filing: In order to file an international application with a national or regional patent office or the WIPO, you must do so in a single language and in accordance with PCT formality rules. Additionally, you have to pay a single filing cost.

International Search: The "International Searching Authority" (ISA), one of the biggest patent offices globally, searches for published patent documents and technical publications (also referred to as "prior art") that may have an impact on your invention's patentability and issues a written opinion on the matter.

International Publication: This is the time, ideally within 18 months of the earliest filing date, that the specifics of your overseas application are made public.

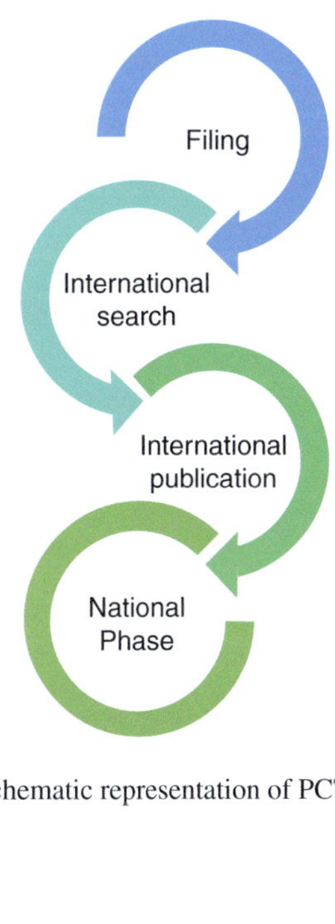

Fig. 18.2 Schematic representation of PCT procedure

National Phase: This is when you begin directly pursuing the grant of your patents before the national (or regional) patent offices of the countries in which you want to obtain them. Typically, this happens 30 months after the PCT procedure concludes and the earliest filing date of your initial application from which you claim priority.

18.6.3 Patent Filing Eligibility (WHO)

If you are a citizen or resident of a PCT Contracting State, you are qualified to submit an international patent application. Only one of the candidates included in the international application has to meet this condition if there are many applicants.

18.6.4 Location for International Patent Application (WHERE)

In most situations, you can apply for an international patent through your national patent office or, if your State's national security laws let it, directly through WIPO. These two offices serve as "receiving offices" under PCT. Residents and nationals of India may submit an international application to the Indian Patent Office at the Receiving Office (RO/IN) in Delhi, Chennai, Mumbai, or Kolkata.

18.6.5 US Patenting Vs Patenting in India

The United States defines what CAN be patented in a more demonstrative manner. Conversely, India's patent regulations specify what is NOT eligible for patent protection. While Indian patent law prohibits even little alterations or extensions to already granted patents, US patent laws permit such modifications. While there is no such provision in India, the United States permits the patenting of discoveries of machines or processes as long as they are new, practical, and obscure. Additionally, software cannot be patentable in India. For software to be patentable, hardware or computer invention must be used in conjunction with it. In the United States, it is legal to patent software as well as new plant discoveries and inventions.

18.6.6 Electronic Filing (E-Filing)

PCT applications are often submitted electronically by applicants. Any capable receiving office that accepts electronic filings will receive PCT applications. The WIPO web tool (ePCT-filing) for preparing PCT applications aids in the preparation of your applications by automatically evaluating the entered data and calling your attention to incomplete or inconsistently filled components. Additionally, it aids in managing your apps, for instance, by monitoring time restrictions for pertinent tasks. When submitting electronically, you are also qualified for several PCT fee exemptions. On www.wipo.int/pct-services, you may find more information on PCT electronic filing.

18.7 Patent Landscaping Analysis

18.7.1 Description

As a public service, the different patent office databases make patent information available so that technical and scientific issues can be resolved in a more effective, systematic, and all-encompassing manner. Health-related inventions come in many forms, and the majority of them are covered by intellectual property (IP) rights [13]. Numerous patent analyses have been carried out using these patent data to come up with new solutions for different technical issues. A patent landscape analysis is a futuristic patent search that shows the top patent grantees, current patenting trends, technology assessments, alliance partners, and other information from search results in symbolic or diagrammatic form [14]. Around the world, there are several databases for searching and analysing patents that are open to the public, including Lens.org, Google Patents, Espacenet, the USPTO Web Patent Database, and Patentscope by WIPO [11]. Different types of advancements in craniofacial imaging have been covered by global patent rules. Here we have performed a patent landscaping analysis to give an examination of current patenting trends and actions in the craniofacial imaging industry globally.

18.7.2 Methodology and Results

A study was undertaken to retrieve and analyse data on craniofacial imaging patents using a tool from the website www.lens.org. The website offers an open access to academic information and patent-related data from across the world as a free resource to help with problem-solving involving science and technology [15, 16]. It provides open access to about 144.3 million global patent documents and over 252.1 million scholarly papers. With such a big collection of academic papers, it is one of the largest patent search databases [17, 18].

Typically, specific keywords were used in patent searches. The keywords that were chosen were dental radiology, oral radiology, oral radiodiagnosis, and craniofacial imaging. The range of the date filter is 1840 to 2022.

The following parameters were primarily chosen for investigation in this study:

- Top countries based on the number of patent documents.
- Top dental patent applicants and owners worldwide.
- Top jurisdictions overall.

As of December 31, 2022, a patent search conducted at lens.org using keywords such as dental radiology, oral radiology, oral radio diagnosis, and craniofacial imaging returned a total of 49,307 patent entries.

Table 18.4 Distribution of craniofacial imaging patents [16]

S.No	Patent applicants worldwide	Patent owners worldwide	Patent documents sorted according to jurisdictions
1	University of California	Immunomedics INC	United States
2	Genetech INC	The Regents of University of California	WO-WIPO
3	University of Texas	Conformis INC	European patents
4	Human Genome Sciences INC	Bristol Myers Squibb Company	China
5	Immunomedics INC	Human Genome Sciences INC	Russia
6	Bristol Myers Squibb Co	Align Technology INC	Republic of Korea
7	Align Technology INC	President and fellows Harvard college	Germany
8	Amgen INC	Board of regents University of Texas	Japan
9	University John Hopkins	Express Scripts Strategic Development	France
10	Zymogenetics INC	The John Hopkins University	Spain

According to the selected parameters, the findings of the patent landscape analysis were illustrated and expanded. The distribution of patents according to patent applicants, owners, and jurisdictions is given in Table 18.4.

1. Top 10 craniofacial Imaging-Related Patent Applicants Worldwide

   With 669 patent applications, the University of California tops the list, followed by Genetech INC company with 589 patent applications.
2. Top 10 craniofacial imaging-related patent owners worldwide

   According to the number of patent filings, with 348 patent documents, Immunomedics INC tops the list, followed by The Regents of the University of California with 313.
3. Patent documents sorted according to jurisdictions

   With 33,243 documents, the United States holds the top spot, followed by WO-WIPO with 10,662 documents.

18.8 Summary

Intellectual property is an area of recent interest to the common man. Complete knowledge of IPs is very much essential for the augmentation of the economic growth of our country. A solid understanding of intellectual property rights facilitates the recognition, conception, execution, and ongoing preservation of innovation more rapidly and straightforwardly. Specialized procedures have been adopted to safeguard applications, species of plants, traditional wisdom, and geographical designations. As far as patents in craniofacial imaging are concerned, India needs to increase its number of patents related to craniofacial imaging.

References

1. Singh R. Law relating to intellectual property (A complete comprehensive material on intellectual property covering acts, rules, conventions, treaties, agreements, case-Law and much more), vol. 1. New Delhi: Universal Law Publishing Co. Pvt. Ltd.; 2004.
2. Saha CN, Bhattacharya S. Intellectual property rights: An overview and implications in pharmaceutical industry. J Adv Pharm Technol Res. 2011;2(2):88–93. https://doi.org/10.4103/2231-4040.82952.
3. Anonymous. Research and development statistics. New Delhi: Department of Science and Technology (DST), Government of India; 2002.
4. Anonymous. Research and development in industry: An overview. New Delhi: Department of Scientific and Industrial Research, Government of India; 2002.
5. Quintero JC, Trosien A, Hatcher D, Kapila S. Craniofacial imaging in orthodontics: historical perspective, current status and future developments. Angle Orthod. 1999;69:491–506.

6. World Intellectual Property Organization (WIPO). What is intellectual property. Switzerland: WIPO Publication. https://www.wipo.int/about-ip/en/#.
7. Bainbridge DI. Intellectual property. New York: Longman; 2002.
8. The Office of the Controller General of Patents. Designs and Trade Marks. India: Government of India; 2023. https://ipindia.gov.in/writereaddata/images/pdf/oatent-office-procedures.pdf.
9. Tidwell JL, Liotta LA. Inventions and patents: a practical tutorial. Methods Mol Biol. 2012;823:391–408. https://doi.org/10.1007/978-1-60327-216-2_26.
10. The Office of the Controller General of Patents, Designs & Trade Marks [Internet]. India: Government of India;[updated on 2023 January 2019].
11. Yang YY, Akers L, Yang CB, Klose T, Pavlek S. Enhancing patent landscape analysis with visualization output. World Patent Inf. 2010;32(3):203–20. https://doi.org/10.1016/j.wpi.2009.12.006.
12. Manual for patents [updated on 2021 Aug 17, cited on 2023 January 20]. https://ipindia.gov.in/manual-patents.htm.
13. World intellectual property organization (WIPO). Switzerland; Patent Co-operation Treaty(PCT) 2023. https://www.wipo.int/pct/en/faqs/faqs.html.
14. Tulasi GK, Rao BS. A detailed study of patent system for protection of inventions. Indian J Pharm Sci. 2008;70(5):547–54. https://doi.org/10.4103/0250-474X.45390.
15. https://www.greyb.com/patent-databases-best-search-platforms/. Last Assessed 29 Dec 2022.
16. Jefferson OA, Koehllhofer D, Warren B, Jefferson R. The Lens metarecord and LensID: an open identifier system for aggregated metadata and versioning of knowledge artefacts. 2019. https://about.lens.org/news/the-lens-metarecord/.
17. Charting influence. Nature. 2017;548:S6–7. https://doi.org/10.1038/548S6a. https://about.lens.org/. Last Assessed 31 Dec 2022.
18. Tay A.. Lens.org–detailed review of a new open discovery and citation index. Musings Librariansh; 2018. http://musingsaboutlibrarianship.blogspot.com/2018/11/lensorg-detailed-review-of-new-open.html.

MIX
Papier aus verantwortungsvollen Quellen
Paper from responsible sources
FSC® C105338

If you have any concerns about our products,
you can contact us on
ProductSafety@springernature.com

In case Publisher is established outside the EU,
the EU authorized representative is:
Springer Nature Customer Service Center GmbH
Europaplatz 3, 69115 Heidelberg, Germany

Printed by Libri Plureos GmbH
in Hamburg, Germany